THE
HEALING
WORKBOOK

4th Edition

A 12 Week Step-by-Step Program
To Heal Injury and Illness
And Transform the Health of Body & Mind

RICK D. FISCHER

WITH AGA POSTAWSKA

For information contact info@thehealingworkbook.com
or visit http://www.TheHealingWorkbook.com

ISBN-13: 978-1519200457
ISBN-10: 1519200455

4th Edition

Printing History
Softcover 1st edition / December 2013
Softcover 2nd edition / May 2015
Softcover 3rd edition / October 2015

Cover Design: Rick D. Fischer
Interior Design: Rick D. Fischer

IMPORTANT DISCLAIMER: The information in this book is solely for informational purposes. IT IS NOT INTENDED TO PROVIDE MEDICAL ADVICE. The author does not take responsibility for any possible consequences from any treatment, procedure, exercise, dietary modification, action or use of medication which results from reading or following the information contained herein, or from the failure to first consult with your medical professional. The information herein is not intended to be, nor should it be construed to be a cure, antidote, remedy, answer, or otherwise considered to be a substitute for professional therapy or treatment. THIS INFORMATION DOES NOT REPLACE THE ADVICE OF YOUR PHYSICIAN OR OTHER HEALTH CARE PROVIDER. Some of the techniques and remedies mentioned here have not been evaluated in scientific studies and may cause adverse reactions with prescription medication. The author is not responsible for any adverse reactions to recipes, supplements, treatments, exercises, therapies, or other information mentioned in this book. ALL READERS ARE ENCOURAGED TO SPEAK WITH THEIR PRIMARY HEALTH CARE PROVIDER BEFORE STARTING ANY NEW THERAPEUTIC TECHNIQUE OR NUTRITIONAL PROGRAM.

"Our bodies are our gardens -
our wills are our gardeners."

~William Shakespeare

This book is dedicated to

Miya and Lily

For the joy and love you've brought to this world,

Your light shines eternal, forever inside me;

...

To the *health* care professionals

That serve the advancement of wellness

By being open to, not suppressing, nature's wisdom

Thank you for contributing to a healthier world;

AND

To all those suffering from injury or illness

Who courageously choose

To take responsibility for their own healing,

You are <u>all</u> my inspiration.

TABLE OF CONTENTS

FOREWORD

We as a people have reached a point in modern time where we must step back and regain a clear, authentic perspective on what true healthcare means and entails – at its core. Health involves not only the physical body, but also our minds, spirits, and emotions as well, as they are all intimately connected and have a direct influence on one another, just as do the many systems of the human body. Leaving any component of this totality out in our treatment methodologies and considerations means failing to honor and successfully treat the comprehensive health of the Whole Person.

Administering "therapies" to individuals that simply replace one set of symptoms for another, or subject the individual to a plethora of possible detrimental side effects is discounting the human condition in all of its excellence and sovereignty. In addition, simply treating an individual's symptoms is synonymous to putting a Band-Aid on a wound that will never truly be allowed to heal, as it is simply being covered up. Health and healing modalities and methodologies need be just that: healing and healthy. Furthermore, viewing the body as a series of individual, non-connected systems and dis-ease as a spontaneous manifestation that has no underlying cause is also problematic. Our anatomy can very accurately be described as an interdependent patchwork that is operating in a harmonious flow in order to maintain homeostasis and balance. This notion must be recognized and adhered to in order to accurately and appropriately treat any imbalances that may arise – for this is essentially the root of dis-ease, an imbalance in the harmonious flow of the Whole Person.

The human body is a self-righting vessel that was magnificently and brilliantly designed to heal autonomously when given the proper support, of which our natural world has already provided for us in great abundance. This fact can be clearly seen when analyzing the lifestyles and healing modalities of our early ancestors. Hardly any of the chronic illness that is ubiquitous today existed back then, and for good reason. Yes, the advent of "modern medicine" has been a brilliant development in many respects, however we cannot lose sight of the extremely helpful and efficacious healing agents that are already available to us within our exquisite and generous natural earth.

In order to regain our hold and get back to the root and heart of what true healthcare genuinely means, these concepts must emerge as axiomatic amongst all treatment modalities within the macro field of healthcare. Failing to do so will simply perpetuate these aforementioned, counterproductive and enigmatic practices which are antithetical to the acquisition and maintenance of sincere and lasting health and healing.

It is time we emerge into a societal landscape that is freed from limiting, parochial, and rigid dichotomies that catalyze marginalization and welcome a human social world that is characterized by the common goal

of helping and healing others (as well as ourselves), as we must work together in order to facilitate understanding, personal strength, and true and lasting health. Both "allopathic" and "alternative/holistic" modalities must join together to form a unified front, which will in turn strengthen the forces and efficacy behind overall, true healthcare, in its most real form. Marrying these two modalities and/or developing a mutual respect amongst the two enables us to provide broad-spectrum, comprehensive healing that is subjective and relevant to each idiosyncratic case and individual.

Furthermore, the profoundly vital and important fact that nutrition, in and of itself heals, can simply not be left out of the equation. Nutrition has everything to do with how and what our body metabolizes, therefore it is paramount in shifting our physiological state toward a more balanced operation. Nutrition is health.

It is time to open our eyes, without judgment, to the undeniable, spectacular nature of holistic health, as this methodology has kept in the forefront that the optimal well-being and nurturing of the individual is the primary goal, upholding the reverent paradigms and facts behind what true healthcare means and entails.

Holistic healing is effective, and it is only for that reason that I, and so many others, strongly advocate for its viability and acceptance within the "field of healthcare" umbrella. These notions have been ineffaceably solidified within me throughout my own arduous personal healing odyssey with Copper Toxicity, one of many conditions discussed in this book. Throughout this journey, my own deep-rooted, insatiable intrinsic passion for holistic health and nutrition has been instilled, as I have experienced first-hand the incredible cogency and miraculous transformations that holistic healing perpetuates and imparts. The quest to optimal health and wellness is certainly a humbling one: as we must face our own personal limitations with honesty, integrity, and compassion. We must also make the personal choice to truly want to make the necessary changes to inherently better ourselves and agree to adhere to these essential steps in achieving our health and wellness goals. This involves a great deal of courage, dedication, and openness, yet the exquisite gifts that are born from realizing one's own personal responsibility in achieving total wellness are undeniably incredible, and far surpass and outweigh the sometimes arduous task of initially embarking on your excursion.

The honesty, clarity, and veracity that is exhibited by Rick Fischer in the expanded, 3rd edition of The Healing Workbook is so welcomed and needed within our current realm of health education, and truly makes large strides toward perpetuating the prudent navigation toward efficacious and indelible healing and personal growth of which we all seek. Seeing as this realm can be quite overwhelming, especially for someone who is new to taking responsibility for their own health and healing, Fischer's work indubitably provides a practical, well-rounded, proactive, sedulous guide to the insightful, introspective, liberating, and

empowering task of embarking on your own personal comprehensive healing journey. The content is concise and assuredly catchall of the most paramount elements that one must address on this journey. Fischer's work honors and recognizes the highly salient truth that healing and treatment must be conducive and paralleled with the whole human condition in order to be all-inclusive and effective – as we are each versatile and unique beings, embodying a multifarious mind/body/spirit/emotional framework and henceforth our healing programs must reflect this structure, taking into account each of these equally important components as a means of thoroughly leading us to a state of optimal balance and vitality. Fischer fervently presents a copious array of daily tools and exercises and gives an expansive, wide-variety of information to enlighten you, in identifying some of the most important components of achieving and maintaining wellness. This is exemplified in his inclusion and analysis of the profoundly important (yet less well-known) component that minerals/micronutrients/mineral ratios are an absolutely vital area to focus on when truly addressing the underlying cause of our physiological and psychological imbalances. Additionally, Fischer provides incredibly valuable content regarding gut health (the root cause of most illness), tools and resources to address your emotional/spiritual/intellectual inner landscape, a wide variety of nutrition/dietary guidance, naturally sourced treatment methods and agents to target many different maladies, and additional helpful and insightful articles.

Health is the essence behind who we are as people, and it is for this reason that it should be in the forefront of our conscious, daily lives. Fischer's 12-week, practical program aids and impels the reader throughout the process of achieving wellness to the degree that it becomes a solidified way of life. This work firmly upholds one of the most important paradigms within holistic healing: that our healing is dependent upon realizing the root cause of the problem and working from there, as opposed to alleviating or covering up symptoms. That is where true, deep healing is achieved and maintained. In addition, the paramount notion is upheld that optimal wellness involves the Whole Person, as we are an interdependent compilation of our emotional, intellectual, spiritual, and physical Selves.

Feel sincerely grateful that The Healing Workbook has come into your possession, as it can and will serve as an all-encompassing renewal for you on a spiritual, emotional, intellectual, and physical level, as it honors each component that is most predominant within the brilliant, multifaceted assemblage that comprises your Whole Being. As Fischer so eloquently states, "You have the power within you to make magic happen. We all have it within us. Let this book be your guide to awakening the natural and powerful healing abilities within you."

-Megan B. Westbrook

INTRODUCTION – SETTING THE STAGE

"I believe it's imperative that each one of us takes responsibility for the health of our minds and bodies so that we may live life embracing our passions rather than battling disease; I believe the health of our body is influenced greatly by the health of our mind, while the health of our mind is affected by what we feed our body-we must work on both for optimal health to prevail."
~ Rick Daniel Fischer

Most people don't think about their health until they lose it. Then they realize that, without health, they have nothing. Many then turn to their doctor for some magic pill that will fix everything - a magic pill that will somehow fix overnight the damage they've been causing their body continually over many decades. Magic pills don't work, certainly not in the long run and, between side effects and lack of addressing the source of the problem, most often just make things worse. If prevention is too late, then we must find a way to treat the illness, or injury, in a safe holistic way that does not further jeopardize the health of the individual, and ideally one that can resolve what caused the issue to develop in the first place.

Health and healing begins inside us, not in some pill. The miracle of good health is within each of us, and so we all have the ability to make that miracle reappear, by looking within. Whether your setback is in the form of an injury or illness, the choice is yours how you handle it. In other words, you are in control. While this concept might be hard to accept at first, it is true, you are in control of your healing. Let me ask you, if you knew *exactly what* to do in order to heal, would you do it? Whether your answer is yes or no, you are in control. Understanding this is a first step toward your recovery. It is in taking full responsibility for your healing - understanding that doctors and therapists have tremendous specialized knowledge and tools they can assist you with but that there is work you must also do yourself - that long term health can be restored. As you do this work and advance through your recovery, you may discover that this current health setback isn't the end of the world, but may in fact have been a blessing in disguise.

I believe everything we need to live healthy and prevent or cure illness is already provided to us in nature, and within us. The problem is that we pollute our body and our mind with unhealthy things - food, chemicals, thoughts, hurts, etc. It's not that we purposely try to poison our bodies, but the fact is that most of us do, every day. That head of

lettuce you think is healthy can contain over 50 toxic pesticides. The way your mind interpreted some otherwise trivial event when you were a baby may subconsciously be causing a self-destructive pattern that's running your entire adult life. The drug your doctor gives you with good intention can superficially help one symptom but cause dis-ease elsewhere. We end up playing Wack-a-Mole with our health. A health problem appears and we whack it with a drug, a drug that then makes another health issue appear later, and for which another drug is prescribed. That's when we see people with a whole shopping cart full of pills on their kitchen counter, a different one for all their different ailments, never once having stopped to look at the underlying cause, or to consider that there may be more natural and safer alternatives for healing, or that the drugs themselves are contributing to their symptoms.

"Our figures show approximately four and one half million hospital admissions annually due to the adverse reactions to drugs. Further, the average hospital patient has as much as thirty percent chance, depending how long he is in, of doubling his stay due to adverse drug reactions."
~ Milton Silverman, M.D. (Professor of Pharmacology, University of California)

According to Barry Sears, author the "the Zone Diet", "more people die every year in America from taking the *correct* dosage of anti-inflammatory drugs than die from AIDS!" If that isn't shocking enough, consider that iatrogenic disease is the third highest cause of death in the U.S., right behind heart disease and cancer. If you've never heard the term iatrogenic before, it's because the media never talks about it, even though it claims the lives of more people than if a jumbo jet were to crash every single day! Iatrogenic means "accidentally caused by a physician or medical care".

Drugs therefore, in my opinion, are not the answer. I believe there's a better way - and this is what you'll learn - and apply experientially - as you go through this book. I need to forewarn you though, there is a lot of information in this book that goes against the message of conventional medicine; this includes a lot of information that the pharmaceutical industry doesn't want you to hear. This book is going to shake things up for you; it may challenge your beliefs, especially if you're of the belief that your doctor has all the answers. I ask only that you keep an open mind as you go through the journey this book offers. This book has been written to serve you, and with your heart and mind open, it will.

I believe the health of people will change when they learn to take responsibility for their own health and healing – this means being proactive in lifestyle and diet rather than reactive only after years of destroying their bodies. It also means diligently doing the actions steps this book outlines. You can read all the health and healing books you want, but just reading isn't going to change the condition of your body – you must take action on what you read. You must do the work; no one can do it for you. The knowledge is here. It's up to you to apply it. The layout of this book is created to help you do just that – breaking down what could otherwise be an overwhelming undertaking and delivering it in actionable daily steps.

The discussion of responsibility also means becoming aware that our beliefs about health become largely formulated by the marketing messages of various interest groups and industries that best serve the mission of those groups, but not necessarily our health. After all, there is no money in 'health' - (when was the last time you saw a commercial on TV promoting healthy mushrooms, raw kale, or the importance of magnesium?). Money is made off packaging and manufacturing processed foods, and later on in selling medications and 'healthcare' to manage all the illness that results. (Even many hospitals perpetuate this cycle, with about 40% of hospitals in the U.S. having fast food restaurants on their premises![1,2]). It shocks me when I pick up a health publication found in hospitals and medical offices that promotes Splenda as the 'healthy alternative', or promotes sugar-laden high-fructose-corn-syrup-containing artificially-colored drinks like Minute Maid as being healthy. This is not health care!!! Health care would be teaching the public how to live healthy, putting advertising dollars behind real foods and natural remedies, instead of the billions of dollars that are put into marketing sugar saturated soft drinks, cigarettes, processed foods, and then, as a result of all that, pills. Dr. Andrew Weil sums it up perfectly when he states, *"We don't have a "health care" system, we have a "disease management" system!"*

"Unfortunately, most physicians are taught very little about the use of food for healing when they're in medical school, and many never take the time to learn even the most basic nutritional principles. This is why most conventional doctors cannot guide you in nutritional healing, and why many are outright suspicious about claims that food can heal." ~ Dr. Mercola

---

[1] Cram P, Brahmjee KN, Fendrick AM, Saint S. Fast food franchises in hospitals. JAMA 2002; 287: 2945–6.
[2] http://www.jabfm.org/content/19/5/526.full

We can't blame the doctor though, for he's just passing on what he was taught. The problem starts in the schooling, with a serious lack of education on nutrition and preventative medicine. As written in the following article by the American Medical Association itself:

"While physicians encourage patients to make healthy food choices, only 27 percent of U.S. medical schools actually offer students the recommended 25 hours of nutritional training, according to a recent perspective piece in Academic Medicine. Modern medicine maintains the importance of proper nutrition, yet on average, U.S. medical schools only offer 19.6 hours of nutrition education across four years of medical education, according to the perspective authors. "This corresponds to less than 1 percent of estimated total lecture hours," they wrote. "Moreover, the majority of this educational content relates to biochemistry, not diets or practical, food-related decision making." ..."No standardized patient examination tests the knowledge or skills of medical trainees to advise a patient seeking guidance with regard to evidence-based diet and lifestyle modification," they wrote. Training at the postgraduate level has followed suit, they said. They pointed to how the word "nutrition" isn't included in board examination requirements for internal medicine certification, and cardiology fellows don't need to complete a single requirement in nutrition counseling. Once in practice, fewer than 14 percent of physicians believe they were adequately trained in nutritional counselling,"" [3]

Let me be clear right from the start. I am a certified health coach with many thousands of hours of study and training in nutrition and mineral balancing and years of experience in psychology and mindset development techniques - I am NOT a doctor. And this is exactly WHY I am able to offer you this information and say a lot of the things I do in this book - because I am not bound by industry and special interests who's agendas often place profits over health. Sadly, as shown above, and despite their good intentions, many doctors graduate from medical school with tunnel vision based on the years of influence that the pharmaceutical companies have had over them since the day they entered academia. It's not uncommon for doctors to be wined and dined by drug corporations during their school years, and the influence continues into private practice where some doctors receive millions of dollars from pharmaceutical companies to promote their drug (you can even view some of these payouts in the U.S. at https://projects.propublica.org/docdollars/.) I know too of cases where certain drug companies would offer prizes (concert tickets, free trips, etc) to the doctors who sell the most of their drug! How could such bribery and practice ever be in the best interest of the patient?

Further public confusion comes from the stamp of "FDA Approval", making some unsafe drugs sound safe (because they're "FDA approved"), while many safe natural remedies are made to sound

---

[3] https://wire.ama-assn.org/education/whats-stake-nutrition-education-during-med-school

unsafe just because they've not been FDA approved. As one example, at the time of this update, the FDA has just launched a crackdown to *"protect consumers from potentially harmful, unproven homeopathic drugs"*. Whether one believes in homeopathy or not, there seems to be a double standard when heavily promoted FDA-approved drugs have proven dangerous side-effects (and sometimes more side effects which aren't even being disclosed). Perhaps if so much of the FDA's budget didn't come from pharmaceutical companies there would be a little less bias in what gets approved vs what gets attacked! To make matters worse, doctors can potentially lose their license by prescribing something that is 'not FDA approved'. Sadly, as most natural cures, hormones, and alternative remedies existing in nature are usually not patentable (and thus not profitable), they are the ones that risk not getting that fancy stamp of approval.

Added to this fiasco are the opinions and commentaries (of which you'll find no shortage of on the Internet, and even amongst the medical field for that matter), lambasting natural and alternative therapies because they are not 'scientifically proven' or 'approved'. Let's not forget that every drug that's been recalled by the FDA was once proven to be "safe and effective" by the FDA. Yet the sad reality is that many of the greatest medical minds today practicing alternative forms of medicine, though they have healed and saved many, are scathingly attacked for the natural medicine they practice. Science (along with mainstream medicine) most certainly has its place and can save lives, but it is far from perfect. It is also not free from causing harm - just look at the number of drug recalls, the 2.2 million or so U.S. hospital patients who experience adverse drug reactions to (science based) prescribed medications[4], the manipulation of studies based on profits (more on this in a moment), and contradictory scientific studies that seem to come out every week dispelling the findings of the previous study. There is also much that science does yet understand. The fact is, many things in this world, and in medicine, have not been scientifically proven, yet we know them to be true (take for example the concept of the Chinese meridian system of energy channels in the body – scientifically 'unproven' in Western medicine and sometimes called a 'pseudoscience' or 'quackery' by skeptics, yet it has existed for thousands of years as the basis to the traditional and very effective Chinese way of healing). If a treatment is presented that is shown to have helped people, even if the shortcomings of 'science' have not yet found a way to 'prove' it, why should such treatment be denied to those who could benefit by it? The view to offer and promote only scientifically proven and 'FDA approved' Western treatments while dismissing and attacking everything else is, to me, not only extremely closed minded and

[4] *Lazarou J, Pomeranz BH, Corey PN. Incidence of adverse drug reactions in hospitalized patients: a meta-analysis of prospective studies. JAMA . 1998 Apr 15;279(15):1200-5.*

completely ignorant of wisdom that has existed for millennia, but, even more importantly, it also closes the door to gaining a greater understanding of the energy-mind-body connection and that which might not always be visible yet still exists and can offer profound healing and help to people.

"Modern Medicine would rather you die using its remedies than live by using what physicians call "quackery". ~ Dr. Robert Mendelsohn, M.D.*

There are big profits to be made by the drug industry, and when money is involved, the seeds of manipulation grow. The public has been led to believe that drugs are generally safe, because studies show them to be so; even doctors are often blindsided by the extent of the manipulation. Doctors usually rely on what is known as a meta-analysis to assess the clinical effectiveness of a treatment or drug. The meta-analysis combines data from multiple randomised control trials. It's always been thought that pharmaceutical companies don't fund these papers. However, as was recently published in the Journal of Clinical Epidemiology, it was found that 1/3 of the papers (in a 185 paper study) were written by pharmaceutical employees.

"We knew that the industry would fund studies to promote its products, but it's very different to fund meta-analyses," which "have traditionally been a bulwark of evidence-based medicine…It's really amazing that there is such a massive influx of influence in this field." ~John Ioannidis (epidemiologist at Stanford University School of Medicine and co-author of aforementioned study)

The drugs, which are marketed to help ease conditions, in turn often cause harm in other areas – and these harmful effects are often not published, or are concealed. Obviously a manufacturer driven only by profit is not going to design a study that looks for the adverse effects.

"The medical profession is being bought by the pharmaceutical industry, not only in terms of the practice of medicine, but also in terms of teaching and research. The academic institutions of this country are allowing themselves to be the paid agents of the pharmaceutical industry. I think it's disgraceful." ~Arnold Seymour Relman (1923-2014), (Harvard Professor of Medicine and Former Editor-in-Chief of the New England Medical Journal)

"Medical school should be renamed Pharma school. Doctors only learn to treat symptoms with drugs while ignoring the cause. Real health won't be found inside a doctor's office." ~Brandy Vaughan, ex-sales rep for Merck Pharmaceuticals

Consider also that:

"There is not a single disease every identified caused by a lack of a drug, but there are diseases caused by a lack of vitamins, minerals, and nutrients. Why, then, do we consider the former - chemical medicine - the standard of care, and food-as-medicine quackery? Money and power is the obvious answer."
~ Sayer Ji

As controversial as this information may be, my intention is not to dance in a fire of political and industry agendas. Nor is it to attack all doctors, as <u>many doctors do outstanding work every day saving lives</u>; and those who are making a difference and furthering the advancement of medicine through good intention and learning rather than silencing that which they don't understand deserve to be greatly commended. My intention with this book is to get back to the simple basics of what each one of us can do as individuals to help ourselves heal and live healthier. I've simply seen far too many people, including loved ones closest to me, have their lives shattered (or ended) by some doctors who didn't understand safer, more prudent options, or who failed to recognize that the body and mind are an integrated system, not individual parts functioning independently. Dr. Mark Hyman says it perfectly,

"The body is one integrated system, not a collection of organs divided up by medical specialties. The medicine of the future connects everything."

Sadly, modern medicine tends to treat only symptoms and not the underlying cause. Allopathy serves an important purpose when it comes to healing symptoms. It falls short however when it comes to addressing/healing the causes. We need to heal our bodies at the source, not at the upstream effect. The source will always be there, and if the source is polluted, it will continually affect what happens downstream. Allopathy and alternative medicine need to marry their strengths for a fuller service to the health of humanity. Personally I want you to be aware of what your healthier and natural options are because, more often than not, they are not discussed. I certainly don't claim to have all the answers, nor do I claim that this book addresses every single possible health concern out there, or every single remedy for that matter. The field of medicine and body systems is infinitely complex. However, I would confidently argue that almost all illness begins in the mind and the gut, and this is where our focus ultimately needs to be for healing and health. Some of the ideas you are about to learn may challenge what you've been taught to believe. I ask that you be open. My purpose is to help people become more

conscientious of their actions and options, and through offering natural holistic guidance and opening their awareness of themselves, make a healthy lasting difference in people's lives. My hope is that this book, without being overly scientific in jargon, gives the reader practical and accessible tools and inspiration to thrive in their healing and health.

The illustration below presents the basic concept to this book. Our mindset, our gut health, our adrenals and other organs, they are not only all interconnected, they are also all affected by stress (widely acknowledged) and minerals (an area less understood). Each of these individual connections will be addressed in the course of this book. When we understand the powerful role that minerals and other micronutrients play on our health – in fact their delicate balance dictates both our health and personality – we can begin to understand how important nutrition is for all aspects of well-being.

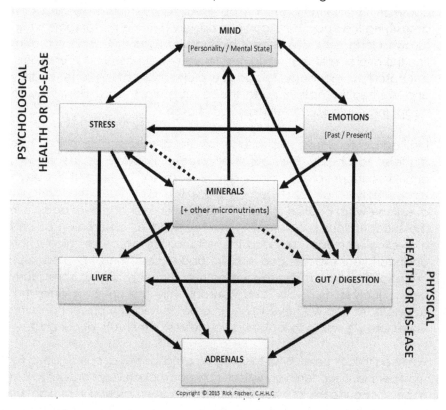

Any book that focuses solely on diet/nutrtition however fails to ignore the all important element of the mind and the role it has played in your health. Likewise, a psychology book on emotional healing can help in

that one particular area but ignores the influence of diet and how micronutrients can affect not only the body but also the mind. Diet also plays a key role in healing, as up to 85% of our immune system is in our gut! For this reason this book heavily emphasises both mindset as well as nutrition. Furthermore, I want to introduce you to a unique collection of treatments and therapies (some you've heard of, many perhaps you've not) that can further help in your healing.

In terms of diet, there are basic principles that most anyone can apply. Certain foods have specific healing properties, while other foods are known to cause dis-ease within the body. This is not a diet book that insists you switch to any one particular diet. As you go through these coming weeks you'll notice that raw food and greens are quite important for health, and yet, in no way am I advocating a vegan or vegetarian lifestyle. I've seen first hand the dangers such a choice can cause. A vegetarian diet can be great for short term healing and detoxifying the body, but it can also be very detrimental for some when followed long term. Everyone is bio-individually unique, and you must find the overall diet that works best for you – not based on your beliefs, but based on your body. This book explains many of the super-healthy and not-healthy options (and the reasons why), and allows you to adopt these into your lifestyle as you choose.

Diet can cure illness; it can also create disease – everything from diabetes to obesity, allergies, liver disease, headaches, depression, arthritis, cancer, pretty much any disease (or at least the body's susceptibility to disease) can be traced to diet. *But here's the key question – what caused the diet?* The answer over and over again is in the subconscious programming we received as children. Not only marketing messages, but also the trauma, the abuse or ridicule, the abandonment experienced in childhood – these show up in our diet, our addictions, and the way we both consciously and unconsciously treat ourselves as adults, and consequently the illness or pain that develops. And so we have to ask, in order to heal the present and the future, are we willing to look inside ourselves at the truth of our past.

We need to look carefully at this programming, as well as our mindset. For most people, a sudden diagnosis or injury can make it very hard not to lose hope. Of course this isn't helped when care givers around you might be saying your life will never be the same, that it may be months or years before you are able to fully return to your activities, or even, that your days are numbered. Depression, despair and hopelessness can very quickly sink in. In these dark moments when the unthinkable seems to be happening,

how do you carry on? How do you keep a positive mindset when the prognosis is dim, or the recovery phase daunting? What role has your inner world (thoughts, emotions, programming) played in creating your current situation? How do you go about shifting yourself from 'disaster' onto a path that is truly conducive for optimal healing and health? Why is it that some people make miraculous recoveries, and others succumb? It all starts in the mind.

The mind is one of the most powerful tools we have available when it comes to healing ourselves from illness and pain. Looking at health from a holistic approach, our physical, mental, emotional, and spiritual states are all interconnected. When 'dis-ease' or injury shows up in the physical realm, it is often a result of tension or conflict in the other realms (as I mentioned on the previous page). And while drugs and operations may temporarily alleviate the symptoms of the dis-ease (or the pain from injury), if we do not look at and work on our mental, emotional and spiritual states then the underlying cause of the dis-ease still exists. An adverse event that may have happened 40 years ago in childhood didn't just happen 40 years ago - it's happening now, living in your cells, living in your fat, living in your illness and symptoms. Until one deals with the deeper issues, all the medicine taken, diets tried, and treatments attempted can only offer a temporary fix. Eventually the problem lying beneath will resurface because there's an emotional pain that hasn't been addressed, a subconscious program that's running the show. This is why mind-body medicine is so imperative. Without it, only the superficial is touched.

Consider the fact that the body is, at all times, in a state of continually repairing and replacing itself. The only guidance the body has to do this are the messages sent to it from the mind. If we want to heal, we must therefore begin with the mind. Positive thoughts actually strengthen the immune system (while negative thoughts weaken it).

In the words of Napoleon Hill, "It is a well-known fact that one comes, finally, to believe whatever one repeats to one's self, *whether the statement be true or false.* If a man repeats a lie over and over, he will eventually accept the lie as truth. Moreover he will believe it to be the truth."[5] If you therefore continually say you are in pain or ill (because you have been for some time), then your body will learn to accept that pain or illness as the state of your body; and even after your body is physically healed, the trained mind will allow the sensation of pain

[5] *Hill, N. (1960). Think & Grow Rich. U.S.A.: Fawcett Books.*

and illness to continue. Conversely, even if you truly are in pain or ill, and yet continually tell yourself that you are pain-free (or phrased more positively "I'm in perfect health and comfort"), then your mind will work to manifest that notion and the physical sensations of pain will dissipate.

There is also something known as the 'Nocebo Effect'. Just as with the better known placebo effect where the mere belief that something will heal you can make you feel better, the nocebo effect is the allowance of negative messages to take root and manifest. The negative expectation that something will harm you (such as side effects listed on a drug bottle) can actually induce those very symptoms even if the drug is replaced with a plain sugar pill. This has been proven in a number of clinical trials. The important thing to note here is that, whether you have positive or negative beliefs, they often become a self-fulfilling prophecy.

The Law of Attraction sums the concept up simply; "what we focus on expands". If we focus on the pain, or illness, we will attract more pain and illness. If we are negative and fearful in our thoughts, we will tend to attract the very things we are trying to avoid. Everything we create physically we create first in thought. If we go deeper, we realize that those thoughts come from our beliefs, many of which are formed in childhood, or even earlier. (As you go through this book you will be doing exercises that will help you reshape those thoughts and beliefs).

Ironically most people have a very negative and non-supportive dialogue going on their minds. This mind chatter (that little voice in your head) rarely seems to obey the 'off' button. This inner dialogue is what creates our outer reality, and then we wonder why things aren't going the way we want. Sceptics will say 'well, simply thinking positively about it isn't going to cure my condition'. While it's true that a fleeting positive thought will not cure you (the thought needs to be continually repeated with conviction (ie: belief!)), it's also true and has been shown that blisters can be produced simply by the power of hypnosis. Consider that if the mind can produce negative symptoms and ill health through *negative focus*, then the mind can also produce good health through *positive focus*.

In order to truly effect change in the state of one's health, positive *thinking* therefore is not enough. There is a big difference between positive thinking and positive *focus*. One can, on the inside, feel negative and hopeless about a situation, and yet still think and verbalize positive thoughts. Saying to yourself "I'm going to be OK" is

positive thinking and yet afterward you retreat back to the voice inside you saying "There's no hope". This kind of thinking will not affect positive change. Positive focus on the other hand is when your inner voice, beliefs, thoughts and daily actions are in alignment and congruent with the positive outcome you're seeking. Positive focus is more than just saying and thinking positive thoughts. It's about wholeheartedly feeling and truly believing in those thoughts, focusing 110% on the positive outcome, and allowing no space for negative alternatives. Not only does positive focus help you feel better, it also significantly boosts the immune system.

You have purchased or have been given this workbook because you are wanting to heal. You first deserve to congratulate yourself for taking this first step, and for being open to taking responsibility for your own healing, starting within you. You might be asking, "Is this workbook right for me?" and "Is it going to work?". Well, this book was originally created for people dealing with illness or injury serious enough to potentially alter one's life – anything from serious sports injuries to life threatening illness. This book is for those who refuse to take their situation lying down; who are either determined to do whatever it takes to recover or who are seeking the motivation to get to that state of mind. It is not meant to replace any professional medical advice or treatments you are currently receiving, but rather supplement it to further increase the effectiveness of what you are doing. As such, this book is also a fantastic resource for all practitioners of holistic health as a tool to empower their patients towards more complete healing.

The way this book has evolved however now makes it also a very effective resource for any individual seeking to make a permanent and positive healthy lifestyle change; as it is too for those seeking a preventative and proactive approach to maintaining good health. It is for those open to healing themselves emotionally (as all illness starts from within). It is for those that are open and willing to take responsibility for their own healing and health, understanding that healing (and good health) is not some end goal but an ongoing journey.

If this sounds like you, then the pages of this book truly do have the power to take your life to a whole new level, a place of wellness you may only currently be able to dream of and hope for at present.

HOW TO USE THIS BOOK

There are 2 ways to most effectively use this book. The way this book is structured it offers a 12 week program to creating overall health and healing. Ideally, each day you will read the Health Tip and complete the Action Step(s) given to you for that day. Improving overall health and well-being from the inside out can be an enormously daunting task, if not broken down into bite size bits. That's the benefit of being guided daily to take one manageable action step, in a progressive order where appropriate. Consistently and diligently following this book over the next 12 weeks will create an astonishing transformation in your overall health. This is the method I suggest when there is no dire urgency to heal a specific condition. For a chronic long term condition that may be uncomfortable but that isn't going to 'kill you', it's best to go through the entire 12 weeks to approach your healing holistically and systemically. I highly recommend that if you use this method of approaching the book, you commit to doing it daily. Set aside a block of time each day to invest in your health. Without this commitment, people often start off strong and with good intention, but by the second week they start skipping days, and pretty soon they're down to reading just a page a week, or sporadically whenever they remember. Even if this happens it is still better than doing nothing at all, however it will simply take you that much longer to transform your health. There are invaluable transformative tools in this book, and the sooner you can apply them, the quicker you'll restore your health and be feeling better.

As a convenient second method, this book is fully indexed at the back so that you can quickly and easily refer to any topic you might want immediate access to.

If you choose to go through this book progressively for the 12 weeks, you'll notice that each day of the week has a general theme. Day 1 is generally related to mindset, the brain, thought patterns, etc. Day 2 is generally to do with eliminating unhealthy foods from your diet. Day 3 is about adding in healthy foods. Day 4 tends to relate to therapies and treatments, while Day 5 is more concerned with lifestyle activities. Day 6 is a bit of a mixed bag of useful suggestions, and Day 7 is a review of the past week. If you missed a day during the week or didn't get to quite finish an action step, Day 7 is your chance to catch up.

For each of the first 6 days, you'll see a simple guided journaling box. Journaling is a lot more powerful than you may at first think, and doing so is an important part of the healing process. You will get out of it what you put in. This book is meant to be written in. Don't be afraid of marking up the pages, and no one needs to see what you write except for yourself. What matters is only that you do the exercises. The journaling sections for the first 6 days are as follow:

TODAY'S INTENTION: Write a short sentence about how you want to see your health. Write it in the present, using only positive words (ie: avoid words such as 'not', 'don't', etc), and feel the intention as if it is your reality now. Alternatively, you can also choose to write an intention for an action you'll commit to doing that day that will get you closer to the health you want.

POSITIVE OUTCOME(S): Search for signs in your life, or your day, where you have made positive progress and/or you are a step closer to realizing your intention. If nothing comes to you as obvious, dig a little deeper. Have you taken an action step today that will serve you well? Have you been working on your mindset? Is there something, no matter how small, that you're able to do today that you didn't or couldn't do yesterday? How about your thoughts, have they improved? Even if you're experiencing a set-back, always find at least one positive thing that has happened today as evidence in your improvement.

AFFIRMATION: Choose an affirmation for today and write it in this space. You may choose an affirmation from the list provided in Part II of this book. Instructions are also provided on page 243 how to write your own affirmations in case you choose to create your own. In either case, whether you choose one of the ones provided or your own, make sure you write it down in the space provided. This helps to cement your mind's attention on this particular affirmation for the day. Focus on this affirmation throughout the day, repeating it to yourself as often as possible.

GRATITUDE: Gratitude is the magic ingredient that brings you more of whatever it is you want in life. When you become grateful for something you are (a) focusing positive energy on it and, by the Law of Attraction, what you focus on expands, (b) creating a more positive energy vibration in your body which improves your thoughts, energy levels, immune system, and quality of life, (c) letting the universe know that

you are not taking whatever it is you're grateful for for-granted, and therefore (d) you are open to receiving more of it, When you think about it, there are an infinite number of things to be grateful for. Think of all the things you ARE still able to do; all the kind things people in your life have done for you; all the conveniences you have access to that make your life easier; the people who are here for you and love you; the miracle of your body and how it's kept you alive without you even thinking about it on a day to day basis; all the things you've achieved, lessons you've learned, and the opportunities that lay ahead for you. Write at least 2 or 3 things you are grateful for each day.

~

On the 7th day of each week, your instructions are a little different. As mentioned, this is your day to catch up on any action steps you may have missed during the week. It's also a time to do more complete journaling work. The journaling for day 7 includes:

1. CELEBRATE THE LITTLE WINS: It's the little steps you do each week that, when done consistently, bring about big results. When suddenly we have an injury and even the smallest, simplest tasks seem challenging, it can become quite frustrating and discouraging. The key is not to fight it. Accept that this is the way things are right now. It does not mean this is who you were, or will be. It's simply this moment in time. The actions you take now may not seem like big things, they may even seem inconsequential. Under the surface however it all has an effect. It doesn't matter how small the feat, celebrate it. Be proud of your progress, even if you can't see it yet. It will help shift you into a more positive mindset, a mindset that then becomes conducive to healing. Each week, celebrate something you've done toward your healing journey that you're proud of. It may be something as simple of exercising an extra 10 minutes on Tuesday when you really didn't feel like it, finding a good physiotherapist, being able to sit up in bed without pain, or discovering your flexibility has improved a few more inches. The list is endless. What accomplishments are you proud of?

2. AREAS I CAN IMPROVE ON: It's always easy to do what's comfortable, to let the voice of laziness over speak the desire for greatness, or let ego overshadow your higher self. Look at the steps you've taken during the past week on your road to recovery. Were there things you could have done better, or with more focus? Have you diligently done all your daily

action steps? Did you take a shortcut in any of your exercises by not doing as many reps or sets as you had set out to do? Did you postpone seeking out a new therapist? By being honest with yourself here you'll be able to more clearly pinpoint those things which are holding you back from getting back on your feet faster. Then use these areas as commitments to follow through on during the coming week.

3. GRATITUDE: A big part of the healing process begins after you're able to find gratitude in the things around you, even in difficult situations. In fact, feeling gratitude is so important that we include it on this 7th day as well. As you've already been doing, taking a few minutes to write down things you're grateful for forces you to reflect positively and further helps to develop a positive mindset. Attitude is everything. What are the things in your life right now, big or small, that you're grateful for?

4. MAKING USE OF YOUR DOWN TIME: For many of us our days run into the next with an infinite 'To Do' list and a finite number of hours in the day. So many of the little projects get put on the back-burner as more pressing matters take precedent. Well, here's your chance to get back to those smaller projects, the simpler things. Illness or injury (yes, even sometimes those injuries caused by fluke accident) are our body's way of letting us know that we need to slow down, and this is our wake up call. During the acute stage of your injury or illness you may very well be confined to home, or even the hospital. Even if you're not, it's unlikely you're at the gym or playing soccer with your beer buddies during this time. You'll likely find you have some extra time on your hands. Don't fight the fact that you can't be out there doing all the things you normally would be. You'll get your chance again. Right now though is your chance to reflect on things, catch up on those little projects at home you've been putting off for months or years (this does not mean fixing the roof!) - possibly read some books, do goal setting, whatever it might be. These same things you can do in the hospital. What are some of the things you've been too busy to do that you can now use this down time for?

5. OPENING DOORS: When one gets a serious injury or illness it's easy and natural to at first see all the doors that have suddenly been seemingly closed on us. In fact, *we don't just see those closed doors, we stare at them!* So much so that often we aren't aware of new doors that are constantly opening for us. A large part of the healing process begins as soon as we stop staring at the doors that have closed on us

and start looking at the new doors which are opening. Each new door that we see opening gives us not only a new reason to heal faster, it also inspires and motivates, and most importantly, helps us find gratitude. It also helps us to 'let go'. With an open mind look inside and around you. What new doors do you see potentially opening for you as a result of what you're currently experiencing? What new possibilities could be opening up for you?

6. WHAT'S WORKING: Use this section to record what's working for you and what's not. This can be in terms of exercises (perhaps a certain movement or exercise gives you pain or doesn't feel 'right',) or in terms of attitude (are you still fighting what you cannot change this moment?), or even self-discipline (are you not following through on what you know you should be doing?). Not only will this information help your therapist diagnose and adjust exercises and treatments accordingly, but it may also give you insight into areas where you may be sabotaging your own progress.

This workbook will help you reprogram your mind to a more positive, hopeful, healing way of thinking, while simultaneously walking you through daily action steps to holistically restore the health of your physical body. The approach is multifaceted, as the shift to a positive focus strong enough to overcome all odds requires the following elements:
- ✓ Daily health-improving action steps
- ✓ Positive (and believable) self-talk
- ✓ Embracing gratitude
- ✓ Accepting the lesson(s) your body is trying to tell you
- ✓ Creating a clear picture of the bright future that lies ahead
- ✓ Clearing mental blockages and subconscious programs
- ✓ 100% commitment and determination to overcome your injury or illness
- ✓ Daily repetition of the above

As you progress through the health tips and action steps over the next 12 weeks (Part 1 of this Workbook), you will often be referred to additional worksheets and resources found in the latter parts of this book. It's important to act on each step as they are presented to you.

This includes the journaling. This is no time to be lazy or make excuses; it is your life and health on the line after all. The few minutes you spend each day doing the assigned exercises will have profound effects. You can literally transform the state of your entire body's health by following this 12 week program.

You will get out of this workbook what you put into it. Please allow yourself to trust in these steps, and the daily journaling exercises, even if right now you aren't able to see the benefit, or the connection. While nutrition and therapy can seem the obvious route to healing, the journaling and self-reflection process is equally crucial to any transformation. It will help you discover and validate your thoughts, awareness and experiences, and will subconsciously begin to re-program your mind for better health. Chances are your ego will appear from time to time, convincing you there are better and more important things that you could be doing than completing your workbook exercises and action steps. Do not be fooled though, as giving up does no good to anyone. Stay committed, and remind yourself why you began this journey. What is your health, and a whole new way of living and feeling healthy, worth to you?

Remind yourself that nothing is impossible. Miracles happen every day. Let your determination to heal be stronger than any negative external (or even internal) messages you hear. Never allow anyone's opinion of you or your condition determine your reality. You have the power within you to make magic happen. We all have it within us. Let this book be your guide to awakening the natural and powerful healing abilities within you.

To Your Health, and Successful Recovery!

BEFORE WE BEGIN

It is important that you begin this journey with the right frame of mind, and with the commitment of following through. Too many people begin a new undertaking with the best of intentions of following through, but a few weeks or months later their commitment is nowhere to be seen. Just think of New Year's Resolutions and gym membership as an example (how full gyms are in January and how empty do they get by March or April!). This Workbook should not be started as a fleeting commitment that can be broken. The information herein and the journey guided by this Workbook is powerful – but you MUST do the work and you must follow through. Some of the action steps may feel uncomfortable to you, and they demand you make adjustments to certain areas of your life, including your diet. When resistance comes up for you, remember that you purchased this book because your injury or illness is either putting your lifestyle, or life, on the line, that it's causing suffering; and it is not just you that you need to think of, but also those who love you and depend on you. Nothing should be more important than restoring your health. Please commit to following this program DAILY and diligently, including all the 'Action Steps', for the next 12 weeks. (I need to repeat though that you should first have the consent of your health care practitioner before making any changes to diet, medication, or exercise).

While it's not imperative that you do your journaling at the same time every day, doing so can be beneficial. If you set a certain time each day to do your journaling, it will soon become a positive habit for you, and you will be less prone to forgetting or scheduling in other things during this important time.

An important caveat to take note of: Sometimes, in the course of healing, once the acute phase of the pain is behind us, we can get lazy and settle for 'good enough'. You're able to do certain activities again, and the constant daily reminder of pain is gone. At this point the average person tends to get lazy and skip out on the exercises and work that brought them to this point in their recovery. HOWEVER, are

you someone who settles for mediocrity? Is your healing truly complete inside? Are you able to physically do <u>everything</u> you'd like to be doing? If any of these answers brings up a 'no 'response, then stopping at 'good enough' is not good enough. For optimal healing you need to follow through fully. This is why, even if you are feeling better after a few weeks or a month or two, it's imperative that you complete the full 12 weeks of this Workbook. By doing so, you will discover not only better health, but also a grand transformation of who you are, physically, as well as mentally.

And so, before you begin, your first assignment is to simply read with conviction the 'My Commitment to Healing' on page 192 in Part II of this book. Read it now, and read it again as often as you want whenever you need a reminder of why you picked up this Healing Workbook.

PART 1:

12 WEEK HEALING PROGRAM

HEALTH TIP:

There is a saying that goes 'What you resist persists'. Accepting yourself by letting go of resistance to what currently is can be the missing link to getting back to the health you want. Acceptance of what is *now* does not mean you cannot change what *will be*. These next 12 weeks are going to change your life, and you'll be taking a number of vital action steps toward improving your health. Change is not about doing one big "healthy" thing today and then nothing tomorrow. Change comes about through your habits - adopting healthy actions that are manageable, and doing them consistently, daily. As you embark today on this journey, first accept now as it is - a moment in time - knowing that who and where you are today won't be, with the right habits, who and where you can be tomorrow!

ACTION STEP:

Today you are being given three simple yet very important action steps. First, in the top box on the following page, record your 'starting point'. Write down your condition, the state of your health, pains and aches, your attitude and outlook, and how you're feeling. This will give you a measuring tool that you'll be able to refer back to weeks from now to gauge how far you've progressed. Secondly, if you've not read aloud the Commitment to Healing on page 192, please do so today, and do so with full commitment.

TODAY'S INTENTION:

_____

_____

_____

POSITIVE OUTCOME(S):

_____

_____

_____

AFFIRMATION:

_____

_____

_____

GRATITUDE:

_____

_____

_____

_____

My Starting Point:

My Why:

Your third action today is to record your 'WHY'. Depending on your condition and health goal, the journey to get there will likely involve some sacrifices, maybe giving up some unhealthy foods that you enjoy, or adopting healthier habits which might not come easy. To keep you motivated, it's absolutely imperative that you have a compelling reason to achieve your goal. This is what will get you there! When your reason for doing something, anything, is immensely strong, you will usually find a way to make it happen. Put another way, the BIGGER your 'Why', the SMALLER the 'HOW' becomes. Find that emotional reason inside of you that will drive you and motivate you as you take on the challenge ahead. How will it feel when you've remedied your illness/healed your injury/have more energy/aren't suffering the way you might be now? What's at stake? Who's lives are affected? What will it give you, and your loved ones? What is your BIG reason for healing? Write down your WHY below. (You can include a picture too if you'd like).

My Why:

"Your present circumstances don't determine where you can go;
they merely determine where you start." ~Nido Qubein

WEEK 1 / DAY 2- DATE: _____

HEALTH TIP:

Did you know that sugar contributes to osteoporosis, weakens eyesight, causes food allergies, cardiovascular disease, kidney disease, anxiety, interferes with the absorption of protein, increases cholesterol, uses up magnesium (which in turn increases the negative stress response and in turn leads to another long list of health conditions), feeds cancer, and weakens the immune system? It is also largely responsible for the obesity and diabetes epidemic that we are currently experiencing today. Refined, processed sugar is very hard on the liver (just as damaging as excess alcohol) and much of it is stored as fat. While much of the media has blamed obesity on fat consumption and/or laziness, the fact is sugar is the primary cause. Between 1977 to 2000, Americans doubled their daily sugar intake. With 80% of foods lining grocery store shelves containing excess sugar, it's no wonder we're experiencing such growth in these chronic conditions. At the current rate, 95% of Americans will be overweight or obese within 20 years!

Too much refined sugar can also lead to muscle imbalances and in turn trigger points that cause pain in other parts of the body. To heal any number of infections, diseases, and ailments, we must first loosen the grip on our addiction to sugar. Yes, for many people, sugar is an

TODAY'S INTENTION:

_____

_____

_____

POSITIVE OUTCOME(S):

_____

_____

_____

AFFIRMATION:

_____

_____

_____

GRATITUDE:

_____

_____

_____

_____

addiction. In fact, it's just a few molecules different from the chemical composition of cocaine, and has a similar addictive effect on the brain!

Your body only needs roughly 1 tsp. of sugar to operate the entire bloodstream, yet the average American consumes 26 spoonfuls of refined sugar every day. That's 135 pounds per year! For many, that number is even higher. Many people are consuming the equivalent of their entire body weight in sugar in a year. A single bottle of soda contains the same amount of sugar as what people consumed in their entire lifetime 400 years ago!!! We look at these figures and wonder why we are seeing rising rates of cancer and obesity and diabetes. The answer is clear. We need to cut back.

> While sugar is sugar, even that which is found in natural fruits, at least fruits also provide a healthy dose of fiber (which takes time to digest), allowing the sugar to be released gradually into the body and offering a more sustained form of energy rather than a sudden (and hard on the body) sugar spike. Over time, sudden sugar spikes damage the pancreas and liver and can lead to diabetes, heart disease and liver disease.

ACTION STEP:

Start reducing your sugar consumption. Reducing this one ingredient alone can have a dramatic effect on your overall health. Starting today become aware of how much sugar you're taking in by reading labels (don't just look for the word sugar – high fructose corn syrup, dextrose, maltose, dextrin, fructose, fruit juice concentrate, galactose, glucose, hydrogenated starch, mannitol, polyols, sorghum, sucrose, sorbitol, and xylitol are all other forms it masquerades as), and make an effort to reduce your sugar intake as much as possible. A few notes on this though… if you try to quit cold turkey, expect the first 2 to 3 days to be quite difficult, and you'll likely experience symptoms of headache, digestive upset, and mood imbalances, just as you would with any addiction detox. These symptoms will subside after a few days to a week. If quitting cold turkey is too hard and you must have sweet things, here are my top 8 suggestions for reducing your sugar consumption:

- ❖ Substitute sugar for either stevia or coconut sugar, both of which are healthier alternatives.
- ❖ Focus on non-starchy carbs such as kale, cauliflower, green beans, zucchini, mushrooms, tomatoes, artichoke. (Complex

carbs such as sweet potatoes & yams can help alleviate sugar cravings, but they are starchy and should be avoided at least initially while trying to get off sugar).

❖ Protein with every meal will help balance insulin and make your sugar reduction challenge easier.

❖ When selectively reducing sugar, aim to reduce (ideally eliminate) liquid sugar, such as what you'll find in energy drinks, fruit juices, sodas, and sports drinks. This is the most dangerous type of sugar, as well as the leading source of added sugar in the Western diet. Artificial sweeteners are just as bad. (You'll learn more about both of these nasty culprits in the weeks ahead).

❖ Each time you have a sugary snack, combine it with a healthy option. For example, if you reach for that chocolate bar, have an apple with it, or some almonds. This will get you used to eating healthier options and will help over time to eliminate the bad stuff.

❖ Eat smaller and healthier meals throughout the day. When you're not hungry, the desire for sugar subsides.

❖ Food cravings are often a sign of a lack in some other area of life. Start becoming aware of your emotional state when those cravings appear... are you substituting sugar for some unfulfilled emotional need?

❖ Remove temptation. It's easy to grab those sugar-filled snacks when they're staring at you in the cupboard sweetly calling your name. Toss 'em! If they're not in the house it will make it a lot harder for you to cheat on those cravings.

(www.sugarscience.org offers a great resource for further study on sugar).

"People are fed by the food industry which pays no attention to health, and are treated by the health industry which pays no attention to food."
~ Wendell Berry

WEEK 1 / DAY 3- DATE: _____

HEALTH TIP:

The topic of water might sound basic, but we're laying the groundwork these first few days for deeper healing in the weeks ahead. Humans are 55%-78% water. Without water our entire body suffers and can cause everything from headaches to back pain, dry skin, heart and kidney problems, etc. A good idea is to fill up a washable water bottle (many are marked with the ounces on the side) with your daily 'to drink' amount and bring it with you throughout the day and drink as you go. Make sure you finish it each day. How much should you drink? A general guideline is 7 to 10 cups (56oz – 80oz) of water per day for men and 6 to 9 cups (48oz – 72oz) for women. How can you tell if you need more water? Look at your urine. Clear is good. The darker it is, likely the more dehydrated your body is.

TODAY'S INTENTION:

_____

_____

_____

POSITIVE OUTCOME(S):

_____

_____

_____

AFFIRMATION:

_____

_____

_____

GRATITUDE:

_____

_____

_____

ACTION STEP:

Ensure you drink your 6-10 cups of water today, and start making it a daily habit. When choosing your water, go mainly for spring / artesian water which contains a wide variety of essential trace minerals. Trace minerals, as you'll learn later, are the spark plugs of life. Branded spring waters include Evian, Arrowhead, Volvic, Poland, and Fiji. You can also go online and find your own natural spring water sources close to your home at www.findaspring.com. (Avoid reverse osmosis water, though common as it is. It does not hydrate the body as well as spring water,

and may even contain plastic particles from the plastic membrane the water is forced through in the filtration process. Furthermore, with reverse osmosis or distilled water, the body tends to leach minerals out of the bone to put 'back into' the water. If you do drink reverse osmosis, then it's certainly a good idea to add some Himalayan sea salt or trace minerals to the water). Tap water meanwhile may contain heavy metals, fluoride, chlorine, and even medicines (which are not monitored or filtered). Carbon filtering removes chlorine, but it doesn't remove fluoride. Fluoride (discussed more on page 100) is linked to a long list of damaging health effects, including osteoporosis and cancer.

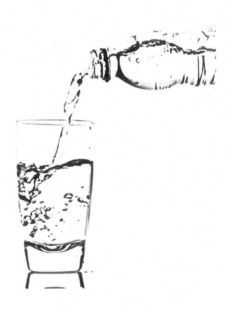

"As a retired physician, I can honestly say that unless you are in a serious accident, your best chance of living to a ripe old age is to avoid doctors and hospitals and learn nutrition, herbal medicine and other forms of natural medicine... Almost all drugs are toxic and are designed only to treat symptoms and not to cure anyone. Most surgery is unnecessary.
In short, our mainstream medical system is hopelessly inept and/or corrupt."
Dr. Allan Greenberg (12/24/2002)

WEEK 1 / DAY 4- DATE: _____

HEALTH TIP:

It can be said that all illness first begins in the mind, but from a physiological perspective, all illness begins in the gut. An unhealthy gut leads to a dizzying array of medical conditions, and much of the connection between gut-body-mind is little understood among many in the medical community. In fact, the brain and the gut are inseparably connected, and gut issues can lead to the failing of the brain, just as brain dysfunction can lead to serious gut issues. Additionally, all autoimmune disease begins in the gut (and there are over 200 such disorders, including Celiac Disease, Rheumatoid Arthritis, Multiple Sclerosis, Crohn's Disease, Alopecia, Hashimoto's Thyroiditis, just to name a few). 85% of our immune system is also in our gut. If we want to heal major chronic illness or degenerative disease, even our brain, we cannot ignore examining the health of our gut.

TODAY'S INTENTION:

_____

_____

_____

POSITIVE OUTCOME(S):

_____

_____

_____

AFFIRMATION:

_____

_____

_____

GRATITUDE:

_____

_____

_____

_____

Our entire gut is lined with beneficial gut flora. These gut flora help synthesize nutrients and place nutrients in the right amounts into the blood. The flora also protect and help move enterocytes (intestinal absorptive cells) which, when their movement is impaired, can mutate and form cancer. Normal gut flora will never allow a cancerous process to begin in the digestive tract.

Antibiotics are one major cause of impaired gut flora. We must realize that even if we have not recently taken antibiotics directly, we are indirectly ingesting antibiotics through the meat we eat (85% of all antibiotics used in the U.S. are given to slaughter animals to keep them alive in their horrid living conditions). And it's not just antibiotics. Any long term medication will also lead to damaged gut flora.

(Incidentally, babies born through C-section also have less than ideal gut flora, leading to higher incidences of autism, ADHD, dyslexia, and learning disabilities.)

Damaged or impaired gut flora can not only lead to cancer as already mentioned, but it also impairs our immune system, is a major cause of many allergies, and opens the door to pathogens taking over our digestive tract which then (through being absorbed into the blood stream) go on to create mental disorders in the brain and disease wherever else they end up in the body.

ACTION STEP:

While it can take 6 months to a couple of years to properly heal a damaged gut, there are simple things that you can start doing today to get an upper hand on gut pathogens and strengthen your good gut flora. A good quality probiotic (or even probiotic drinks such as "Good Belly") is something everyone can benefit by. Coconut (in any form) has antimicrobial and antiviral properties and is great to take. Also aromatic herbs such as oregano, rosemary, turmeric, cayenne are antimicrobial and beneficial, with oregano (especially oil of oregano) leading the pack. Foods such as sweet potato, pumpkin, squash, turnip, cantaloupe, green tea, honey, bee pollen, and artichokes all help feed the good bacteria. Bone broth and gelatin are also highly beneficial to the integrity of the gastrointestinal tract and healing the gut. Of the items mentioned above, which can you start consuming more of? Choose at least 3 that you can commit to consuming regularly.

_____

_____

_____

Additionally, when healing the gut and dealing with small intestinal bacterial overgrowth (also known as SIBO), you'll want to eat low FODMAP foods as much as possible, at least in the short term for easing of symptoms. FODMAP stands for Fermentable Oligo-Di-Monosaccharides and Polyols, a list of which is included for reference in Part II of this book (page 194).

One of the most in depth gut healing protocols available today is known as the GAPS Nutritional Protocal Diet (GAPSdiet.com). To properly follow through with GAPS however takes a big commitment, and as such it might not be for everyone.

As an alternative, Part 3 of this book provides an elimination diet (including recipes) by health coach and gut healing expert Aga Postawska that will help you start pinpointing some of the foods that might be causing you gut-related issues, as well as symptoms that extend far beyond the gut. While we're on the topic of gut health, read her article on page 330 that will walk you through the leaky gut – brain health connection and the vital importance of healing your gut flora.

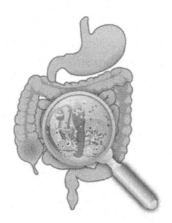

"The human body has every mechanism for self-healing and self-repair programmed into it. All you have to do is just feed it properly and not bombard it with toxins."
~ Natasha Campbell-McBride

HEALTH TIP:

"Every stress leaves an indelible scar, and the organism pays for its survival after a stressful situation by becoming a little older." ~ Dr. Hans Selye

Entire books can be filled on the detrimental effects of stress alone. Stress has far reaching effects on nearly every system in the body. As stress increases, cortisol and aldosterone are released, in turn increasing sodium and copper retention in the kidneys. As sodium increases over potassium, magnesium (the primary calming mineral) is lost, and the tendency for anger, anxiety, and addictive behaviors increase. The rising stress weakens the liver and the adrenals, increasing fatigue and a number of adrenal-related health issues (I discuss this further in my article on page 362 in Part 2 of this book). Zinc gets depleted, which increases the risk of allergies, immune issues, and even leaky gut. Candida (from rising bio-unavailable copper) can take hold, and emotions and outlook can become negatively affected. Virtually every system in the body is affected by stress, and one of the most important things you can do for your health and healing is to reduce stress. This includes reducing or eliminating stressors in all forms, including physical trauma, emotional trauma (both real and imagined), toxic and heavy metal toxicity, lack of sleep, anxiety, poor diet, infections and illness, prescriptions drugs, and even excessive exercise.

TODAY'S INTENTION:

_____

_____

_____

POSITIVE OUTCOME(S):

_____

_____

_____

AFFIRMATION:

_____

_____

_____

GRATITUDE:

_____

_____

_____

_____

There are many ways to reduce stress, breath-work being just one such way. Breathing is not only a great way to help relieve stress, it is also the fundamental basis of all healing, and all life. Breathing deeply allows more oxygen into our bodies which helps cellular respiration and metabolism, brain function, energy levels, healing, relieving anxiety and, of course, stress, Here are a few simple breathing techniques you can use whenever you feel stressed. For each of these, try not to breathe using your chest muscles, but rather with your diaphragm. When you do this correctly, your abdomen will extend outward on the exhale.

a) Sit or stand in a comfortable position. Breathe in through your nose, counting to 4. Exhale slowly, as if blowing a bubble through a wand, until your lungs are empty.

b) Stand. Bend at the waist. Put your hands on your knees. Breathe in through your nose. Exhale hard in one breath.

c) Stand or sit. Exhale fully to begin, and place your tongue at the roof of your mouth. Inhale to the count of 4, hold for a count of 7, and then exhale forcefully for a count of 8. Repeat this 4 times only, twice a day.

d) Sit. Place your hands on your thighs. Breathe in through your nose while you bring your hands up to your chest. Then push your hands straight out in front of you and exhale at the same time.

ACTION STEP:

Take a few 5 minute breaks today and practice the above breathing techniques. Then pick your favorite and work it into your daily routine.

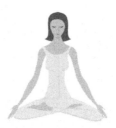

"Slow breathing is like an anchor in the midst of an emotional storm: the anchor won't make the storm go away, but it will hold you steady until it passes."
~Russ Harris

HEALTH TIP:

Garlic is one of nature's best antibiotics, containing anti-bacterial, antiviral, & antifungal properties. Garlic stimulates the body's entire immune system & is effective against strep, staph, & even anthrax bacteria! It helps clear mucus from the lungs, can be useful in treating upper respiratory infections, & helps in the support of the urinary, circulatory, & digestive systems. It's also effective against heart disease, kidney disorders, diabetes, & many cancers. Aged garlic extract (AGE) has even higher antioxidant properties than regular garlic, protecting even further against heart disease, blood cholesterol and high blood pressure. The key to garlic's antibiotic effectiveness is its magical ingredient 'allicin' - created through an enzyme reaction which occurs only after the garlic clove is crushed or chopped. It reaches maximum potency about 10 minutes after the clove is cut, & then diminishes rapidly after an hour. Therefore, the crushed uncooked garlic should be eaten within this time frame to achieve the maximum healing benefits. *(For more on how garlic and other herbs can help various conditions, review the **Herbs & Supplements Guide** at the back of this book).*

TODAY'S INTENTION:

_____

_____

_____

POSITIVE OUTCOME(S):

_____

_____

AFFIRMATION:

_____

_____

_____

GRATITUDE:

_____

_____

_____

_____

ACTION STEP:

Find a way to incorporate garlic into one of your meals today.

While Kyolic is an odorless and 'sociable' alternative that offers most of garlic's benefits, it's also beneficial to get used to chewing raw garlic. While this may sound horrific to some, it's really not as bad as it sounds (although it may take a few tries to get used to it). This method really allows the allicin to hit those germs most effectively. Cut about 1/6 of a clove to start (you can do more as your tolerance increases). Cut this small piece as finely as possible and let it sit for 10 minutes. Then put it in your mouth and let it sit between your teeth as you absorb the juices from it. Eventually you'll swallow it. As you feel a slight burning sensation in the back of your throat, be conscious of all those bad bacteria that it's killing.

This is not a practice you need to do every day. But anytime you feel a respiratory / throat infection coming on, this is a great thing to do. Even otherwise, garlic has so many benefits as mentioned in today's Tip, that making this a daily habit is not a bad thing. (Of course probably a good idea to plan this activity several hours away from any important social activities!)

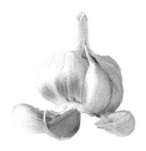

*"What lies behind us and what lies before us are tiny matters
compared to what lies within us."*
~ Ralph Waldo Emerson

THIS WEEK'S REVIEW:

Today is your chance to go over the action steps of this past week, reincorporate any activities you may have forgotten, and complete any activities yet unfinished. Use today to catch up and take stock.

Check off the items you've completed below:

☐ I've written my 'Why'.

☐ I've looked at how much sugar I'm consuming and am reducing my sugar intake by doing _____

☐ I'm drinking 6-10 glasses of water each day.

☐ Into my daily diet I've incorporated at least 3 low-FODMAP food or other ingredients to help strengthen my gut and benefit my good flora.

☐ I've at least read the articles in Unit 3 on regarding Gut Health and the Elimination Diet.

☐ I am doing at least 1 focused breathe exercise daily.

☐ I bravely explored chewing raw garlic

☐ I completed all my daily journaling exercises, including today's which are on the following 2 pages.

Of the tips I've learned so far this week, 3 action steps that I commit to doing consistently going forward are:

1. _____

2. _____

3. _____

1. This week I'm proud of:

_____

_____

_____

_____

_____

2. This coming week I commit to following through on the things I didn't fully do this past week (health-wise or other) which include:

_____

_____

_____

_____

_____

3. I'm grateful for:

_____

_____

_____

_____

_____

4. Now that I have some down time, a few things I've been meaning to do that I could do now are:

_____

_____

_____

_____

5. I choose not to stare at the closing doors but rather new ones which are opening. These are:

_____

_____

_____

_____

6. What's worked this week and what's not?

_____

_____

_____

_____

7. General notes and thoughts:

_____

_____

_____

HEALTH TIP:

You set goals in life, in business, in projects, in finances. The same should be done with your health. Now, setting a date for a complete recovery may be risky depending on your condition as some things you simply can't force the timing of. However, there are steps you can take toward your healing that can and should become your mini milestones – your goals. Having an effective goal setting system for your health will keep you on track and will certainly aid in your healing sooner rather than later.

Equally important to the end goal is the action you will consistently take to get there. Rather than stating your goal as "to have my torn tendon completely healed by August", it is better to state the goal as "to spend 30 minutes every day doing the exercises my physiotherapist has given me."

To truly succeed with goal setting, accountability is also key. While healing is an individual (internal) process that no one can do for you, the miracle of healing becomes so much easier when the journey is shared with someone else. Someone you can open yourself up to with love and/or someone to hold you accountable. Whether it's an early morning wake up call to encourage you to work-out, checking in to make sure you're doing your daily rehabilitation exercises, or holding you accountable to doing your daily actions in this book, that 'accountability partner' should believe in you, be positive, and won't take any crap when you

TODAY'S INTENTION:
_____
_____
_____

POSITIVE OUTCOME(S):
_____
_____
_____

AFFIRMATION:
_____
_____
_____

GRATITUDE:
_____
_____
_____
_____

present excuses. They should be there with tough love for one purpose – to help you get better.

ACTION STEP:

Included in this book on Page 195 is the My H.E.A.L.T.H Goals Worksheet (and instructions), a powerful goal setting and tracking tool for you to use each month. Begin today (making today the first day of the month) by filling in goals for each of the six areas.

Secondly, in the box below, write down the name of 1 or 2 close friends or colleagues that you can ask to be your accountability partner. Contact those people within the next 24 hours, tell them the goal you're working toward, and ask if they'd be willing to hold you accountable in your action steps.

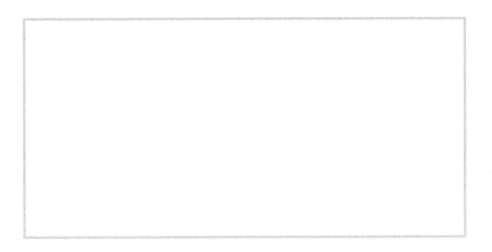

"If you don't know where you're going, you'll end up someplace else."
~ Yogi Berra

HEALTH TIP:

Many allergies don't come with obvious symptoms such as rashes, swelling, or nausea. Often, the symptoms are subtle, yet profound, resulting in conditions ranging from overall feelings of fatigue, lack of focus, indigestion, headaches, sinus infections, psoriasis, eczema, congestion, gastrointestinal problems, insomnia, and arthritic problems to name but a few. The best way to heal food allergies is to (a) remove the food that causes the reaction and (b) heal the lining of the gut (which you've already begun work on last week).

So, how do you find out if you have a food allergy (short of obvious and immediate reactions)? Well, blood tests and skin tests don't always work. The best way is through dietary testing.

TODAY'S INTENTION:

_____

_____

_____

POSITIVE OUTCOME(S):

_____

_____

_____

AFFIRMATION:

_____

_____

_____

GRATITUDE:

_____

_____

_____

_____

ACTION STEP:

Last week you were introduced to the Elimination Diet in Part 3 of this book. I've you've not yet tried it, make today the day you start. You might choose to follow the full diet for the full 3 weeks, or start off slowly by even eliminating 1 food item for a week and seeing how you feel. The more you can commit to the program the more you'll be able to see the results. Often by the end of the first week you'll

begin seeing differences in how you feel (if the eliminated food(s) is indeed having an effect on you. Take notes on how you feel. You can use the Food Journal provided on page 204 to help you with this. Granted this challenge may not be easy, as we are often allergic to foods we crave the most! However eliminating those foods will not only reduce the obvious negative symptoms, it will also give your gut lining a chance to rebuild itself. This in turn will strengthen your immune defenses, increase your ability to absorb good nutrients, increase your body's tolerance to allergens, not to mention make you feel better all around.

A faster approach for understand one's food sensitivities, if the budget allows, is to do a Mediator Release Test (MRT). It is a very reliable and comprehensive assessment for getting to the root of food allergies.

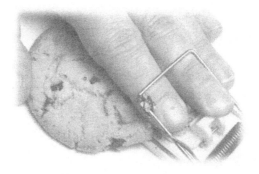

"Health is a state of complete physical, mental and social well-being, and not merely the absence of disease or infirmity."
~World Health Organization

HEALTH TIP:

Mushrooms are one of the greatest healing foods on earth. They offer immune and energy support, and because they also act like sponges, are excellent for helping to absorb toxins and metabolic waste (helping the body to detox). Chaga mushroom is the king of all medicinal mushrooms. According to David Wolfe, one of the world's leading authorities on nutrition, chaga mushroom is the most powerful immune boosting and anti-cancer substance on earth. It also contains the most powerful radiation removing properties of any substance on earth.

Reishi mushroom, the most widely studied herb on earth, is a great immunity booster against the flu, and is useful in treating prostate cancer. In fact, the Japanese government even recognizes reishi as a cancer treatment!

Maitake mushroom is recognized by the American Cancer Society to limit and even reverse tumor growth.

It is hard to comprehend the millions of dollars that go into cancer drug "research" and pink ribbon awareness campaigns (everyone already knows cancer exists) when the real awareness should be on the simple every day healthy alternatives people can use to protect and heal themselves.

TODAY'S INTENTION:

_____

_____

_____

POSITIVE OUTCOME(S):

_____

_____

_____

AFFIRMATION:

_____

_____

_____

GRATITUDE:

_____

_____

_____

_____

Even the lowly white button mushroom is powerful. According to nutritional expert and best-selling author Dr. Joel Furhman, eating mushrooms every day (even just white button mushrooms) reduces the risk of breast cancer by 64%.

Other powerhouse mushrooms for healing include:

Lion's Mane - has shown effectiveness against Parkinson's disease.

Shiitake – helps protect against inflammation and harmful viruses. It also attacks tumors.

Cordyceps – enhances energy and stamina and is useful in recovering from adrenal fatigue.

Note: Chaga mushroom has been used safely for thousands of years. It may however interact with diabetes medications like insulin resulting in low blood sugar and should be used cautiously by those on diabetes medication.

ACTION STEP:

What mushrooms can you start taking to help with your condition? Some possible ideas may include:

- ➢ Incorporate button mushrooms into your salads & meals
- ➢ Make a tea from chaga mushroom and drink it daily. You can always add cacao or another tea to make it more flavorful.
- ➢ Sprinkle some chaga mushroom powder into a daily smoothie
- ➢ Go to your local health food store and inquire into what mushroom tinctures or capsules are available.

"The doctor of the future will give no medicine but will interest his patients in the care of the human frame, in diet, and in the cause and prevention of disease."
~ Thomas Edison

HEALTH TIP:

We've already touched on the importance of a healthy gut. Today's tip is a continuation of that topic, focusing on candida (yeast infection / parasitic fungus). Candida can lead to a number of conditions including depression, moodiness, brain fog, spaciness, OCD, anxiety, gas, excess mucous, memory problems, personality changes, infertility, urinary tract infections, asthma, impaired immunity, and eating disorders.

"Over time, candida grows from a yeast form into a fungal form and starts creating waste products known as mycotoxins. Among the mycotoxins produced is acetaldehyde, a poison that is converted by the liver into alcohol. As alcohol builds up in the system, symptoms associated with alcohol intoxication develop. This is why one of the most common symptoms of candida is brain fog... In its fungal form, candida also grows long roots called rhizoids that puncture the intestinal lining, leading to a condition called leaky gut syndrome. This creates holes in the digestive tract, allowing candida to pass through into the bloodstream." ~Brenda Watson, N.D.

Everyone with autism, rheumatoid arthritis, MS, lupus, chronic fatigue, fibromyalgia, gluten intolerance, even Alzheimer's has elevated levels of yeast. Birth control pills also feed yeast. High levels of bio-unavailable copper in the body (you'll learn more about this silent epidemic in week 5) also allow candida to flourish. Copper, in its bioavailable form, is a natural fungicide that helps in the control of candida. However when

TODAY'S INTENTION:

_____

_____

_____

POSITIVE OUTCOME(S):

_____

_____

_____

AFFIRMATION:

_____

_____

_____

GRATITUDE:

_____

_____

_____

_____

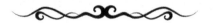

copper becomes bio-unavailable (due to copper toxicity/deficiency, weakened adrenals, low ceruloplasmin production), it is rendered incapable of controlling candida. Other contributing factors that can lead to high levels of candida include stress, excessive sugar, coffee, alcohol, infections, and a high non-organic meat diet.

Bringing yeast under control will not only help the above conditions, it can also help with psoriasis and eczema, and even prevent and/or reverse autism in children! The Elimination Diet offered in this book is a good starting point. For further research in this area to fully tackle candida head-on, the Body Ecology Diet (as created by Donna Gates) is an excellent resource (www.bodyecology.com). A live blood analysis (as you'll learn about in week 5) is a great method for determining candida and parasite levels in the body. Hair Tissue Mineral Analysis (coming up tomorrow) provides telling indicators as to one's copper level which can then be quite indicative of a candida problem.

While it will take a committed effort over several months to cleanse from candida, some simple steps you can begin doing now include:

- ✓ Eliminating or reducing yeast, gluten, sugar, white flour, and soft drinks
- ✓ Minimizing sweet fruits like bananas and tropical fruits which can spike blood sugar which in turn can lead to candida.
- ✓ Limit complex carbohydrates to gluten free grains (millet is a great one) and root vegetables
- ✓ Eat organic meats
- ✓ Focus on healthy fats such as avocado & coconut butter
- ✓ Supplement with Pau D'arco tea, oregano oil, grape seed extract
- ✓ Incorporate bone broth into your diet
- ✓ Take a good multi-strain probiotic
- ✓ Strengthen your liver and adrenals (as you will do in the coming weeks) which will assist in making copper bioavailable which in turn greatly helps combat candida.

ACTION STEP:

In addition to implementing ways as mentioned above to reducing your candida levels, it's also time to start prioritizing. Use the scheduling exercise on page 205 in Part II to ensure you start making time for the things that are most important to you in life.

"It's not about prioritizing your schedule, but scheduling your priorities."
~ Steven Covey

WEEK 2 / DAY 5- DATE: _____

HEALTH TIP:

There are two simple screening tests that I believe everyone can benefit enormously from. Today we look at one of these tests. It's called a Hair Tissue Mineral Analysis (HTMA).

"[HTMA] may be the most important health test that exists... Only when you and your doctor know for sure your mineral status and important ratios can you adapt your diet, minerals and supplements to work toward proper balance."
~ Dr. Robert Thompson, MD

The health of both your body and mind is greatly affected by the delicate balance of minerals in your system. Blind supplementation of vitamins or minerals we think is good for us, may in fact be quite harmful. Minerals do not operate independently from each other. Increasing the level of one can throw off the levels of others. Let me give you an example. Let's say you supplement with calcium (or even copper). Both will lower magnesium levels. This in turn decreases potassium and increases sodium. The ratio of sodium to potassium affects our ability to handle stress, and the health of our adrenals. As sodium increases, blood pressure increases, the tendency for anxiety, panic and anger increase, and the negative ego mind takes precedence over the higher spiritual mind. Meanwhile the drop in magnesium lowers energy production and can lead to a sudden fatal heart attack if it's allowed to go too low. As you can see, even a simple and common supplement can lead to drastic physical and psychological changes. This example is *not* to say that calcium or copper supplementation is bad for all people – certainly not. For some people the supplementation of these minerals is beneficial, depending on the existing

TODAY'S INTENTION:

_____

_____

_____

POSITIVE OUTCOME(S):

_____

_____

_____

AFFIRMATION:

_____

_____

_____

GRATITUDE:

_____

_____

_____

_____

balance of other minerals. This is why it's imperative to understand the mineral levels in your body before supplementing, and HTMA is the best way of assessing such levels. Unfortunately, a wide-spread lack of understanding leads many practitioners to continue testing mineral levels via blood. Blood serum tests can be very misleading as they only show the level of circulating minerals, NOT the level of minerals in cells and stored in organs. Let's look at magnesium and copper as cases in point.

Less than 1% of the body's magnesium is in the blood, and only .3% is in the blood serum. A blood serum test therefore offers a very inaccurate reading of the body's overall magnesium status. Furthermore, serum magnesium levels can actually change depending on how the blood is drawn. As the tourniquet is applied longer, magnesium rises due to hypoxia. The blood magnesium can also rise (showing as a normal or high level) during an intracellular loss of magnesium, leading to depletion of the nutrient.

Turning to copper, blood serum tests again are very misleading. Due to the tight homeostatic balance blood must maintain, blood serum testing most often will not show elevated copper (or other mineral levels for that matter). Excess copper is stored in tissues and cells, not the blood, and so a blood test can show normal copper levels even though stored tissue copper may be dangerously high. A blood test is also only reliable in a very short window of time. For example, if a patient is exposed to copper daily and has a blood serum test performed during such time, the test might catch the high circulating copper level. However, if the source of the exposure is removed and a week or two later a new blood test performed, it could very well show perfectly normal levels of copper, even though this ignores all the accumulated bio-unavailable copper stored in tissue.

Unlike blood testing, the Hair TMA is able to detect much more accurately the levels of stored minerals in the body – both essential nutrients and toxic minerals. The testing involves sending in a tablespoon-size amount of hair sample to a clinical laboratory (under specific guidelines to avoid contamination) which then uses spectrophotometry to determine the levels of about 30 minerals and 8 toxic metals in your hair.

Minerals are known as the spark plugs of life, and imbalance can be linked to almost every health condition. This is why it's so important to understand your mineral levels. You can bet with almost 100% certainty that there are mineral deficiencies in YOUR body. Why are mineral deficiencies so prevalent, even if you live 'healthy'? Here are just a few of the many reason:
- With each passing decade, the soil in which our food is grown is becoming more and more deplete of minerals.
- Food processing
- Fluoride in drinking water
- High consumption of sugar, coffee, alcohol, and soda drinks (all of which waste magnesium)

> ➤ Wide-spread use of glyphosate (herbicide) on crops
> ➤ Use of pharmaceutical drugs, birth control, diuretics, antacids and acid blockers, and certain antibiotics
> ➤ Increasing levels of stress in a fast-paced world
> ➤ The Standard American Diet as well as vegetarian / vegan diets
> ➤ Supplementing with the wrong vitamins and minerals which antagonistically lower the levels of other minerals
> ➤ Unhealthy gut environment leading to poor mineral absorption

"99% of the American people are deficient in minerals, and a marked deficiency in any one of the more important minerals actually results in disease."
~(Senate Document 264 74th Congress, 1936)

Note the date of the quote above. The situation has certainly worsened even more since that time! Now, having a Hair TMA done is one thing, having it properly interpreted is another. It's not enough to simply look at individual mineral levels and diagnose your status on that basis alone. Many psychological (and physical) symptoms present themselves when <u>ratios</u> between mineral levels are out of balance, even though levels of the individual minerals might appear in standard testing to be in the "normal range". This is why it's so important to work with someone who specializes in HTMA, and doesn't just pass on an automated lab report to you. Only once you have a clear picture of the mineral levels and possible imbalances in your body can proper supplementation (vitamins and minerals) then be intelligently recommended. A number of serious conditions can be corrected (or avoided) by simply supplementing with the correct minerals in the correct amounts.

"Mineral deficiencies are responsible for a host of health problems, which are incorrectly treated by drugs," Dr. Robert Thompson, M.D.

ACTION STEP:

Today you're encouraged to learn more about how minerals are affecting your health. Two great resources to start are (i) the HTMA article included on page 340, and (ii) the book 'The Strands of Health', by Dr. Rick Malter, 2003. As a specialist in this field I truly believe HTMA is a screening test everyone should have done. I've included below a coupon which will give you a $40 discount should you decide to test your minerals.

"Natural forces within us are the true healers of disease." ~Hippocrates

WEEK 2 / DAY 6- DATE: _____

HEALTH TIP:

It's very important that your doctor is on board with your healing, and shares your commitment to finding a way. Although all doctors have a lot of training, not all share the same treatment protocol, and many are focused on the one area in which they studied, limiting their understanding of other approaches. Finding a doctor who promotes a holistic approach is a good start. Many naturopathic doctors are now covered under medical plans. If you're happy with your doctor, stay with him or her. Otherwise, a second opinion can't hurt.

ACTION STEP:

Healing emotional wounds and shifting towards a more positive and empowering mindset is equally as important as any diet or therapy you do. While you'll be doing a lot of work in this area over the coming weeks, your step today is to complete the Victim vs Victor exercise on Page 210.

TODAY'S INTENTION:

_____

_____

POSITIVE OUTCOME(S):

_____

_____

_____

AFFIRMATION:

_____

_____

GRATITUDE:

_____

_____

_____

_____

"As my sufferings mounted I soon realized that there were two ways in which I could respond to my situation - either to react with bitterness or seek to transform the suffering into a creative force. I decided to follow the latter course."
~Martin Luther King Jr.

WEEK 2 / DAY 7- DATE: _____

THIS WEEK'S REVIEW:

Today is your chance to go over the action steps of this past week, reincorporate any activities you may have forgotten, and complete any activities yet unfinished. Use today to catch up and take stock.

Check off the items you've completed below:

☐ I've completed the My H.E.A.L.T.H. Goals worksheet

☐ I've found myself an accountability partner.

☐ I've begun allergy testing on myself using an elimination diet.

☐ I've added medicinal mushrooms into my diet.

☐ I've completed the scheduling exercise on page 205.

☐ I've completed the Victim vs Victor exercise.

☐ I've looked into having a Hair Tissue Mineral Analysis test done. (www.htmatest.com)

☐ I completed all my daily journaling exercises, including today's which are on the following 2 pages.

Of the tips I've learned so far in this book, 4 action steps for my health that I **commit** to doing consistently going forward are:

1. _____

2. _____

3. _____

4. _____

1. This week I'm proud of:

_____

_____

_____

_____

_____

2. This coming week I commit to following through on the things I didn't fully do this past week (health-wise or other) which include:

_____

_____

_____

_____

_____

3. I'm grateful for:

_____

_____

_____

_____

_____

_____

_____

4. Now that I have some down time, a few things I've been meaning to do that I could do now are:

_____

_____

_____

_____

5. I choose not to stare at the closing doors but rather new ones which are opening. These are:

_____

_____

_____

_____

6. What's worked this week and what's not?

_____

_____

_____

_____

7. General notes and thoughts:

_____

_____

_____

HEALTH TIP:

Emotional healing can have powerfully profound effects, especially when dealing with things such as cancer or even heart disease. When we keep negative feelings (resentment, hate, regret, anger, unforgiveness) trapped within our bodies, cortisol levels rise causing stress, suppressing the immune system, and allowing more easily normal cells to mutate into cancer cells. For heart conditions, often dealing with emotional issues is a first step in healing the physical organ. In terms of overall healing, it's important to forgive ourselves, and others. We need to identify and then release those false beliefs that we have been carrying with us (sometimes through generations) and by doing so, our immune function will improve.

ACTION STEP:

Turn to page 213 and work through the Emotional Clearing Exercise #1. The exercises in this section are some of the most important ones you may ever do, so please do not skip this assignment! You might also want to read the article on page 356 at this time.

TODAY'S INTENTION:

_____

_____

_____

POSITIVE OUTCOME(S):

_____

_____

_____

AFFIRMATION:

_____

_____

_____

GRATITUDE:

_____

_____

_____

_____

"Many people live their lives punishing those closest to them (and inevitably themselves) as subconscious retribution for the injustice done to them by someone else. This pattern needs to stop. It begins with awareness."
~Rick D. Fischer

WEEK 3 / DAY 2- DATE: _____

HEALTH TIP:

Heart disease and cancer remain the leading cause of death in developed countries. We can reduce the risk of both these diseases by our lifestyle choices and by limiting the amount of inflammatory food we eat. Some key inflammatory foods to avoid include sugars (as well as aspartame and Splenda, both of which have been linked to leukemia and have numerous other side effects I won't even get into here), common cooking oils, trans fats, gluten, dairy products, red and processed meats and all processed foods, sodas, alcohol, refined grains, and artificial food additives.

ACTION STEP:

Take a look at your diet. Are you consuming large amounts of any of the above items? Write what you feel are your major inflammatory food culprits in the box below. Your action step is to eliminate at least one of these from your diet for the next 30 days. Choose at least one! The more of these you can avoid the better.

TODAY'S INTENTION:

_____

_____

_____

POSITIVE OUTCOME(S):

_____

_____

_____

AFFIRMATION:

_____

_____

_____

GRATITUDE:

_____

_____

_____

_____

"Optimal health is a journey taken one step, one habit, and one day at a time"
Dr. Wayne Scott Andersen

HEALTH TIP:

Yesterday you learned about inflammatory foods and (hopefully) have eliminated at least a few from your diet. On the other side of the coin, many foods are anti-inflammatory – foods you want to add to your diet to decrease inflammation and promote better health. Diabetes for example can be reversed in as little as one month with an anti-inflammatory diet.

Some anti-inflammatory foods include water, kelp, wild salmon, green tea, papaya, pineapple, blueberries, broccoli, organic extra virgin olive oil, garlic, and high grass fed protein (grass fed cows as opposed to corn fed cows). Omega 3 is one of the most important anti-inflammatory nutrients we can consume. Walnuts, flaxseed, sardines, soybeans, and the aforementioned salmon are all great sources of Omega 3. Lastly, no anti-inflammatory diet would be complete without turmeric, which is one of the most potent anti-inflammatory agents in nature!

I realize that eating healthy and organically can be more expensive that eating non-organically, or fast / processed food. It's true that the initial outlay might be higher, but really it's an investment in yourself, and the extra money to spend to eat healthy today can save you medical costs in the future. One great idea (if you live in North America)

TODAY'S INTENTION:

_____

_____

_____

POSITIVE OUTCOME(S):

_____

_____

_____

AFFIRMATION:

_____

_____

_____

GRATITUDE:

_____

_____

_____

_____

is visit www.localharvest.org. There you'll find farms in your region from which you can buy direct, at huge cost savings! (www.doortodoororganics.com is another option available in certain parts of the U.S.). In terms of eating organic produce, not everything you buy needs to be organic. Certain produce contain more pesticides than others. The chart on page 224 lays out which fruits and vegetables should be given priority when buying organic. While we're on the topic of organic, another link I think you'll find useful is www.eatwild.com/products/. There you'll find the most comprehensive source for grass-fed meat and dairy products in the United States and Canada.

ACTION STEP:

In the box below, choose 3 – 5 of the previously mentioned anti-inflammatory items that, starting today, you will commit to making a part of your daily or weekly diet.

In addition to the above, (and looking into LocalHarvest.org), I also want to help you get guidance today from the people in your life (or perhaps people you've heard of) that inspire you the most. How would they handle your current situation? Turn to page 225 and do the exercise.

"Health is the proper relationship between microcosm, which is man, and the macrocosm, which is the universe. Disease is a disruption of this relationship."
~Dr. Yeshe Donden

WEEK 3 / DAY 4- DATE: _____

HEALTH TIP:

If you're reading this while healing from cancer, or want to proactively avoid it, here are some great natural methods for healing and prevention. Avoid charred foods (including breads & meats) which are carcinogenic. Processed meats & rotisserie chicken skin is especially bad, as is corn beef. So too is pork which thickens lymphatic fluids and is a toxic binder attracting heavy metals and produces free radicals. The World Health Organization has now officially stated that processed meats, especially bacon, sausages and ham, do cause cancer.

Optimize your insulin levels & avoid white sugar & high fructose corn syrup. Look into treatment using antineoplastons (peptides & amino acids that turn off the genes that cause cancer). Take curcumin which has anticancer properties & is effective when combined with the alkaloid piperine. Several drops daily of yew tip oil has also shown great benefit against cancer. Alkalize your body – this is key! Take those medicinal mushrooms as discussed last week. Load up on broccoli, an anticancer superfood. And finally, focus on the mind-body-spirit-stress connection. Emotional clearing as you learned about earlier this week can have profound healing effects.

TODAY'S INTENTION:

_____

_____

_____

POSITIVE OUTCOME(S):

_____

_____

_____

AFFIRMATION:

_____

_____

_____

GRATITUDE:

_____

_____

_____

_____

If you're looking for ways to prevent specifically prostate cancer or ways to fight it, here are some tips (ladies, I'll get to breast cancer in the next paragraph). Eat seeds, nuts, green leafy vegetables, vegetable oils, cooked tomatoes, and whole grains, all of which contain vitamin E (high levels of which have been shown to reduce the risk of developing prostate cancer). As well, eat a low fat diet, maintain optimum (not excessive!) levels of vitamin D, drink daily cups of green tea which contains antioxidants called polyphenols which can help protect against several types of cancer, stay active & exercise, and avoid gaining weight especially after the age of 50. If you have prostate cancer, studies have shown that following an Ornish Diet (a 100% plant whole food diet...) can actually change gene expression, turning on disease preventing genes and turning off prostate cancer genes. More information on the Ornish Diet and program can be found at www.ornishspectrum.com.

For breast cancer, some great foods for fighting it include mushrooms (as discussed in Week 2), broccoli (contains carotenoids and sulforaphane which slow tumor growth), flax seeds (which fight estrogen fueled cancer which breast cancer is), chia seeds (which bind to excess estrogen and pull it out of the body), beets (which help oxygenate the blood), iodine, and artichokes (which contain enzymes that stop the replication of cancer cells). The book 'Saving Tatas' by Christine Austin provides an excellent first-hand account and guidance in breast cancer healing and prevention.

As cancer is such a major topic, a special unit is included starting on page 315 which outlines a more complete anti-cancer strategy and discusses a number of alternative (and successful) treatment modalities.

ACTION STEP:

If cancer is something on your radar, natural medicine and alternative therapies offer a vast array of effective treatment choices. If you haven't yet explored the therapy resources at the back of this book yet, please do so, along with the aforementioned special unit on Cancer.

Taking suggestions from the previous pages as well as the more complete anti-cancer strategy on page 315, list 5 things you can and will start doing this week as either a cancer healing or preventative strategy.

My cancer prevention / healing strategy will include:

_____

_____

_____

_____

_____

_____

_____

_____

_____

_____

"The profit margins in conventional cancer therapeutics are immense. As such, doctors are trained to think only in pharmaceutical terms. Rarely are they even aware of non-patentable alternatives other than hearing from their peers they are 'useless', 'dangerous' and 'quackery'. Amazingly, in spite of the fact that the human body becomes what it absorbs, doctors receive no formal training in nutrition, yet it is nutrition which lies at the heart of cancer prevention and recovery. When a cancerous body cries out for a nutritional solution, damaging pharmaceuticals are administered instead, leading many patients to a worsening of their condition, and often death."
~ Phillip Day

WEEK 3 / DAY 5- DATE: _____

HEALTH TIP:

A poor physical environment – as a result of being stressful, noisy, unhealthy, toxic, dangerous, or uninspiring, can be detrimental to your health and healing. On the other hand, a good physical environment can help create good health, and lead to a faster recovery as well as feelings of inspiration, calmness, safety, and freedom.

ACTION STEP:

How conducive to healing is the environment you're in? Is it stressful? Are you around dangerous toxins and chemicals? Are the people around you supportive or unsupportive? Do you have access to nature and fresh air? Analyze your immediate environment today and make notes of what changes you can make. Even if the changes are small, try to consistently improve your environment to one that is healthy, positive, and healing.

TODAY'S INTENTION:

_____

_____

_____

POSITIVE OUTCOME(S):

_____

_____

_____

AFFIRMATION:

_____

_____

_____

GRATITUDE:

_____

_____

_____

_____

In addition, turn to page 226 for an introduction to wellness wheels and your own Personal Wellness Score. (I've included a bonus too!)

*"I find it a lot healthier for me to be someplace
where I can go outside in my bare feet."*
~ James Taylor

HEALTH TIP:

Almost all disease can be traced to the liver. In the weeks ahead we'll look more closely at improving the adrenals along with mineral balances, among other topics. However much of that work can only be effectively done once the liver is functioning properly. Various toxins (including toxic levels of minerals) bombard the liver, the body's 'filtration plant', daily. Though the liver is fantastic at regenerating itself and can function at even less than half capacity, too many toxins will eventually overburden the liver. This will in turn cause the adrenals to weaken, which then affects the bioavailability of minerals, which then exacerbates the burden on the liver even more. A toxic liver is one of the most common reasons behind chronic fatigue. If you are waking up in the morning feeling like you haven't even slept, or are chronically fatigued throughout the day, there's a good chance your liver is overburdened with toxins. The liver is also tied to emotional disturbances, and so ongoing mood swings, including depression, irritability, anger, and over-reacting to certain events are additional indicators of a potential liver problem (not really surprising as healthy hormone levels (including thyroid hormone) are dependent on healthy liver function). Brain fog is also one of the common symptoms of a toxic liver.

TODAY'S INTENTION:

_____

_____

_____

POSITIVE OUTCOME(S):

_____

_____

_____

AFFIRMATION:

_____

_____

_____

GRATITUDE:

_____

_____

_____

_____

As mentioned, as toxins accumulate in the liver, the adrenal system weakens, and this can eventually lead to adrenal burnout (with symptoms including complete physical exhaustion, anger, resentment, apathy, withdrawal, dizziness, tendency to panic, and changes in personality, including bi-polar). Conversely, as the adrenals 'burn-out', the liver is able to produce less and less of a protein called ceruloplasmin, which in turn lowers the bioavailability of key nutrients such as iron and copper.

Everything that enters your body is chemically broken down and filtered by the liver. When the liver gets overwhelmed with toxins, in addition to the above symptoms mentioned, it can also affect:
> digestion (in fact one of the liver's primary roles is to produce bile which is necessary for the digestion of fats),
> blood sugar (the liver creates GTF (glucose tolerance factor) which acts with insulin to control blood sugar),
> weight (a toxic liver makes it harder to lose weight as a toxic liver cannot properly convert the thyroid hormone T4 into T3 which then leads to the hypothyroidism). You may experience difficult to lose belly fat especially *above* the waistline.
> menstrual regularity
> insomnia (the liver tends to work hardest at night (in Traditional Chinese Medicine the liver is most active from 1:00am-3:00am) and yet the overburdened liver can't keep up with filtering the toxins. This can lead to night sweats, racing mind, liver pain, and trouble falling or staying asleep)
> the functioning of every cell in the body – that even includes the malfunction of cells or abnormal growth of cells (ie: cancer).

Is your liver toxic? Chances are it is if you:
> Have had exposure to heavy metals such as mercury, copper, aluminum either through diet, birth control, dental fillings, or other environmental factors
> Have taken long term consumption of alcohol or drugs (both street as well as prescription and OTC such as Acetaminophen)
> Eat diets high in fatty or processed foods, low in fiber, or high in protein
> Have a history of hepatitis, chemotherapy, antibiotics, or gallbladder problems.

Just as a car functions better with a cleaned out oil filter, or as you clean out the lint filter in your dryer, the liver too needs to be cleaned out in order for you to have best performance. The liver excretes toxins via the kidneys → urine, and via the gallbladder → bile → bowel action. Often the bile ducts and gallbladder get congested, and proper toxin elimination can't happen. In these cases, a gallbladder flush can help open up the bile ducts, allowing bile to flow more smoothly, which then allows more oxygen to reach the cells, which in turn kills cancer cells and re-establishes proper communication links with the brain, nervous system, immune system, endocrine system, and the body as a whole. A full gallbladder flush can be tricky for some people and should only be done under supervision. However there is a lot you can do even without a flush to strengthen and recharge your liver. (Be careful though with some of those over the counter liver detoxes. The liver needs to be nourished before an intense detox. What happens is that the fat, which is burned during the detox, holds many of the toxins in the body. These toxins go into the blood and then the liver, but without being properly nourished the liver cannot properly activate the essential phase 1 and phase 2 elimination pathways, and instead the toxins go back into circulation and this can end up long term causing all sorts of problems).

ACTION STEP:

As almost everyone can benefit from detoxifying their liver, today's action step presents a basic liver detox program that you can follow as a guideline. If you're considering doing any sort of detox, starting with a liver detox is really important. So long as the liver is toxic, the body is unable to properly cope with new toxins, or with flushing them out. No other cleanse (except a colon cleanse which could be done prior – optional but not necessary) will work optimally until the liver is cleared and functioning properly. It's a good idea to do a liver cleanse/detox once a year.

(It's always recommended that you check first with your doctor before beginning any such program, especially if you're on any medication or have been diagnosed with an illness).

There are many liver detox programs out there, some very specific and regimented, some much harder than others. The one presented here is not the only method, but it is relatively simple to follow and is great as a first time liver cleanser. Tomorrow, you can start your liver cleanse. Today, here is your shopping list to get prepared....turn the page.

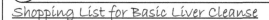

Shopping List for Basic Liver Cleanse

Liquids:
Water, Unsweetened Apple Juice, Unsweetened Cranberry Juice, Apple Cider Vinegar

Fruits and Vegetables (organic whenever possible):
Apples, Beets, Lemons, Oranges, Broccoli, Sprouts, Asparagus, Artichoke, Avocado, Kale and other dark green leafy vegetables, Sauerkraut, Cabbage

Spices:
Nutmeg, Cinnamon, Ginger, Turmeric, Cilantro, Garlic

Teas (choose one or two):
Fennel, Stinging Nettle, Dandelion Root, Peppermint, Wormwood, Green tea

Supplements (all are not necessary but aim for as many as you can get):
Psyllium husk, Flaxseed, Probiotic, Food-Grade Diatomaceous Earth, Milk Thistle, Yellow Dock, Spirulina, Blue-Green Algae, B-Vitamin complex, Desiccated Liver (organic), He Shou Wu, Magnesium, Schisandra berry, Nettles

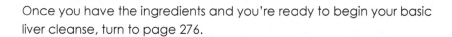

Once you have the ingredients and you're ready to begin your basic liver cleanse, turn to page 276.

Once you have the ingredients and you're ready to begin your basic liver cleanse, turn to page 276.

"The art of healing comes from nature, not from the physician. Therefore the physician must start from nature, with an open mind."
~ Paracelsus

WEEK 3 / DAY 7- DATE: _____

THIS WEEK'S REVIEW:

Today is your chance to go over the action steps of this past week, reincorporate any activities you may have forgotten, and complete any activities yet unfinished. Use today to catch up and take stock.

Check off the items you've completed below:

☐ I've worked through the Emotional Clearing Exercises

☐ I've eliminated at least one major inflammatory food from my diet

☐ I've added at least 3 anti-inflammatory foods to my diet and am committed to keeping these in my diet regularly for at least the remainder of this program.

☐ I'm doing at least 5 things to heal from, or prevent, cancer.

☐ I've made at least one positive and healthy change to my environment.

☐ I've completed the introductory Wellness Wheel exercise on page 227

☐ I've begun a basic liver detox.

☐ I completed all my daily journaling exercises, including today's which are on the following 2 pages.

Of all the tips I've learned so far in this book, 5 action steps for my health that I fully **commit** to doing consistently from now on (the most important tips I'm taking forward with me) are:

1. _____

2. _____

3. _____

4. _____

5. _____

1. This week I'm proud of:

_____

_____

_____

_____

_____

2. This coming week I commit to following through on the things I didn't fully do this past week (health-wise or other) which include:

_____

_____

_____

_____

_____

3. I'm grateful for:

_____

_____

_____

_____

_____

_____

4. Now that I have some down time, a few things I've been meaning to do that I could do now are:

_____

_____

_____

_____

5. I choose not to stare at the closing doors but rather new ones which are opening. These are:

_____

_____

_____

_____

6. What's worked this week and what's not?

_____

_____

_____

_____

_____

7. General notes and thoughts:

_____

_____

_____

HEALTH TIP:

Are you noticing patterns in your life that may be sabotaging your ultimate happiness, or even your health? So many people are subconsciously running off patterns that were formed in childhood (or even earlier), and these patterns not only lead to emotional upset but can also negatively affect one physically. Sometimes patterns are imitation patterns - repeating things you've seen or heard. Other times patterns are revenge patterns - acting in certain ways towards oneself or others as a way to make up for pain caused in the past by someone else. This week you'll be given several tools that will help you uncover - and heal - those patterns. First however, the passage on the following page from Osho's book "Being In Love" offers an appropriate explanation of how one lives out patterns. I include this here only for your own contemplation.

TODAY'S INTENTION:

_____

_____

POSITIVE OUTCOME(S):

_____

_____

AFFIRMATION:

_____

_____

GRATITUDE:

_____

_____

_____

_____

"...And children learn the ways of their parents – their nagging, their conflict. Just go on watching yourself. If you are a woman, watch – you may be repeating, almost identically, the ways your mother used to behave. Watch yourself when you are with your boyfriend or your husband: What are you doing? Are you not repeating a pattern? If you are a man, watch: What are you doing? Are you not behaving just like your father? Are you not doing the same nonsense that he used to do? ...People go on repeating; people are imitators. The human being is a monkey. You are repeating your father or your mother, and that has to be dropped...

The first step is, get rid of your parents. And by that I don't mean any disrespect towards your parents, no.... I mean you have to get rid of your parental voices inside, your program inside, your tapes inside. Efface them... and you will be simply surprised that if you get rid of your parents from the inner being, you become free. For the first time you will be able to feel compassion for your parents, otherwise not; you will remain resentful...

If you want to become a human being and not a machine, get rid of your parents. It is hard work, arduous work; you cannot do it instantly. You will have to be very careful in your behaviour. Watch and see when your mother is there, functioning through you – stop that, move away from it. Do something absolutely new that your mother could not even have imagined. For example, your boyfriend is looking at some other woman with great appreciation in his eyes. Now, watch what you are doing. Are you doing the same as your mother would have done when your father looked at another woman appreciatively? If you do that, you will never know what love is, you will simply be repeating a story. It will be the same act being played by different actors, that's all; the same rotten act being repeated again and again and again. Don't be an imitator, get out of it. Do something new. Do something new that your mother [father] could not have conceived of. This newness has to be brought to your being, then your love will start flowing."

~ Osho

ACTION STEP:

In this book we purposely deal a lot with the inner world (mental, emotional and spiritual) because it is this inner world that creates our outer (physical). You're also coming to understand that healing begins in the mind. Last week you began doing exercises in emotional clearing. Today we take that a step further by looking at negative patterns that repeatedly show up in our lives, contributing to everything from stress to heartache to disease. What messages did you pick up that are subconsciously running your mind and creating patterns in your life?

As well, this week is an opportunity to examine any negative thoughts you have (and we all have them!). If we have negative thoughts of sickness, we continue to manifest that. Positive and supportive thoughts meanwhile help us achieve positive outcomes... and positive health.

Today you're being given three action steps:

1. Turn to page 236 to examine your patterns (at least the conscious ones – you'll be given tools to accessing the unconscious ones soon).
2. Turn to page 235 and begin completing the exercise on unsupportive thoughts. If you're not able to finish it all today, you will have a chance tomorrow as well.
3. Read the article on page 356 on how childhood events affect mineral balances and adult programming.

"You cannot control what happens to you, but you can control your attitude toward what happens to you, and in that, you will be mastering change rather than allowing it to master you."
~ Sri Ram

HEALTH TIP:

As you make necessary changes to your lifestyle and diet, one more thing you'll definitely want to avoid is high fructose corn syrup (HFCS). It can be found in certain baked goods, canned fruits, dairy products, soft drinks, and many sweetened beverages. It's pretty much everywhere these days, in fact thanks to government subsidies our intake has increased nearly 1000% since the 1980s! Unfortunately it can help worsen diabetes, lead to heart disease, obesity, damage your immune system, punch holes in your gut (causing leaky gut), increase iron buildup in the liver, speed up the aging process, and even lead to mercury poisoning as some HFCS contains mercury. Even worse than sugar, it keeps your body from producing key hormones that inhibit hunger and regulate your energy cycle. HFCS also scars the arteries, and it is a must for anyone with heart disease, cancer or diabetes to avoid HFCS completely.

ACTION STEP:

Go through your weekly diet and record below all the unhealthy foods and snacks you eat. Also, finish the exercise from yesterday on unsupportive thoughts if you've not done so already.

TODAY'S INTENTION:

_____

_____

_____

POSITIVE OUTCOME(S):

_____

_____

_____

AFFIRMATION:

_____

_____

_____

GRATITUDE:

_____

_____

_____

_____

"It's choice, not chance, that determines your destiny."~ Jean Nidetch

HEALTH TIP:

Our body's pH ("potential of hydrogen") balance can play an important factor in our overall health. If our body is either too acidic or too alkaline, a host of health complications can ensue. Unfortunately most Americans are over-acidic because their diet is high in processed foods, meats, sugars, salt, caffeine and alcohol. The aforementioned, along with cheeses, eggs, unsoaked beans, white flour and soft drinks are all acid-forming foods. Toxins we eat and breathe in also create an acidic environment in our body, and our important alkalizing minerals are then used up in an effort to deal with those toxins.

While we absolutely DO need our stomach to be acidic (ie: antacids are NOT a good idea!), ideally we want our body as a whole to be slightly more alkaline than acidic, with a pH measurement of between 7.35 to 7.45. In fact, maintaining a slightly higher alkaline level in our body is a natural cancer cure (while a maintained acidic state can lead to cancer). Very few people remember that back in 1931, medical Nobel Prize winning Dr. Otto Warburg proved that while cancer flourishes in an anaerobic (acid) environment, it cannot survive in an aerobic (oxygenated - alkaline) environment!

TODAY'S INTENTION:

_____

_____

_____

POSITIVE OUTCOME(S):

_____

_____

_____

AFFIRMATION:

_____

_____

_____

GRATITUDE:

_____

_____

_____

_____

Furthermore, vast numbers of people today are complaining of low energy, constant fatigue. While there can be many reasons behind this, one of the key factors is based on the pH of your blood. Properly flowing blood smoothly transporting oxygen to our cells allows for higher and more sustained energy in our bodies. However acidic blood slows down this transport of oxygen to the cells, leading to constant states of lethargy. If you want more energy, your pH level is a great place to start!

A few of the many foods that help balance our bodies to a more alkaline state include: Alfalfa sprouts, Apples, Asparagus, Avocados, Bananas, Broccoli, Cucumber, Flax Seed Oil, Garlic, Ginger, Green Tea, Kale, Lettuce (dark), Lemons, Melons (honeydew, cantaloupe, watermelon...), Olive Oil, Parsley, Peaches, Pineapple, Seaweed, Spinach, Tofu, Watercress... and water!

Do keep in mind though that the stomach needs to be kept very acidic, and anything that tries to lower stomach acidity should be questioned. Most people in fact are not acidic enough in the stomach and could benefit by taking an HCL (hydrochloric acid) supplement.

ACTION STEP:

For a more complete breakdown of acidic vs alkaline foods, turn to the graphic on page 240. Also, on page 238 there is a simple pH test you can do at home to determine your level.

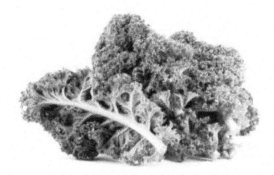

"The fork is your most powerful tool to change your health and the planet; food is the most powerful medicine to heal chronic illness."
~ Dr. Mark Hyman, M.D

WEEK 4 / DAY 4- DATE: _____

HEALTH TIP:

Today we look at osteoporosis, and how you can protect yourself against it. Although it is a condition most often diagnosed later in life, the health of your bones is predominantly built during your first 30 years. If you're young (and especially if you're a woman and Caucasian - those most at risk), it's never too early to start thinking about strengthening your bones, So what do your bones like?

Calcium is probably the first thing that comes to mind, especially as it's promoted widely as the 'maintainer of good bone health'. Good sources include whole grains, beans, kale and other dark green leafy vegetables, and almonds and other nuts. Limited supplementation may be fine. Sadly however, we've been conditioned to believe that the more calcium we have, the healthier our bones will be. The truth is, excess calcium, with a lack of other minerals, actually <u>increases</u> the risk of bone fracture! Let me explain. High calcium intake blocks the absorption of magnesium, creating potential magnesium deficiency. Magnesium is necessary for calcium to be properly deposited into bone (where it should be) as opposed to soft tissue (where its effects become harmful). So, while calcium is beneficial, it's imperative that before supplementing with calcium you first ensure that your magnesium levels are high enough. Otherwise, the very thing you are supplementing (calcium) will create a condition (magnesium deficiency) which results in the calcium being deposited in the wrong place...leading to a host of conditions, including osteoporosis! In fact, studies have shown that high calcium intake doubles the risk of hip fractures – my guess is that many of

TODAY'S INTENTION:

_____

_____

_____

POSITIVE OUTCOME(S):

_____

_____

_____

AFFIRMATION:

_____

_____

_____

GRATITUDE:

_____

_____

_____

_____

these people were probably low in magnesium. Most people are, indeed, low in magnesium...and over-calcified.

> *"People in the United States consume more dairy products and other foods high in calcium per capita than the citizens of any other two nations on earth put together...we also have the world's highest rates of osteoporosis and bone fractures among elderly people."*
> ~Phyllis A Balch, CNC, Prescription for Nutritional Healing, 2006

So, if extra calcium isn't the answer, what can help your bones? Magnesium as mentioned (low levels negatively affect bone mineralization and increases the loss of calcium through the urine), the mineral strontium, boron (very important as a magnesium cofactor and helpful against osteoporosis and arthritis), potassium, chromium, soy isoflavones. Vitamins C, D, E, and K, silica (helps deposit the calcium into the bones), and collagen (a protein that improves the fracture resistance of the bone by adding an element of elasticity). Think about it, calcium is hardening (brittle), while collagen is soft (flexible). Silica and collagen go hand in hand. According to a study by the School of Public Health at the University of California, silica-supplemented bones have a 100% increase in collagen over bones with low-silica. When we are young are bodies have lots of silica, but as we age, silica levels decrease). You can also add sea salt to your diet, which contains a great mix and proportion of essential minerals. Finally, reduce your body's acidity. To buffer acidity, your body leaches calcium (and other minerals) from the bones. This calcium, which now has entered the blood, encounters cholesterol, which then causes arteries to harden and leads to atherosclerosis. On that note, be cautious if your blood test shows your calcium 'within range' – when the blood calcium drops too low, calcium is leached from the bone to prop the blood level back up!

> Did you know that silica supplementation can offer many additional benefits against the effects of aging? Beyond bone strength and flexibility, it can also help keep skin cells looking youthful, strengthen soft fingernails, protect against muscle injury, help prevent kidney stones, heal urinary tract infections, regulate high blood pressure, and also improve memory in the aged.

ACTION STEP:

If you`re concerned about osteoporosis or aging, make an appointment to talk to your doctor about silica supplementation, or visit your local natural health store and inquire about the various options available depending on what you`ll be taking it for. A Hair Tissue Mineral Analysis (www.htmatest.com) can also give a much better assessment of mineral imbalances in your bones than the typical bone density test. And finally, stay physically active with actvities that involve both footwork as well as load bearing movements/ exercise.

> *"What the caterpillar calls the end of the world, the master calls a butterfly."*
> ~ Richard Bach

WEEK 4 / DAY 5- DATE: _____

HEALTH TIP:

Meditation and other relaxation techniques have powerful health benefits. Take at least a few minutes each day to meditate. Among the proven benefits of meditation, it: improves immunity (including in those recovering from cancer), improves fertility, lessens IBS, lowers blood pressure, helps reduce inflammation, reduces anxiety, enhances energy, increases levels of serotonin, strengthens the mind, helps reduce heart disease, and lowers stress.

ACTION STEP:

There are many ways to meditate, from sitting quietly without thought, to focusing on a single thought, to performing simple tasks slowly and mindfully. Starting today, give yourself for at least 5 to 10 minutes per day, or longer, the gift of meditation. As well, how are you coming along on your 'My H.EA.L.T.H. Goals' worksheet that you filled out in week #2? What actions do you need to take in order to meet the goals you set?

TODAY'S INTENTION:

_____

_____

_____

POSITIVE OUTCOME(S):

_____

_____

_____

AFFIRMATION:

_____

_____

_____

GRATITUDE:

_____

_____

_____

"What is necessary to change a person is to change his awareness of himself."
~ Abraham H. Maslow

WEEK 4 / DAY 6- DATE: _____

HEALTH TIP:

Today I'm excited to share with you a healing method that I believe can revolutionize the concept of healing. It works with all 5 dimensions of our human existence simultaneously: the body, mind, emotions, spirit, and consciousness. and in doing so is in perfect alignment with the message of this book – that healing begins within oneself, and that our thoughts, patterns and past conditioning play a big role in our health.

This method of healing can be used to not only heal humanity, but also yourself as an individual - to release lifetimes of trauma and pain that's causing suffering - both internally in the emotions as well as manifesting itself physically. It's called the Self-Healing Dalian Method. Using the power of one's innate consciousness to facilitate healing, it works to release self-sabotaging beliefs and

TODAY'S INTENTION:

_____

_____

_____

POSITIVE OUTCOME(S):

_____

_____

_____

AFFIRMATION:

_____

_____

_____

GRATITUDE:

_____

_____

_____

thought patterns from the body's cellular memory and clears energy blockages that are responsible for inner unrest and external physical manifestations. By releasing repressed thought forms and emotions (which dwell in our cells and organs), many physical ailments, even so called 'incurable ones', have been shown to disappear permanently. To guide you through the Self-Healing Dalian Method is beyond the scope of this book and would not do the Method the justice it deserves, however it is certainly a technique that one can do oneself once

learning the Method. It is a simple, yet delicate, process. My intention is simply to introduce this gift to you so that you can choose to pursue it further if it resonates with you. If you are truly ready to do deep healing work, I cannot emphasize enough how highly I recommend you to try the Self-Healing Dalian Method for yourself or work directly with its creator, Mada Eliza Dalian. For more information you can visit www.madadalian.com. (This method is also mentioned in the Therapies Resources Section where many of the conditions it can help improve are listed.)

ACTION STEP:

You have two action steps today:

1. Look further into the Self-Healing Dalian Method if it resonates with you. The "Healing the Body & Awakening Consciousness with the Dalian Method: An Advanced Self-Healing System for a New Humanity" book and 2 CD set can be used as a practical tool that can help you release and transform many layers of unconscious belief patters, deepen your self-awareness, and heal your body at the same time.

2. Ho'oponopono is an ancient Hawaiian healing practice based on reconciliation and forgiveness. Your second 'challenge' is to mindfully practice Ho'oponopono. Turn to page 241 to begin.

"If we can accept that we are the sum total of all past thoughts, motions, words, deeds and actions and that our present lives and choices are colored or shaded by this memory bank of the past, then we begin to see how a process of correcting or setting aright can change our lives, our families and our society."
~ Morrnah Nalamaku Simeona

THIS WEEK'S REVIEW:

Today is your chance to go over the action steps of this past week, reincorporate any activities you may have forgotten, and complete any activities yet unfinished. Use today to catch up and take stock. Check off the items you've completed below:

☐ I've worked through the exercises to clear unsupportive thoughts and negative patterns...and I will continue this important work.

☐ I've taken an inventory of the major unhealthy foods I've been eating, and will consciously lessen my intake of those foods.

☐ I've done a pH test and have an idea of how acidic or alkaline my body is.

☐ I've discussed with a health professional if I would be a good candidate for silica and/or collagen supplementation to help protect the health of my bones.

☐ I am making meditation part of my daily practice, even if just for a few minutes a day.

☐ I've visited www.MadaDalian.com to learn more about the Self-Healing Dalian Method.

☐ I have practiced Ho'oponopono.

☐ I completed all my daily journaling exercises, including today's which are on the following 2 pages.

Of all the tips I've learned so far in this book, 6 action steps for my health that I fully **commit** to doing consistently from now on (the most important tips I'm taking forward with me) are:

1. _____

2. _____

3. _____

4. _____

5. _____

6. _____

1. This week I'm proud of:

_____

_____

_____

_____

_____

2. This coming week I commit to following through on the things I didn't fully do this past week (health-wise or other) which include:

_____

_____

_____

_____

_____

3. I'm grateful for:

_____

_____

_____

_____

_____

4. Now that I have some down time, a few things I've been meaning to do that I could do now are:

_____

_____

_____

_____

5. I choose not to stare at the closing doors but rather new ones which are opening. These are:

_____

_____

_____

_____

6. What's worked this week and what's not?

_____

_____

_____

_____

_____

7. General notes and thoughts:

_____

_____

_____

WEEK 5 / DAY 1- DATE: _____

HEALTH TIP:

Affirmations are positive declarations said to oneself stating that something is true. The more you tell yourself positive, supportive, and expansive thoughts, the more positive your outer reality will become. The more conviction and feeling with which you express the affirmation, the better it will transform into reality. Therefore, to promote healing, begin the habit of stating empowering and healing affirmations to yourself. *Afformations*, a term coined by Noah St. John, are similar to affirmations except that they ask a positive question instead of using a statement. For example, instead of the affirmation "I feel great", the affirmation could be "Why do I feel so great?" This forces your mind to find the answer that will in turn create the reality you want.

ACTION STEP:

Turn to page 243 in Part II and beginning today incorporate affirmations (or afformations) into your daily routine.

TODAY'S INTENTION:
_____
_____
_____

POSITIVE OUTCOME(S):
_____
_____
_____

AFFIRMATION:
_____
_____
_____

GRATITUDE:
_____
_____
_____
_____

"A belief is only a thought you continue to think. A belief is nothing more than a chronic pattern of thought, and you have the ability -if you try even a little bit- to begin a new pattern, to tell a new story, to achieve a different vibration, to change your point of attraction." ~ Abraham-Hicks

HEALTH TIP:

Are you suffering from any of the following: anxiety, depression, racing thoughts, chronic fatigue, moodiness, brain fog, poor concentration, insomnia, PMS, irritability, digestive disorders, lowered immunity, iron deficiency, or abnormal amounts of energy and can't figure out why? It could be you have heavy metal toxicity, where the levels of a mineral or heavy metal (such as lead, copper, mercury, aluminum) is dangerously high in your body.

Lead and mercury toxicity are quite often talked about, and pretty much everyone has some level of these metals in their body affecting their health... along with aluminum and arsenic which are also common. However, there is also copper toxicity, something that is far less talked about or known, but affecting people at epidemic levels. Sources such as drinking water through copper piping, adrenal insufficiency and stress, occupational exposure, copper sulfate sprayed on crops, estrogen dominance, and congenital inheritance from mother to fetus in utero are contributing causes, vegetarians and those on a birth control pill or using a copper IUD are at especially high risk of copper toxicity. The vegetarian/vegan diet is high in copper, the copper IUD of course contains copper, and the Pill raises copper retention as estrogen rises (anything that raises estrogen raises copper retention!). Many people today unknowingly have elevated levels of copper in their systems. At extreme levels, it can burn out the adrenals and lead to very damaging physical, emotional and social complications. Extreme personality changes can also occur. Unfortunately, very few in the medical and nutritional fields understand the psychological (or physical) implications of copper toxicity.

TODAY'S INTENTION:

_____

_____

_____

POSITIVE OUTCOME(S):

_____

_____

_____

AFFIRMATION:

_____

_____

_____

GRATITUDE:

_____

_____

_____

_____

Tragically, testing for copper toxicity is quite often botched by doctors who are focused on blood tests and don't know what to look for (ie: copper toxicity in most cases won't show up in a blood test). People are being wrongly diagnosed or given harmful medication when the key to healing in a lot of cases of physical impairment as well as psychosis begins with properly rebalancing minerals. Certainly not everyone is affected by copper, or will be affected the same, yet vast numbers of women (men too, but women especially) have had their lives completely altered by the damaging effects of excess copper in their bodies. Makers of birth control devices or copper containing 'health' products will vehemently deny any connection exists, and young women especially fall victim to the astounding lack of public education in this area. Those being put on the Pill or IUD are not being given proper informed consent when being prescribed these birth control methods, and this needs is something that needs to change.

Copper toxicity in later stages is directly attributed to mental illnesses such as paranoia, schizophrenia, and anxiety. Even at less severe levels, left untreated long term copper toxicity can lead to chronic fatigue, brain fog, poor concentration, fibromyalgia, endometriosis, I.B.S., candida, Alzheimer's, diabetes, thyroid issues, rheumatoid arthritis, & cancer. Although copper is an essential mineral in the human body, at high bio-unavailable levels it becomes both toxic as well as bio-availably deficient. I have dedicated much of my practice to helping those with copper toxicity and bringing awareness to its implications, and much of my research is available at www.coppertoxic.com. I have also included summary article on copper toxicity on page 350.

ACTION STEP:
Hair Tissue Mineral Analysis is the most accurate way of assessing the extent of copper toxicity in the body. Today, your suggested action steps are:
1. Familiarize yourself more with this topic by reading the full article beginning on page 340.
2. Arrange to book an HTMA test to determine if copper...or for that matter any other essential mineral or toxic metal, may be out of balance in your body and potentially adversely affecting your health.

"I really do think that any deep crisis is an opportunity to make your life extraordinary in some way." ~ Martha Beck

WEEK 5 / DAY 3- DATE: _____

HEALTH TIP:

Adrenal fatigue occurs when your adrenal glands can no longer meet the demands of stress. This can occur as a result of illness (especially serious respiratory infections), surgery, a life crisis, copper toxicity as discussed yesterday, a buildup of other toxins in the body which constantly bombard the immune system, or any ongoing difficult situation that causes prolonged production of cortisol along with stress either physically and mentally.

Unfortunately, many doctors refuse to acknowledge the concept of adrenal fatigue, and it's not something that can be seen as black or white in a blood test either. An HTMA test, or an adrenal saliva test can provide much greater evidence of one's adrenal state.

Adrenal fatigue / exhaustion can wreak havoc in life, leaving one constantly tired and feeling rundown or overwhelmed. When your adrenals are exhausted, your previously heightened cortisol levels drop, opening the door to inflammatory diseases, mood disorders, chronic fatigue, fibromyalgia, chronic pain, a weakened gut and low stomach acid, hypothyroidism, and a weakened immune system more vulnerable to parasites, toxins, allergens and bacteria. In fact, adrenal exhaustion is like a waiting room in the office of serious disorders.

If you've been following along in this book, you've already by now taken steps to support the liver, as this is a first step for healing the

TODAY'S INTENTION:

_____

_____

_____

POSITIVE OUTCOME(S):

_____

_____

_____

AFFIRMATION:

_____

_____

_____

GRATITUDE:

_____

_____

_____

_____

adrenals. You've also looked at your mineral levels. If you've discovered that copper is high, or some other metal, then that internal stress must be dealt with in order for restoration of the adrenals. We've also talked about external stress reduction and breathing – this is key in terms of allowing your adrenals to recharge. Today, we look more specifically at dietary adjustments that can help with healing worn out adrenals.

If you have adrenal fatigue, it's important to eat a healthy breakfast before 10am, an early lunch, and dinner between 5pm-6pm. Avoid fruit, especially in the morning. Try to combine fat, protein & complex carbohydrates at every meal & snack. Hydration (between meals) is essential. Most importantly, to recharge your adrenals, they need to be allowed to rest; this means avoiding stimulants (and stimulating foods/herbs). Would you like to know which foods can be good for your adrenals and which might actually be hurting you? I've included this for you on the next page!

Calming activities, meditation, avoiding stress, and adequate sleep all are helpful when it comes to restoring adrenal strength. Stimulating activities and supplements are contraindicative. In fact, the more you need that 'caffeine boost' to get you through the day, the more you probably need to let your adrenals rest. However, the most important element is having a healthy gut – this is key when it comes to improving adrenal issues. This is why your diet is so important, and why we looked at improving candida and gut issues earlier in this program.

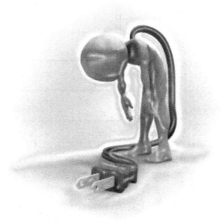

It's Time to Re-Charge!

Adrenal Restoration Diet

ADD (Good for Adrenals)	ELIMINATE (Bad for Adrenals)
✓ Dark greens (including seaweed, kale, and spinach) ✓ Sprouts ✓ Ginger ✓ Sea salt in a glass of water with lemon ✓ Sesame seeds, nuts (walnuts, cashews, & almonds which are all high in magnesium) & whole grains ✓ Salmon or char ✓ Organic animal meat / protein ✓ Apple cider vinegar ✓ Red and orange vegetables (5-6 servings per day) ✓ Broccoli ✓ Oils: coconut, almond and olive ✓ Teas: licorice, peppermint, chamomile	▪ Sugar ▪ Alcohol ▪ Coffee/ caffeine/ black tea ▪ Deep fried foods ▪ Soda ▪ Processed meats ▪ White flour (bread, cookies) ▪ Gluten (if at all possible) ▪ Cow's milk ▪ Artificial sweeteners ▪ Fast food ▪ White rice ▪ Sodium ▪ Asian ginseng (too stimulating for severe adrenal fatigue)

Some supplements that can also help with your energy and adrenal restoration include: GABA, L-Theanine, L-Tyrosine (assists adrenal function while relieving stress), Ashwaghanda (an adaptogen that is both stimulating and relaxing and can assist with insomnia), Magnesium Chelate, Cordyceps, Rhodiola (adaptogen that reduces the stress response, improves mental function, reduces fatigue, anxiety and depression), Holy Basil, Schisandra, Suma, Wild Yam, Milk Thistle (excellent in aiding liver function which aids adrenals), B-Complex Vitamins especially Vitamin B5, Vitamin C (this is essential), DHEA, R-lipoic acid, Eleuthro (adaptogen that assists with immune function and physical stress), Adrenal Glandulars, Rehmannia (Chinese herb that is great for depleted adrenals), Astragalus (great tonic and adrenal support herb), Dried Nettles, Licorice (use with caution if you have high blood pressure), and EPA/DHA fish oils. Food-grade Diatomaceous Earth is great for detoxifying and killing off any parasites that might be robbing you of energy. Probiotics and Turmeric are also good all around. Speak with your doctor or health store professional for the best dosages for you. Keep in mind that the more exhausted the adrenals, the less you may be able to tolerate herbs and glandulars.

Adrenal Tea Recipe: Boil HeShouWu for 25 minutes. Then add Rehmannia (hard black pancake) and continue simmering for another 20 minutes. Drain this water into a cup and add licorice, peppermint, or chamomile tea. Add a squirt each of Eleuthro tincture, Astragalus tincture, and Schisandra drops. Drink and enjoy! (Feel free to experiment with adding coconut oil, a little stevia, or chicory root to adjust the flavor).

Nettle Infusion: Stinging nettle infusion (not the same as nettle tea) is excellent for the adrenals, while also nourishing to the kidney and liver. To make an infusion, into an empty bottle or large canning jar pour a quart of boiling water over 1 cup of dried nettles. Allow to stand for at least four hours before drinking. Drink 1 to 2 cups per day, storing the remainder for drinking on subsequent days.

ACTION STEP:

Be kind to your adrenals, and your body, by giving them a chance to recover. Today's actions steps are:

1. Test your adrenals. Maybe you already know your adrenals are shot. But if you're not too sure, you can do a simple at home experiment. Lay down and rest for five minutes. Then take your blood pressure. Then stand up and immediately again take your blood pressure. If the systolic number in your reading (the first number in the measurement (ie: 120/80) is lower than the number when you were laying down, chances are you have sluggish adrenals. Alternatively, if you've had your HTMA test done, the ratio between sodium to magnesium is also representative of adrenal strength. The higher the Na/Mg ratio is over 4:1, the more hyper-adrenal you are, while a reading under 4:1 is a sign of adrenal insufficiency. Low HTMA sodium and potassium together are also a great sign of adrenal insufficiency.
2. Read the article on Adrenal Fatigue starting on page 362 to better familiarize yourself with this condition and its relationship with stress.
3. Evaluate how you can reduce: stress, intense physical exertion, the need to be in control of everything, negative self-talk. Evaluate how you can increase: rest, mindful chewing and eating, patience, healthy relationships, positive self talk.
4. Add the ingredients on the previous page to your shopping list and begin your own adrenal improvement diet.

"There is a predisposition in this country to kinds of virtuous extremes, and I lived this life myself. I was a vegan, I was a vegetarian, I was non-fat, I was low-fat, I was anorexic, in short I thought that if animal foods would kill you and fats would kill you, the less the better and zero must be ideal. This is obviously nonsensical thinking. It's black its white. It's rigid. It's extreme. And it's not virtuous...
Little by little I started to eat these foods (traditional - meat, poultry, raw milk, etc) again and in time came back to being a moderate omnivore, a conscientious carnivore, a traditional foods person, and restored my health along the way.... ...
I was...gloomy and irritable, I was depressed in the winter, in short I was a sickly person with a big personality and I had no idea that my virtuous diets were making me sick until little by little I added traditional foods back."
~ Nina Planck (Food Writer)

HEALTH TIP:

Dark Field Microscopy (also known as live blood analysis) is a technique that allows you and the doctor to look inside your living cells to assess your digestive, eliminative, immune and circulatory functions, as well as the presence of bacteria, viruses, parasites, fungus, toxins, and candida – information that is very helpful when it comes to healing the gut and working on adrenal strengthening. In my opinion it's one of the more important examinations of holistic medicine as it can offer an early warning to problems before they ever fully develop (including such things as rheumatoid arthritis, colitis, even cancer). This isn't the typical blood test your family doctor is familiar with – the one that gets sent off to a lab somewhere. Instead, Darkfield allows the practitioner to look in real time inside your living blood cells and even into the smaller bodies not visible in normal hematology slides. A single drop of blood is taken usually from the tip of your finger (or the earlobe as is often used in Europe), and from this single drop you will discover the state of the miraculous universe that exists within your body.

TODAY'S INTENTION:

_____

_____

_____

POSITIVE OUTCOME(S):

_____

_____

_____

AFFIRMATION:

_____

_____

_____

GRATITUDE:

_____

_____

_____

_____

ACTION STEP:

No matter where you are in your healing, a live blood analysis is great to have done, allowing you to see your present state and what may be lying ahead so that you can take proactive steps. Your task today -book an appointment at a clinic that offers live blood analysis testing.

"Action is the foundational key to all success". - Pablo Picasso

HEALTH TIP:

No matter what your age, movement is of prime importance. Tests have shown that people at any age, regardless of physical ability, can improve their health and well-being by taking up some gentle, regular exercise. Movement helps prevent weight gain, keeps your heart healthy, alleviates stress, increases energy, boosts feel-good endorphins, has psychologically positive benefits, and helps in the development and protection of your body.

Walking is something most people can do – it can be a great source of quality time for you and your pet, your spouse, and the entire family. It's also a great way to keep your heart healthy, reduce stress and back pain, wear off those dinner calories, reduce the risk of osteoporosis, dementia, and type 2 diabetes and release feel-good endorphins.

ACTION STEP:

Your action step today, literally, is movement. Plan to talk a walk today... either during the day or after dinner. You can do this no matter where you are. No excuses! As well, do what you can to incorporate movement consciously into your daily habits. If movement is something you already do lots of, then challenge yourself by creating a "movement plan" for the week ahead. Write in when you'll do your walks, runs, gym workouts, tennis games, etc. Write in what you would normally do, then increase either the frequency, duration, or intensity.

TODAY'S INTENTION:

_____

_____

_____

POSITIVE OUTCOME(S):

_____

_____

_____

AFFIRMATION:

_____

_____

_____

GRATITUDE:

_____

_____

_____

_____

"If you can't fly then run, if you can't run then walk, if you can't walk then crawl, but whatever you do you have to keep moving forward."
~ Martin Luther King Jr.

HEALTH TIP:

Are you recovering from surgery to a broken bone or torn tendon or ligament? If so, chances are you've been wearing a cast. Ask your doctor or surgeon about having a Range-of-Motion brace instead. Some doctors might not allow it and there could be good reason, but a second opinion can't hurt. A range of motion brace can speed up your recovery time by allowing you to build up your range of motion incrementally during the time that you would otherwise be confined to a hard cast. As long as you're careful wearing it & don't overdo it, you'll be a lot further ahead after 6 weeks than if you were wearing a cast that whole time.

ACTION STEP:

You're now a solid month into this program and it's time to revisit two important steps to keep your momentum going. Your first action step today is to re-read your Commitment to Healing that you read at the beginning of this program. Secondly, what is your WHY? It might be the same as you first wrote down, or it might have changed. Either way, write your current WHY below.

TODAY'S INTENTION:

_____

_____

_____

POSITIVE OUTCOME(S):

_____

_____

_____

AFFIRMATION:

_____

_____

_____

GRATITUDE:

_____

_____

_____

_____

"Energy and persistence conquer all things"~ Benjamin Franklin

95

WEEK 5 / DAY 7- DATE: _____

THIS WEEK'S REVIEW:

Today is your chance to go over the action steps of this past week, reincorporate any activities you may have forgotten, and complete any activities yet unfinished. Use today to catch up.

Check off the items you've completed below:

☐ I am saying positive affirmations / afformations daily.

☐ I've ordered an HTMA test to determine the levels of copper and other minerals and metals in my body.

☐ I've made an appointment to have a live blood analysis done.

☐ I've read the article in Part 362 on Adrenal Fatigue, and have taken action steps to improve the health of my adrenals.

☐ I am consciously making an effort to add more movement into my daily routine.

☐ I have re-read my Commitment to Healing and have rewritten my WHY.

☐ I completed all my daily journaling exercises, including today's which are on the following 2 pages.

Of all the tips I've learned so far in this book, 7 action steps for my health that I fully **commit** to doing consistently from now on (the most important tips I'm taking forward with me) are:

1. _____

2. _____

3. _____

4. _____

5. _____

6. _____

7. _____

1. This week I'm proud of:

_____

_____

_____

_____

_____

2. This coming week I commit to following through on the things I didn't fully do this past week (health-wise or other) which include:

_____

_____

_____

_____

_____

3. I'm grateful for:

_____

_____

_____

_____

_____

_____

4. Now that I have some down time, a few things I've been meaning to do that I could do now are:

_____

_____

_____

_____

5. I choose not to stare at the closing doors but rather new ones which are opening. These are:

_____

_____

_____

_____

6. What's worked this week and what's not?

_____

_____

_____

_____

7. General notes and thoughts:

_____

_____

_____

HEALTH TIP:

As important as it is, we tend to take our brain for-granted. That is until we start forgetting things, or suffer a brain injury or concussion. Forgetfulness isn't always caused by the obvious though (injury, Alzheimer's, etc...). Damaged (narrowed, stiffened) blood vessels in the brain are another common cause of dementia and milder memory loss. Risk of this 'cerebrovascular disease' increases with smoking, high blood pressure, and diabetes.

Although less common, selective memory loss can also occur when the zinc to copper ratio is out of balance in the brain. Too much zinc (from supplementation for example) is just as dangerous as too little zinc (which could occur as one example from copper toxicity – a form of heavy metal poisoning where the copper level in the body has risen to damaging levels – I'll go into this in more detail next week). Proper balance is key. Numerous studies show that the cells of the hippocampus (the part of the brain which records and processes important memories) die when deprived of zinc.

TODAY'S INTENTION:

_____

_____

_____

POSITIVE OUTCOME(S):

_____

_____

_____

AFFIRMATION:

_____

_____

_____

GRATITUDE:

_____

_____

_____

_____

Whether you're recovering from a brain injury or just want to keep your brain healthy, it needs the right fuel (food). Keep in mind that the brain sponges up 40% of all nutrients in the blood. So if a particular diet is making you nutrient deficient, the brain will be starving. This, combined with high level toxins in your system means the brain can't function properly, and thinking becomes impaired. In addition to heavy metals, fluoride is another such toxin that impairs the brain.   Dr. Philippe

Grandjean, an environmental health scientist at the Harvard School of Public Health, states *"Fluoride seems to fit in with lead, mercury, and other poisons that cause chemical brain drain."* In fact, 42 human studies have linked moderately high fluoride exposure with reduced intelligence[1]. For the health of your brain, try to limit heavy metal and fluoride exposure as much as you can.

Sodium fluoride is a toxic industrial by-product, classified as a poison, too toxic to be dumped, and is one of the main ingredients in rat poison. It's more toxic than lead and just slightly less toxic than arsenic. And yet, somehow, it's deemed to be safe in the drinking water and toothpaste we use daily! The fact is, it's creating a toxic load within our bodies.

So, what does a brain like to 'eat'? It thrives on high quality fats, antioxidants, and small doses of quality carbs. Recommended foods for your brain are avocado, blueberries, salmon and fish oils, MCT oil, nuts (especially walnuts), seeds, beans, chocolate and/or cacao nibs, garlic, green tea, olive oil, and oysters, to name a few. You can also add Ceylon cinnamon to meals, coffee, etc, as it's been shown in studies to slow the decline of brain cells after brain injury or starvation of oxygen to the brain following a stroke. Turmeric also shows great promise for recovering brain function in neurodegenerative diseases such as Alzheimer's. One of the compounds in turmeric, aromatic-turmerone, has the ability to increase stem cell growth in the brain helping to boost brain repair, while curcumin (another compound in turmeric) helps inhibit inflammation. Turmeric, along with resveratrol and luteolin also can help shutting off the glial cells in our brain (which is beneficial in preventing early brain degeneration).

The health of our brain depends not only on supplementing with the foods listed above, but also on the overall health of our gut. This is another reason why the work you've been doing so far in this program is so important. Numerous studies show that gut inflammation leads to brain inflammation (symptoms of which can include the decrease of brain speed and an increase in brain fog). The Standard American Diet (SAD) is certainly not the brain's best friend. The SAD diet is a leaky gut promoting diet that promotes unhealthy gut bacteria. This leads to gut problems (including leaky gut), and in turn the inflammatory reaction in the gut turns on the glial cells in the brain which in turn leads to brain degeneration. The biggest culprits of all in this unhealthy diet are gluten, GMO foods, and soy.

According to the book 'Change Your Brain Change Your Body' by Daniel Amen, it's actually possible to reverse the aging of your brain.

[1] *http://fluoridealert.org/issues/health/brain*

Here are 12 things you can do that will help in the deceleration of the aging of your brain: (1) protect the brain against injury, (2) be conscientious, (3) surround yourself with a positive peer group, (4) take care of your physical health. (5) go running (studies show running may strengthen the hippocampus region of the brain which is associated with long term memory (6) maintain a healthy weight, (7) eat a healthy diet as noted above, (8) get 8 hours of sleep at night , (9) be constantly learning, (10) avoid toxins, (11) manage your stress, (12) live with gratitude.

ACTION STEP:

Daily stimulation of the brain is important, whether it's reading a book, playing a strategy game, or solving puzzles and problems. There are also apps and online sites that offer game stimulation (for example, www.fitbrains.com). Do at least one activity today that stimulates your brain, and try to make it a daily routine.

In addition, I want you to look today at the thoughts you have toward yourself. Are they loving and supportive, or not so much so. By now you've hopefully already released a lot of the pain and negativity inside through the exercises you've already done. We'll go another step further today and work on self-love. Turn to page 248, read the chapter on Loving Oneself, and begin incorporating as many of the tips as possible.

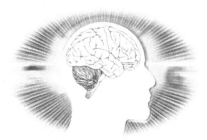

"The truth about childhood is stored up in our bodies and lives in the depths of our souls. Our intellect can be deceived, our feelings can be numbed and manipulated, our perceptions shamed and confused, our bodies tricked with medication, but our soul never forgets. And because we are one, one whole soul in one body, someday our body will present its bill."
~ Alice Miller

HEALTH TIP:

Caffeine is an addictive and can cause dehydration, restlessness, muscle twitching, rapid heartbeat, higher blood pressure, and more. Did you know that for every cup of coffee you drink you need to add an extra 2 cups of water to keep your body properly hydrated? This is over and above the recommended 8-10 glasses of water per day! Caffeine is also a poison and that buzz you feel after a cup or two is your body speeding up its activity to expel that poison from your body.

"But but but... I need it to keep me awake", you say? Caffeine is actually one reason why you're so tired! It gives you a boost in the immediate short term, but over time it weakens your adrenals, affects important mineral levels, and increases the acidity of your blood which slows down oxygenation to your cells, leading to even less overall energy.

TODAY'S INTENTION:

_____

_____

_____

POSITIVE OUTCOME(S):

_____

_____

_____

AFFIRMATION:

_____

_____

_____

GRATITUDE:

_____

_____

_____

_____

While we're on the top of energy, it's good to also be aware of the fact that everything we eat is a form of energy, be it good / bad / positive / negative, what have you. Just do an Internet search for 'Kirlian photographs of food' if you need any evidence of this. Energy is transmitted from the food you eat to your body. Which do you think gives you better energy – chicken meat from a chicken that has lived

it's life on a free range farm playing and clucking with other chickens in the natural outdoors, or chicken meat from an antibiotically-kept-alive chicken squashed tightly in amongst dozens of other chickens in a coop/cage that never sees daylight? You take on the energy of the food you eat.

ACTION STEP:

What are you willing to give up today for the benefits of greater long term energy? If you're addicted to coffee, try slowly cutting down on your consumption. Cutting coffee out cold turkey can lead to unpleasant withdrawal symptoms (although even these usually only last a couple of days). Even just reducing your daily cup by one this week, and one more next week, or choosing decaffeinated, this is a progress in a good direction.

One healthy way to reduce your caffeine consumption is to switch you daily coffee for green tea instead. Green tea still has caffeine, but it's roughly only ¼ that of coffee. The health benefits of green tea are staggering too. It can help people with diabetes regulate glucose levels, protect against free radicals which cause skin wrinkles and aging, improve oral health, reduce the risk of osteoporotic fractures, act as a weight loss stimulant, lessen the severity of asthma, help stop the spread of HIV in the body by stopping the virus from binding to healthy cells, reduce the risk of developing cancer, and boost the immune system.

So, switch your coffee for green tea, or eliminate caffeine all together!

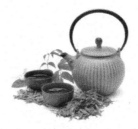

"We can make a commitment to promote vegetables and fruits and whole grains on every part of every menu. We can make portion sizes smaller and emphasize quality over quantity. And we can help create a culture - imagine this - where our kids ask for healthy options instead of resisting them."
~ Michelle Obama

HEALTH TIP:

"The main cause of cardiovascular disease is the instability and dysfunction of the blood vessel wall caused by chronic vitamin deficiency. This leads to millions of small lesions and cracks in the artery wall, particularly in the coronary arteries."
~ Dr. Matthias Rath

Heart disease is the number one killer in the world, and it's largely (and mistakenly) blamed on high cholesterol. Cholesterol is in fact necessary for optimal health, and the body produces it usually in an inverse proportion to the amount you eat. There is 'good' cholesterol (HDL) and what is referred to as 'bad' cholesterol (LDL). LDL by itself however isn't bad, it's *oxidized* LDL that is what damages arteries (thus why anti-oxidants and Vitamin E are so important). LDL is a thick and sticky substance that serves to patch up arteries damaged through poor diet and lifestyle. In other words, it's not even LDL that's the problem, as it's simply the body's protective countermeasure that happens as a result of poor health choices. Without this LDL, we would die from internal bleeding. When enough LDL patches appear, arteries become 'clogged'. The goal of pharmaceutical drugs to lower cholesterol is simply a form of symptom suppression, and it completely ignores the actual cause of what damaged the arteries. Yet millions are taking cholesterol-lowering drugs (which can cause heart attacks) while research has shown time and again that people with higher cholesterol (especially HDL) live longer. Look at the French population as an example. They have the highest consumption of fats in the world, yet

TODAY'S INTENTION:

_____

_____

_____

POSITIVE OUTCOME(S):

_____

_____

_____

AFFIRMATION:

_____

_____

_____

GRATITUDE:

_____

_____

_____

_____

have the lowest rates of heart disease. If you have high cholesterol, see it as a warning that there is inflammation in your body that needs to be dealt with, rather than taking drugs to simply hide the warning signal.

When LDL builds up, it increases the risk of atherosclerosis, coronary heart disease, heart attack, angina, and stroke. While consuming large amounts of egg yolk, processed foods and alcohol can lead to higher LDL levels, there are many foods which can actually help lower your LDL levels. Some of these good foods include whole grains, beans, steamed vegetables, salads, good quality fats, garlic, beets, nuts (especially walnuts and cashews), and raw vegetable juices. Important supplements for the health of your heart include hawthorn (the most recommended supplement for heart health), resveratrol (can help reverse plague deposits), unrefined sea salt, cayenne, alpha lipoic acid, lipotropic factors, flaxseed, blackcurrant seed, primrose oil, coenzyme Q10, glucomannan, niacin, Vitamin B5, Vitamin E, Vitamin C (Nobel Prize winner Linus Pauling suggests 5-6 grams per day for those suffering from any kind of heart problems, or those at high risk), Magnesium, L-Taurine, and grapefruit pectin (which can reverse arterial plaque, lower cholesterol, and widen the arteries). If you're taking extra calcium to avoid osteoporosis (which we learned earlier can be contraindicative), you should also be aware that, as part of calcium's hardening nature, it also hardens the arteries.

> In the event of a heart attack, the priority must be on calling for an ambulance. While waiting for it to arrive, small amounts of L-taurine, cayenne, and/or magnesium can be placed in the victim's mouth near the cheeks to be absorbed.

By the way, while we talk so much about cholesterol, it's just as important to think in terms of acidity. In fact, hyperacidity is an even worse culprit. When the body is in an acidic state, calcium and minerals leach from bones into the blood where, when they interact with cholesterol naturally found in the blood, they form calcium deposits which lead directly to atherosclerosis (again, hardening of the arteries).

ACTION STEP:
What dietary changes can you start making today to improve the health of your heart?

"The degree of responsibility you take for your life determines how much change you can create in it." - Celestine Chua

HEALTH TIP:

Do you have back pain? Did you know that the way you walk could possibly be the cause? If your foot is flat or you have a fallen arch (over-pronation), it can dramatically increase tension in the lower and mid back, resulting in pain. Under-pronation on the other hand limits the lower body's ability to adequately absorb shock, again leading to pain in the lower back. The investment in a good pair of orthotics can be very helpful. There is great technology these days (such as computerized gait analysis and digital video motion analysis) that can pinpoint exact problem areas of your foot. Ask your physiotherapist if they can recommend a good orthotics company in your area.

ACTION STEP:

Today's action step is really an extension of today's health tip. Back pain is one of the leading causes of disability in Americans, and none of us are immune, no matter what your physical condition. This is why it's so important that everyone pay attention to their posture, to help heal back pain, and as a preventative. What follows is a brief guide to proper posture when lifting, sitting, even sleeping – an excerpt from my "Healing Back Pain" book series (available at www.backpainhealingguide.com). As you read it, decide for yourself what adjustments (action steps) you can make in your movements in order to keep your back healthy.

TODAY'S INTENTION:

_____

_____

_____

POSITIVE OUTCOME(S):

_____

_____

_____

AFFIRMATION:

_____

_____

_____

GRATITUDE:

_____

_____

_____

_____

In order to protect your back, proper posture is not only essential when lifting objects, but also in almost everything you do both day and night. Good posture and proper alignment of your body when you stand, sit or walk reduces stress on the spine. Ensuring you move your body in the correct way will help strengthen your lower back and help you avoid further injury in the future.

Following these guidelines is important for everything, whether you're healing a back injury or not. It may sound daunting and tedious at first, but before you know it your body will learn this new way of movement and it will soon become second nature.

When lifting objects, there are generally three safe ways to do this that won't put your back at risk. With all of these it's important to keep a wide stance (feet shoulder width apart with one foot slightly in front of the other); never bend your back (bend with your hips and knees only); keep your shoulders back; move slowly with no jerking or twisting; hold the load as close to your body as possible near your belly button; and never lift a heavy object above shoulder level. If you are turning or twisting with an object, always pivot with your feet.
If you're picking up a box or an item off the floor, stand as close to it as possible with your feet, bend both knees, tighten your stomach, grab the item, and then lift using your legs to lift while keeping your back straight.

For lifting a small child, or an unusual shaped object, again stand close to the object or child with your feet. Bend down onto one knee, and while keeping your back straight slowly lift with both hands as you stand up.

For picking up smaller objects that might be near a supportive structure or, for example, clothes in a wash machine, do the following. Place one hand on the machine or supportive structure. Reach down to grab your object while lifting one leg off the ground. Return to standing in a slow controlled manner while keeping the back straight.

At all times when lifting, remember to recruit your core muscles. And when carrying an object, remember to always hold it close to your body. If you are carrying a package or bag, whenever possible try to distribute the weight between both hands. For example, rather than carrying home one heavy grocery bag in your left hand, split the groceries into two bags, distributing the weight as evenly as possible, and carry one in each hand.

If you are <u>reaching</u> for an object high up, avoid over-reaching. A good rule of thumb is not to reach for anything higher than what you could reach with both hands together.

<u>Sleeping positions</u> are often taken for granted, as are the mattresses you use. However, how you sleep affects your back and can either be beneficial or detrimental to you, depending on your posture. For anyone with a back problem it's recommended that you use a medium-firm mattress for support – not too soft, not too hard. Avoid pillow-top mattresses. They might be comfortable, but they don't provide as much support for your back. Allowing your body to sag unnaturally for several hours each night into a soft unsupportive mattress is NOT a good idea and can actually create back pain by throwing your spine out of alignment. A mattress that is too hard on the other hand creates pressure points where the body makes contact with the mattress (cutting off blood flow to those areas) and gaps where your body does not make contact. Since the support provided by a firm mattress is not evenly distributed to your body (because of the gaps and pressure points), sleep comfort is affected. While a medium firm mattress is best, as a general rule, the heavier the person the firmer the mattress can be.

It's also best for the back to avoid sleeping on your stomach. As much as possible try to sleep on your back, or on one side. If your disc herniation protrudes to one side, your physiotherapist may also recommend that you sleep on a specific side to help speed your recovery. Sleeping on your side with your hips and knees bent is recommended if you have a sway back or lordosis (in other words your spine curves too far inwards). If you're sleeping on your back, place a pillow under your knees. If you're sleeping on your side, place a small pillow under your waist and another one under your neck above your shoulder. For side sleepers, a slightly less firm mattress can be allowed as the mattress needs to be soft enough for the hips and shoulders to sink in while still supporting the rest of the body.

When <u>standing</u>, your feet should be shoulder width apart and your weight distributed evenly between the ball and heel of your foot. Your knees are slightly relaxed. Avoid locking your knees. Keep your shoulders straight. Avoid rounding them forward. Imagine keeping your ears, shoulders and hips in a straight vertical line.

Always be careful when bending over, even if it's just at the sink while brushing your teeth. Never lean forward over the sink with straight legs.

Slightly bend your knees first, then with a firm stance slightly lean forward.

Avoid standing for extended periods. If you must stand for long periods of time, do your best to include the following:
- Walk around periodically
- Rest one foot on a block about 6" high
- Lightly stretch your back backwards (especially if you have been bending forward while standing).

When <u>sitting</u>, ensure your lower back is supported against the back of the chair. If you're sitting for long periods, place a rolled towel or small pillow at the small of your back. To avoid slouching forward, sit upright, keeping your ears aligned with your shoulders. Your core stomach muscles should be lightly contracted, while your shoulder and chest muscles are relaxed. If your feet don't firmly reach the floor, try placing them on a small support stool or block. Your knees should be level with or slightly lower than your hips. If your work finds you sitting for long periods of time, make sure you take frequent breaks, standing up and moving your body every five to ten minutes. When standing up from a seated position, stand by extending your legs, not by bending your waist.

If you are working at a computer all day, position the screen so it is eye-level and adjust your chair to avoid having to lean forward. You want to keep your back and neck as straight and neutral as possible.

One avenue you might want to look into is replacing your current office chair with a ball chair. Balls chairs force you to constantly recruit your core muscles to keep the ball stable. It's not as hard as it sounds. For the most part, your body will do this subconsciously. It's a great way to avoid slouching and maintain proper posture while sitting. Some ball chairs come on a base with wheels so you can glide around like on a regular chair. Some even have a padded bar in the back for extra support. Or, to really work your stabilizing muscles, just sit on the ball itself, without any base. You just might find after using a ball chair for a few weeks you never want to go back to a regular chair!

If you don't have a ball chair, or if you're in your car, make sure the back of the seat is higher than the front. There are foam 'wedges' you can purchase to achieve this.

Be conscious that sitting all day is quite hard on the body. Doing so contributes to collapsed posture, low energy levels, shortened leg and torso muscles, rounded shoulders, stress in the neck, and low back pain. If your job requires you to sit for extended periods, it is even more important to follow the tips outlined above.

Whether you're bending, lifting, exercising, or playing sports, whatever your posture, the importance of recruiting your core can not be overemphasized. A final suggestion to help with core muscle recruiting and support is an investment in Core shorts. These shorts can be worn as often as possible throughout the day when doing any activity to offer your lower back added protection. Many top professional sports teams require the use of Core shorts as standard gear to protect their athletes. These shorts fit tight to your body under your regular clothing. Core shorts were designed to assist in the rehabilitation of core injuries by providing anatomical and functional support to the core area, as well as compression. Whether someone is injury free or not, core shorts offer an extra layer of protection for any number of strains and sprains in the hip and core area and are vital for anyone recovering from a disc injury for example in which the core has been weakened.

"To love yourself right now, just as you are, is to give yourself heaven.
Don't wait until you die. If you wait, you die now.
If you love, you live now."
~ Alan Cohen

HEALTH TIP:

Obesity rates are rising. In the U.S for example, 15% of states had obesity rates of 35% back in 1988. Today, EVERY state has over 35% obesity rates! This will lead to 1/3 of those born since 2000 developing diabetes. And this is just one side effect. (See the back of this book for a more detailed approach to avoiding and curing diabetes).

Did you know that even a 10% reduction in body weight can lower your risk of disease by 50% or more! A healthy weight also gives you more energy, helps you live longer, improves your quality of life, slows the aging process, improves work performance, improves sleep, and lowers blood pressure just to name a few benefits. When deciding your healthy weight range goal, always think in terms of a range 2 or 3 pounds on either side of your 'ideal' weight. Instead of saying "I'd like to weigh 135 lbs.", you would say "My goal weight is between 132 & 137 lbs." Be realistic in your time-frame for weight loss. 1 to 2 pounds per week is healthy weight loss - beyond that may not be sustainable. And remember that weight loss is not the end goal...it is simply the first step to better health.

By the way, a word needs to be said about those fad diets out there. It seems every month there's a new book claiming a diet that will help

TODAY'S INTENTION:

_____

_____

_____

POSITIVE OUTCOME(S):

_____

_____

_____

AFFIRMATION:

_____

_____

_____

GRATITUDE:

_____

_____

_____

_____

you lose weight... the high protein diet, the high carb diet, the high peanut butter diet, the high how else can we spin a book title that will sell millions diet!!!! Here's the thing - any diet that advertises "high" cannot work long term or be sustained for a lifetime. A high protein diet lowers insulin but increases the hormone glucagon which leads to increased cortisol which in turns leads to weight gain. A high carb diet increases insulin while a low carb diet increases cortisol - both of which make you fat. The key in choosing your diet is balance, and remembering that there will never be a one-size-fits-all diet as everyone is bio-individually unique.

ACTION STEP:

If your goal is weight loss, it's not about counting calories. Instead, here are my top 12 Action Steps that work for most anyone!

1. Drink more water. Often you'll feel hungry when all your body really needs is water.
2. Choose healthy fats. Not all fats are bad. In fact, we need fats for healthy functioning and energy. A few good fat sources include nuts (especially walnuts), seeds (especially flaxseed), fish, avocadoes, and extra virgin olive oil.
3. Don't skip breakfast. Think this isn't important? The majority of people who lose weight and KEEP it off are the ones who eat breakfast. Eating breakfast helps jumpstart our metabolism, and gives us fuel to burn off through the day. Include protein with your breakfast as doing so helps increase your metabolic burn rate.
4. Reduce sugar and refined carbs (this includes those white flour breads, crackers, cookies, etc).
5. Eat more often (and regularly). Smaller more frequent meals throughout the day allows your body to burn energy rather than store it as fat. An example meal schedule could be breakfast at 7am, healthy snack around 10:00am, lunch at 1:00pm, a healthy snack around 4:00pm, and dinner at 7:00pm. This way you're feeding your body regularly at 3 hour intervals.
6. Skip the fad laden sugary snacks for some of these healthier snack ideas on page 203.
7. Incorporate more movement. Find ways to stay active and move through partaking in activities that bring you joy. Go for

a walk after dinner, or rather than waste 15 minutes looking for that ideal parking spot right by the mall entrance, park at the back of the lot and walk.

8. Sleep more. No, not all day. 7 to 8 hours is ideal. People who sleep 5 hours or less are on average 5 pounds heavier than those who sleep longer. Sleep deprivation also increases stress which leads to weight gain.

9. Create a healthy kitchen. Remove unhealthy temptation foods and inflammatory foods (sugar being a key one). It's hard to lose weight when you have inflammation all over your body! Stock up on healthy options, and practice cooking more using quality ingredients and spices.

10. Increase your intake of fruits and vegetables. In fact, aim to make half of your meal plate green.

11. Check your thyroid, and your mineral levels. A very high ratio of tissue calcium to potassium indicates a slow thyroid. You might be doing all the exercise and dieting in the world, but if you don't correct this ratio (and in turn your thyroid), losing that extra weight will continue being an uphill struggle.

12. Stop trying to lose weight. If this seems counter-intuitive, it is. When you're overweight and constantly dieting to lose weight, only to then gain it back time and again, chances are there's a deeper emotional issue at play. The healing of obesity is not in the 'fad dieting', it's in loving yourself as you are. With self-love, weight loss will then occur easier as you naturally take better care of your body.

Also today, you're going to get very clear on what your ideal health looks like. Turn to page 252 to do the exercise.

"Weight loss achieved in trials of calorie-reduced diets is so small as to be clinically insignificant."
~ The Cochrane Collaboration, 2002

HEALTH TIP:

Did you know? Adding a drop of unrefined sea salt to your water offers many benefits, including decreasing fatigue, boosting the immune system, helping with adrenal disorders, balancing thyroid disorders, soothing headaches, lowering cholesterol levels, and lowering high blood pressure levels. Want to make that water even healthier? Squeeze in half of a fresh lemon. This helps alkalize, cleanse, and stimulate your body. Starting tomorrow make this a daily habit each morning. (While we're on the topic of salt, today's also a good day to replace all your table salt (not healthy!) with the much healthier alternatives of sea salt and/or Himalayan salt).

ACTION STEP:

It's been just over a month now since you first filled out your My H.E.A.L.T.H. Goals Worksheet on page 195. How did you do? Did you meet your goals or is there room for improvement in the month ahead? Today, if you haven't already, start on a new sheet, filling out your goals for the coming month (making today the first day of the month), and commit to following through. Where did you sabotage progress last month, and how can you improve this time?

TODAY'S INTENTION:

_____

_____

_____

POSITIVE OUTCOME(S):

_____

_____

_____

AFFIRMATION:

_____

_____

_____

GRATITUDE:

_____

_____

_____

_____

"It is never too late to be what you might have been." ~ George Eliot

WEEK 6 / DAY 7- DATE: _____

THIS WEEK'S REVIEW:

Today is your chance to go over the action steps of this past week, reincorporate any activities you may have forgotten, and complete any activities yet unfinished. Use today to catch up and take stock.

Check off the items you've completed below:

☐ I've looked at news ways this week to stimulate my brain.

☐ I have reduced my caffeine consumption this week.

☐ I've taken dietary steps to improve the health of my heart.

☐ I've looked at my posture while lifting, sitting and sleeping and have made at least one important adjustment to help my lower back.

☐ (If my goal is weight loss) I am now actively doing at least four of the action steps listed on Day 5 of this past week.

☐ I have filled out the My H.E.A.L.T.H. Goals Worksheet for the month ahead.

☐ I completed all my daily journaling exercises, including today's which are on the pages that follow.

Of all the tips I've learned so far in this book, 8 action steps for my health that I fully **commit** to doing consistently from now on (the most important tips I'm taking forward with me) are:

1. _____

2. _____

3. _____

4. _____

5. _____

6. _____

7. _____

8. _____

NOTES: Other Important Things I'd Like to Do or Remember:

1. This week I'm proud of:

_____

_____

_____

_____

_____

2. This coming week I commit to following through on the things I didn't fully do this past week (health-wise or other) which include:

_____

_____

_____

_____

_____

3. I'm grateful for:

_____

_____

_____

_____

_____

_____

4. Now that I have some down time, a few things I've been meaning to do that I could do now are:

_____

_____

_____

_____

5. I choose not to stare at the closing doors but rather new ones which are opening. These are:

_____

_____

_____

_____

6. What's worked this week and what's not?

_____

_____

_____

_____

_____

7. General notes and thoughts:

_____

_____

_____

HEALTH TIP:

It's important not to compare your progress to that of someone else's. Their injury or illness may be slightly less complicated than yours, they may be in different physical condition... numerous factors affect how fast people heal. The important thing is to focus on *your* healing journey. Don't give up, no matter hard things might look. Even if after all you've been doing progress seems slow, have faith that, as long as you've diligently been doing your daily exercises, under the surface healing *is* taking place.

ACTION STEP:

Take a moment today to remind yourself that you love yourself and look for areas where you can be more patient.

Your spirit is loving. To the ego mind, nothing is ever good enough. Turn to page 253 in Part II and discover how much you are living into your healthy 'Spirit' as opposed to your unhealthy 'Ego'.

TODAY'S INTENTION:

_____

_____

_____

POSITIVE OUTCOME(S):

_____

_____

_____

AFFIRMATION:

_____

_____

_____

GRATITUDE:

_____

_____

_____

_____

"One cannot tell when he is going to be healed, so do not try to set an exact time limit. Faith, not time, will determine when the cure will be effected. Results depend on the right awakening of life energy and on the conscious and subconscious state of the individual."

~ Paramhansa Yogananda

119

HEALTH TIP:

Eating gluten, the naturally occurring proteins found in wheat, barley, rye, and by contamination most oats, can be life-threatening to people with celiac disease. For the rest of us, while it may not be life-threatening it can trigger numerous health issues such as bloating, heartburn, chronic headaches, skin rashes, fatigue, insomnia, irritable bowel syndrome and brain fog. In fact, because the symptoms are so similar to a variety of other illnesses, it often takes many years before a person is diagnosed with celiac disease, if that indeed is their condition.

Are your joints sore? Gluten can trigger an immune reaction in people who are sensitive that is similar to when a virus enters the body. Killer cells are released to go and break down the virus and get it out of the body. Unfortunately, these killer cells can break down tissues that are similar in the body - one of these is the membrane that lines our joints!

TODAY'S INTENTION:

_____

_____

_____

POSITIVE OUTCOME(S):

_____

_____

_____

AFFIRMATION:

_____

_____

_____

GRATITUDE:

_____

_____

_____

_____

Taking gluten out of the diet can also often help people with Lyme disease, fibromyalgia, Crohn's Disease, Type 1 Diabetes, and especially IBS. Also, if you have hypothyroid, you'll definitely want to eliminate gluten from your diet. Gluten (or it's protein portion gliadin) has a resemblance to that of thyroid tissue, and when the gluten protein

enters the bloodstream (ie: leaky gut), the body then tries to attack it and anything that resembles it...including the thyroid. Over time, this can leads to an impaired in thyroid hormone production. We'll go more into this during week 9.

ACTION STEP:

If you eat a lot of gluten, try cutting back on, or eliminating entirely, those gluten-containing foods for the next few weeks and see how you feel. You can use the Elimination Diet protocol and recipes in Part III for gluten free meal ideas. Some non-gluten grains include buckwheat, quinoa, millet, amaranth, and rice. As for bread, be careful about just jumping over to the gluten-free bread wagon. Gluten free bread often has added sugar and is even less healthy. If you're trying gluten free, go for real foods, unprocessed nuts, vegetables, fruits, meats, herbs, rice, beans, eggs, and fish. (Keep in mind, cutting back or going off gluten for a few weeks may help you notice some positive changes. However, with gluten, the immune response against it can last up to 6 months each time you eat it, so to really determine most effectively how gluten affects you, you would need to commit to eliminating it entirely for 6 months.)

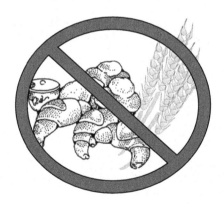

"The food you eat can either be the safest and most powerful form of medicine or the slowest form of poison."
~ Dr. Ann Wigmore

WEEK 7 / DAY 3- DATE: _____

HEALTH TIP:

If you've recently been exposed to higher than normal radiation, perhaps through x-rays, chemotherapy, or even environmentally, there are some foods that can naturally help your body 'detox' from radiation.

First and foremost, chaga mushroom is mentioned again! It contains some of the most powerful radiation removing properties of any substance on earth. It can also be used to help ease the side effects of chemotherapy.

Other foods that help counteract the effects of radiation include wheat grass, micro-algae (chlorella, wild blue green aphanizomenon), kelp, alfalfa leaf tea, basically all green foods, buckwheat groats, apples, and miso. Calcium, magnesium, and CoQ10 help protect the body against radiation, as well as short term use of the herb chaparral. Modified citrus pectin and/or algin are also useful for protecting against radiation exposure, while binding to and helping to eliminate these toxins. Taking baking soda baths can also be helpful.

TODAY'S INTENTION:

_____

_____

_____

POSITIVE OUTCOME(S):

_____

_____

_____

AFFIRMATION:

_____

_____

_____

GRATITUDE:

_____

_____

_____

_____

Other suggestions to limit everyday radiation exposure include using an earpiece or phone guard with your cell phone, a radiation/glare filter screen with your computer, having your home tested for radon, limiting the number of x-rays you have taken, and for women, substituting thermography for mammograms (this topic is discussed more on page 321 in the cancer section of this book).

ACTION STEP:

By now you've been introduced to a number of foods that can help protect against dis-ease and improve your overall health. You may need to make some changes in the way you eat, and understandably for most people these changes aren't easy. To help make this transition, one of easiest ways to start consuming more of the healthy type foods and less of the 'bad-for- us' type is to be aware of which healthy foods we ENJOY eating. You might not be motivated to eat brussel sprouts everyday if you can't stand them, no matter how healthy they are. However by getting clear on which healthy foods you DO like, it will become much easier to alter your eating plan to include more of these healthy foods.

Think of as many healthy foods, snacks, and drinks that you LIKE, whether you currently consume them or not. Use the foods I've mentioned in this book so far to give you some ideas. Record them all in the box below. Which of these can you begin adding to your diet this week? Circle the ones you can see yourself eating more of, and shop for these the next time you're in the store.

"When one door closes, another opens;
but we often look so long and so regretfully upon the closed door
that we do not see the one which has opened for us."
~ Alexander Graham Bell

HEALTH TIP:

Prolotherapy is an effective treatment for chronic pain, especially where tendons and ligaments are involved. "Prolo" is short for proliferation, because the treatment causes the proliferation (growth, formation) of new ligament tissue in areas where it has become weak. Prolotherapy uses a sugar based solution which is injected into the ligament or tendon where it attaches to the bone. This causes a control inflammatory reaction, re-awakening your body's natural healing resources and stimulating the tissue to repair itself. The treatment is excellent for many different types of musculoskeletal pain, including arthritis, back pain, migraine headaches, MS, sports injuries, carpal tunnel, muscular dystrophy, torn tendons and ligaments, tennis elbow, and osteoporosis.

ACTION STEP:

VAKS (short for Visual, Auditory, Kinesthetic, and Spirit) is a way of conditioning the mind through movement and the senses to achieve whatever it is you want. Stating a positive affirmation or desire is important, but when you combine that statement with VAKS, your right brain and left brain become integrated and the conditioning process of your belief is driven deeper into your subconscious. Referring to the VAKS instructions on page 256 in Part II spend 10 minutes today doing your VAKS exercise. Try to make this a new daily habit.

TODAY'S INTENTION:

_____
_____
_____

POSITIVE OUTCOME(S):

_____
_____
_____

AFFIRMATION:

_____
_____

GRATITUDE:

_____
_____
_____
_____

"Always laugh when you can. It is cheap medicine." ~Lord Byron

HEALTH TIP:

Today's tip is to go out shopping for 'Superfoods'! Superfoods generally have low calories but are very nutrient dense, offering superior sources of antioxidants and essential nutrients. We will look at superfoods in two parts, this week and in week 12. This will allow you time to focus on adding a few into your diet at a time. Here's a look at a few you may want to adopt into your regular diet:

Goji berries: are known to be one of the top herbs in Chinese medicine and make a great addition to any smoothie or cereal. It is a superfood that contains 18 kinds of amino acids (six times higher than bee pollen), and up to 21 trace minerals. It is associated with longevity and enhancing the treatment protocol of several diseases including cancer.

Wheat grass: although it comes from wheat seed, it contains no gluten. It is very alkalizing and promotes healthy blood, normalizes the thyroid gland, and helps with digestion, weight loss and cleansing.

TODAY'S INTENTION:

_____

_____

_____

POSITIVE OUTCOME(S):

_____

_____

_____

AFFIRMATION:

_____

_____

_____

GRATITUDE:

_____

_____

_____

_____

Hemp: raw, shelled hemp seeds are one of nature's most complete sources of vitamins, minerals, essential fatty acids, and antioxidants. High in protein it also makes a great substitute for animal protein. This is a true super food that supports optimal health and well-being. A few of the health benefits attributable in part to eating raw hemp seeds include weight loss, increased and sustained energy, rapid recovery from disease or injury, lowered cholesterol and blood pressure, reduced

inflammation, improvement in circulation and immune system as well as natural blood sugar control. Hemp seeds can be added to salads, smoothies, and easily incorporated into your daily diet - aim for three to five tablespoons a day.

Camu Camu: This South American berry offers one of the highest sources of natural Vitamin C from any plant on earth! In addition to its amazing Vitamin C qualities, it offers provides a full spectrum of antioxidants, bioflavonoids, and minerals. Camu camu is a great immune booster and anti-viral. It also has received a lot of praise for its mood-balancing and anti-depressant effects.

Marine Phytoplankton: This food has supported life on Earth for billions of years, in fact it is the basis of the entire food chain on Earth. It is a complete food source, a complete protein source, a high anti-oxidant source, and offers a perfect balance of minerals. To quote Dr. Jerry Tennant, M.D., "One of those rare products that contains almost everything you need for life (and the rebuilding of a healthy life) is marine phytoplankton. It contains the nine amino acids that the body cannot make and must be consumed in our diet (essential amino acids). The essential fatty acids are also present (Omega 3 and Omega 6). Vitamins A (beta-carotene), 81 (thiamine), 82 (riboflavin), 83 (niacin), 85 (pantothenic acid), 86 (pyridoxine), 812 (cobalamin), C, D, and E (tocopherol) and major and trace minerals are all present in phytoplankton. In short, it contains almost everything one needs to sustain life. Therefore, it contains almost everything one needs to restore health by providing the raw materials to make new cells that function normally."

ACTION STEP:
The secret to getting the right answers (in health as well as life) begins with asking the right questions. Turn to page 228 in Part II, choose three to five questions that resonate with you, and answer them.

"Strength is born in the deep silence of long-suffering hearts; not amidst joy."
~ Felicia Hemans

HEALTH TIP:

DHEA is the most abundant hormone in our bodies. Production peaks around the age of 20, and then decreases as we age (by the age of 40 we have roughly ½ of our optimum amount, and by the age of 80 we have less than 5%). As the adrenal glands are responsible for DHEA production, chronic stress, fatigue, and adrenal fatigue will result in lower than normal levels. DHEA helps send the signal to the liver the produce the protein ceruloplasmin (Cp), and if Cp is production is low, then there will likely be a lack of bioavailable copper and iron in the body...which then goes on to affect all the associated symptoms of those minerals. Research has pinpointed low DHEA levels as a marker for many degenerative diseases as well as accelerated aging. At the same time, research is suggesting that DHEA can help reverse, or even prevent, some of the most common diseases associated with aging. These include atherosclerosis, cancer, diabetes, and reduced immunity. While supplementation *may* be something to look into, also to consider is that poor digestion / poor nutrient absorption, adrenal insufficiency, and overexposure to xenoestrogens can all additionally compromise DHEA.

TODAY'S INTENTION:

_____

_____

_____

POSITIVE OUTCOME(S):

_____

_____

_____

AFFIRMATION:

_____

_____

_____

GRATITUDE:

_____

_____

_____

_____

ACTION STEP:

By now you've noticed I emphasize in this book the importance of giving daily gratitude. The more things we can find to be grateful for, the more things we can be grateful for will manifest. Today, give gratitude to someone. Think of a few people who've been the wind beneath your wings, who've given a part of themselves to help you. Perhaps you've acknowledged them for it, or maybe you haven't. Maybe they're no longer in your journey but at one point were an important part of it. Or maybe they are still with you every step of the way. Choose one or more of these people, send them an email, card, or call them, and let them know how much their caring has meant to you. Do it today. You will feel better, and so will they.

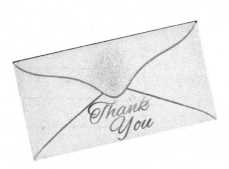

"Gratitude is a vaccine, an antitoxin, and an antiseptic."
~John Henry Jowett

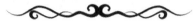

WEEK 7 / DAY 7- DATE: _____

THIS WEEK'S REVIEW:

Today is your chance to go over the action steps of this past week, reincorporate any activities you may have forgotten, and complete any activities yet unfinished. Use today to catch up and take stock.

Check off the items you've completed below:

☐ I've completed the Spirit vs Ego exercise.

☐ I 've taken steps to reduce the amount of gluten I consume.

☐ I've begun incorporating at least a couple superfoods into my diet

☐ I'm eating foods and taking actions that protect me against radiation.

☐ I've done the VAKS exercises at least once this week.

☐ I've let someone important in my life know they are appreciated.

☐ I completed all my daily journaling exercises, including today's which are on the pages that follow.

Of all the tips I've learned so far in this book, 9 action steps for my health that I fully **commit** to doing consistently from now on (the most important tips I'm taking forward with me) are:

1. _____

2. _____

3. _____

4. _____

5. _____

6. _____

7. _____

8. _____

9. _____

NOTES: Other Important Things I'd Like to Do or Remember:

HEALTH TIP:

Fear is a debilitating emotion that can have drastic consequences on your health. Not only does fear add to our stress level which, in of itself can lead to health issues, but fear can also set you up for manifesting that which you are afraid of. As the Law of Attraction states, what we focus on expands; and what we resist persists. If you are afraid of not healing, or a worsening of your condition, those are the very thoughts you are focused on, and where your attention goes, energy flows. By allowing fear to control you, you are subconsciously manifesting that negative outcome. Instead, we need to acknowledge our fear and then, rather than resist it, turn our energy and focus onto more positive outcomes.

TODAY'S INTENTION:

_____

_____

_____

POSITIVE OUTCOME(S):

_____

_____

_____

AFFIRMATION:

_____

_____

_____

GRATITUDE:

_____

_____

_____

_____

ACTION STEP:

Today we take back control of fear. Turn to page 257 in Part II and complete the exercise.

"You will only ever have two choices, love or fear:
choose love and don't ever let fear turn you against your playful heart."
- Jim Carey

HEALTH TIP:

Some artificial food additives like aspartame and monosodium glutamate (MSG) can trigger inflammatory responses, especially in people who are already suffering from inflammatory conditions such as rheumatoid arthritis. Both these ingredients have long lists of negative side effects – avoid them like the plague!

Since we're on the topic of really REALLY bad things in our food, let's also look at trans fats.

"Trans fats are the 'biggest food-processing disaster in U.S. history… In Europe [food companies] hired chemists and took trans fats out… In the United States, they hired lawyers and public relations people."
~ Professor Walter Willet (Harvard School of Public Health).

Artificial trans fats were originally introduced as a means of extending shelf life yet have no nutritional value and are actually harmful to your health, contributing to thousands of cardiac deaths every year. Trans fats clog arteries, increasing the risk of both heart attack and stroke. Trans fats decrease good HDL cholesterol and drastically increase bad LDL cholesterol. Studies indicate that trans fats may raise the risk of diabetes as well as cause insulin resistance. Bottom line - read labels and avoid trans fats whenever possible.

TODAY'S INTENTION:

_____

_____

_____

POSITIVE OUTCOME(S):

_____

_____

_____

AFFIRMATION:

_____

_____

_____

GRATITUDE:

_____

_____

_____

_____

ACTION STEP:

Today you have 2 action steps:

1. Begin reading labels. Go through your cupboards and look for items that contain trans fats, MSG, and or aspartame. Toss 'em! Even though it may feel like you're wasting food, this 'food' is only poisoning your body, so why would you want to keep it around?

2. Be aware of your self-talk, and replace any negative messages with positive ones such as these: "I am human, it's OK to make mistakes"; "I am strong. I can do it"; "I don't have to be perfect"; "I don't owe anyone an explanation"; "I am calm and centered"; "I love myself", etcetera.

"A psychiatrist who refuses to try the methods of Orthomolecular Psychiatry (nutrition as related to mental health) in addition to his usually therapy in the treatment of his patients is failing in his duty as a physician"
~Linus Pauling, Ph.D.

HEALTH TIP:

There is a saying: "dead food does not beget live cells" – in other words dead food (including animal products and that which has been overcooked, or processed and packaged) cannot properly nourish a living organism. The result is a tired body. On the other hand, consuming live foods, (foods that have been left alone in their perfect state), allows your body to be nourished and feel more alive. Juicing is one of the best ways to consume ample amounts of 'live food'. In fact, a glass of vegetable juice has more nutritional value than 3 full meals in a day if those meals have been cooked. Although an old book and now out of print, 'Live Food Juices' by Dr. H.E. Kirschner is an invaluable resource that offers juicing recipes for reversing a variety of diseases. Since juicing strips away the hard to digest fiber of the fruit or vegetable, the nutritional goodness can quickly and easily be absorbed into the body. Juicing is therefore quite beneficial for anyone with compromised intestines, such as those with I.B.S, Crohn's disease, or colitis.

A fruit or vegetable smoothie is another great option. Whether for breakfast or throughout the day, a smoothie is one of the healthiest power meals you can give yourself. A fruit and green mixed smoothie provides you with a full spectrum of essential vitamins, minerals, and

TODAY'S INTENTION:

_____

_____

_____

POSITIVE OUTCOME(S):

_____

_____

_____

AFFIRMATION:

_____

_____

_____

GRATITUDE:

_____

_____

_____

_____

antioxidants, plus it offers lots of fiber (which juicing doesn't), and it empowers the immune system. It also doesn't boost blood sugar the way juicing does. Added benefits are increased energy, weight loss, mental clarity, and reduced junk food cravings, Green smoothies are also a great way to get your daily recommended servings of vegetables without tasting them (as the fruits help disguise the flavor). If you're in the market for a blender (juicers are for juicing, blenders are for smoothies), consider Vitamix - a bit of an investment but it will change your health, the way you eat, and should last a lifetime.

> Fruit is best eaten by itself and eaten raw as the nutrients can be easily destroyed when heated and also because fruit takes less time to digest than most other food. Also, fruits and vegetables that are deeper in colour and smell fresh contain more nutrients. Did you get that? Eat deep colored fruit and darker greens, eat them raw, and eat the fruits separately.

ACTION STEP:

If you have juicer or blender at home, experiment today concoting the healthiest fruit juice or smoothie you can create. If you don`t have blender or juicer, spend some time today looking at your purchase options. A good quality juicer or blender really is a great investment in your health.

I'd also recommend watching the film "Fat, Sick, and Nearly Dead" by Joe Cross. A multi-award winning documentary, it offers a remarkable look at the power of juicing. You can also find a number of great juicing recipes at <u>www.rebootwithjoe.com</u>.

"Knowing is not enough, we must apply. Willing is not enough, we must do."
~ Johann von Goethe

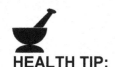

HEALTH TIP:

If you have muscle pain or some other ache, it's possible that the cause of the problem is nowhere near where you're feeling it. The pain may be referred from some distant trigger point. For example, a problem in your foot may cause back or even neck pain. In this case, treating the back or neck will be pointless. Through our kinetic chain (how we move) and the body's fascia, everything is connected, and an imbalance in one area can create a chain reaction somewhere else. If treating the location of the pain hasn't been successful, you may want to look into trigger point therapy which focuses on addressing the source of the pain.

ACTION STEP:

While Trigger Point therapy can be used to heal physical pain, Emotional Freedom Technique (E.F.T.) is a method of using points on the body to help clear emotional pain. It can also be practiced by oneself relatively easily. Turn to page 259 to learn more about, and practice E.F.T. on yourself today.

TODAY'S INTENTION:

_____

_____

_____

POSITIVE OUTCOME(S):

_____

_____

_____

AFFIRMATION:

_____

_____

_____

GRATITUDE:

_____

_____

_____

_____

"Health depends on being in harmony with our souls"
~ Dr. Edward Bach

HEALTH TIP:

Lack of sleep asleep affects our health in a number of ways. Beyond the obvious symptoms of mental and physical drowsiness, not getting enough sleep is also linked to inflammation, cardiovascular disease, and obesity. Generally, for optimum health, women require 6-7 hours of sleep while men require 7-8 hours. To be most effective however, those hours must include several full sleep cycles including REM and non-REM stages of sleep. Hours sleeping before midnight also tend to be more restorative than hours sleeping after midnight. (If you have insomnia, then poor adrenal function / night-time cortisol spikes, and/or an overburdened liver would be initial places of investigation for cause).

ACTION STEP:

In addition to setting your morning alarm, for the next week why not also set an alarm to go to bed? When that alarm goes off, shut off the light and close your eyes.

TODAY'S INTENTION:

_____

_____

_____

POSITIVE OUTCOME(S):

_____

_____

_____

AFFIRMATION:

_____

_____

_____

GRATITUDE:

_____

_____

_____

_____

"To keep the body in good health is a duty... otherwise we shall not be able to keep our mind strong and clear."
Buddha

HEALTH TIP:

Are you habits healthy or unhealthy? Those little things you do every day all add up to having an impact on your health? Do you sit on the couch and watch TV for hours when you come home from work? If so, is that helping the health of your heart? Do you consistently have good oral hygiene? If not, you're allowing bacteria to grow, and when bad bacteria build up in the mouth, they can easily travel to other parts of your body, leading to all sorts of infections and other diseases. Do you allow yourself to lose your temper when you're in traffic? How does that affect your stress level?We need to always be aware of the little things we do every day, understanding that the habits of our daily lives lead to either greater health or lack of it.

TODAY'S INTENTION:

_____

_____

_____

POSITIVE OUTCOME(S):

_____

_____

_____

AFFIRMATION:

_____

_____

_____

GRATITUDE:

_____

_____

_____

_____

ACTION STEP:

I'm giving you 3 action steps to work on today and tomorrow.

1. First, on page 263, go through the list of Unhealthy Habits. How many of these are part of how you live your life? For each one that you do, try to come up with an alternative habit that's healthier. In other words, when you notice yourself about to do the bad habit, what can you quickly shift to doing instead?

2. Secondly, whether religion plays a role in your life or not, praying to a higher power can be used for many types of healing. A few prayers are presented on page 261. Choose and say one today.

3. Finally, how are you coming along on your 'My H.EA.L.T.H. Goals' worksheet that you filled out in week #6? What actions do you need to take in order to meet the goals you set?

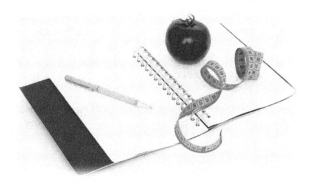

*"There are risks and costs to a program of action.
But they are far less than the long-range risks and costs
of comfortable inaction."*
~ John F. Kennedy

WEEK 8 / DAY 7- DATE: _____

THIS WEEK'S REVIEW:

Today is your chance to go over the action steps of this past week, reincorporate any activities you may have forgotten, and complete any activities yet unfinished. Use today to catch up and take stock.

Check off the items you've completed below:

☐ I've completed the Fear exercise on page 257.

☐ I've been paying attention to my self-talk this week, am catching the negatives, and replacing those messages with positive ones.

☐ I've experimented this week with creating a super-healthy smoothie.

☐ I've practiced the Emotional Freedom technique on myself

☐ I've made an effort to get adequate sleep these past few nights, and will make an even stronger effort in the week ahead.

☐ I've looked at my unhealthy habits and have come up with healthier replacement habits that I am committed to pursuing

☐ I completed all my daily journaling exercises, including today's which are on the pages that follow.

Of all the tips I've learned so far in this book, 10 action steps for my health that I fully **commit** to doing consistently from now on (the most important tips I'm taking forward with me) are:

1. _____

2. _____

3. _____

4. _____

5. _____

6. _____

7. _____

8. _____

9. _____

10. _____

NOTES: Other Important Things I'd Like to Do or Remember:

WEEK 9 / DAY 1- DATE: _____

HEALTH TIP:

Remember to stay focused on your vision of health. *Fighting the illness or injury is fear based,* and as mentioned at the beginning of this program, what we resist persists. By fighting the negative, we are focused on the negative, drawing more of it towards us. Instead of fear based thinking, stay hope based - this means staying focused on your vision of where you want to be. And trust.

ACTION STEP:

No matter where you`re at, looking ahead to a bright future will pull you forward and give you the motivation to carry on. Being clear on your dreams and things you still want to accomplish is an important exercise for everyone to do, whether healing from injury or illness or not. Today you`ll do an exercise in dreams to fulfill. Turn to page 265 to begin.

TODAY'S INTENTION:

_____

_____

_____

POSITIVE OUTCOME(S):

_____

_____

_____

AFFIRMATION:

_____

_____

_____

GRATITUDE:

_____

_____

_____

_____

"I just wish people would realize that anything's possible if they try, that dreams are made if people try."
~ Terry Fox

HEALTH TIP:

If you're a heavy soda drinker, you're not doing any favors to your body, or health. Not only does soda leach important minerals from your bones, it's also been shown to increase your risk of heart attack and contribute to obesity. Soft drinks hugely lower a body's pH and its oxygen content, opening the door for cancer to thrive. Soda contains phosphorus, an epoxy resin called BPA, carcinogens, high amounts of sugar and HFCS, and aspartame - all factors that contribute to health problems and a potentially shorter life.

Think diet sodas are healthier? Not so. Diet sodas contribute to a list of health problems ranging from decline in kidney function, heart disease, obesity (yes, diet sodas contribute to obesity!), and rotting teeth (from the high acidic level). As well, the aspartame found in diet sodas can increase the risk of cancer, non-Hodgkin's Lymphoma, and leukemia. In women it lowers serotonin levels, creating fatigue, irritability, and withdrawal. Aspartame also worsens insulin sensitivity more than sugar. Diabetics take note - diet drinks are not the answer!

TODAY'S INTENTION:

_____

_____

_____

POSITIVE OUTCOME(S):

_____

_____

_____

AFFIRMATION:

_____

_____

_____

GRATITUDE:

_____

_____

_____

_____

ACTION STEP:

Drinking soda while trying to heal your body is like taking two steps forward and two steps back. It's limiting your progress, and potentially making you even sicker. Starting today, reduce your soda consumption. Try replacing it with a healthy glass of water. Remember to be drinking your daily 6-10 cups of water. Also, go through your fridge and cupboards and throw out anything that contains aspartame – after all, it`s poison to your body! Look out for NutraSweet® and Equal®, as they're simply aspartame disguised under other names.

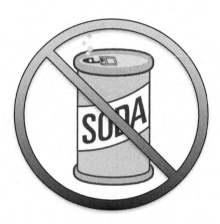

"America's health care system is in crisis precisely because we systematically neglect wellness and prevention."
~ Tom Harkin

WEEK 9 / DAY 3- DATE: _____

HEALTH TIP:

Apple cider vinegar has many health benefits, ranging from helping in weight loss, to lowering blood pressure, liver detoxification, and reducing acne. It can also help increase stomach acid (a good thing) and by putting a few drops on your meat or vegetables can help with the digestion of those foods. For diabetes patients, a couple of tablespoons at bedtime can show favorable changes in blood sugar levels the next morning. Make sure the apple cider vinegar you take is organic and has the "mother" (stringy ball of matter usually at the bottom of the bottle) in it.

ACTION STEP:

There is an old story of a group of thieves that survived a plague in Europe by making and drinking what is today called the Vinegar of the Four Thieves. It works as a great remedy and preventative for colds and flus and, once made, can easily be stored in the fridge for ages. Though you will find many variations to the story (and the recipe), here is one version that is quite effective.

TODAY'S INTENTION:

_____

_____

_____

POSITIVE OUTCOME(S):

_____

_____

_____

AFFIRMATION:

_____

_____

_____

GRATITUDE:

_____

_____

_____

_____

To a 32oz bottle of apple cide vinegar with the Mother, add a tbsp each of thyme, rosemary, lavender, mint, wormwood and sage dried herbs. You can also add a chopped clove of garlic. Seal the jar and let it sit in the fridge for 6-8 weeks, shaking it every so often. Then strain out the herbs, leaving the liquid. Whenever you feel a cold or flu coming on, take 1 tbsp diluted in water every few hours.

"Change your thoughts and change your world."
~ Norman Vincent Peale

145

WEEK 9 / DAY 4- DATE: _____

HEALTH TIP:

According to brain disorder specialist Daniel Amen, 50% of people over the age of 85 will get Alzheimer's. Even more shocking, the causes of Alzheimer's start in the brain 30 to 50 years before symptoms ever appear, and seem to stem from nutritional deficiencies. As there are few treatments and no known cure for Alzheimer's, the focus must be placed on early prevention. Many people with Alzheimer's tend to have low levels of Vitamins B3, B12, A and E, zinc, along with elevated mercury and copper. In fact, copper toxicity is a silent link to Alzheimer's that could likely provide many answers. Yet this link is almost never mentioned to the public. I explain more about this on www.coppertoxic.com, and will include here the following from The Proceedings of the National Academy of Sciences, *"Copper appears to be one of the main environmental factors that trigger the onset and enhance the progression of Alzheimer's disease by preventing the clearance and accelerating the accumulation of toxic proteins in the brain."* The following are all things you can do to minimize your risk of getting Alzheimer's. Avoid gluten, GMO foods, sugar, aluminum, flu vaccinations which contain both mercury and aluminum, and statin drugs. At the same time, make sure you are getting plenty of healthful fats (some sources include ghee, pecans, free range eggs, krill oil, avocado, wild Alaskan salmon), zinc, astaxanthan, alpha lipoic acid, gingko biloba, fermented foods and/or probiotics, vegetables, blueberries, exercise, and mental stimulation. Turmeric is one preventative that deserves special attention. Alzheimer's is an inflammatory disease of the brain, and turmeric is one of the most potent anti-inflammatory agents in nature. Indian's eat turmeric almost every day, and not surprisingly they have the lowest rates of Alzheimer's.

TODAY'S INTENTION:

_____

_____

_____

POSITIVE OUTCOME(S):

_____

_____

_____

AFFIRMATION:

_____

_____

_____

GRATITUDE:

_____

_____

_____

_____

ACTION STEP:

Turn to page 269 in Part II and start writing down what your ideal day looks like.

"The physician treats, but nature heals." ~Hippocrates

HEALTH TIP:

The majority of sunscreens on the market today are more harmful than beneficial. Although sunscreens are designed to decrease your risk of skin cancer, most modern day sunscreens may actually increase your risk of cancer and disrupt the functioning of your hormones. Most 'common' sunscreens on the market today contain parabens which may increase the rate of breast cancer, interfere with the male reproductive system, and wreak havoc on your body's hormones. Oxybenzone and retinyl palmitate are two other harmful ingredients contained in many sunscreen products, the latter being shown to increase the rates of cancer in combination with UV-A rays.

Now, what to do if you get a sunburn? Turn the page for some natural remedies that can help!

TODAY'S INTENTION:

_____

_____

_____

POSITIVE OUTCOME(S):

_____

_____

_____

AFFIRMATION:

_____

_____

_____

GRATITUDE:

_____

_____

_____

_____

* Apply **cool water** (or ice water) as soon as possible. This helps prevent the burn from reaching deeper into the tissue. Take a cool shower for even a minute or two every couple of hours. Pat your skin dry after – do not rub.

* Apply **aloe vera gel** every 3 to 4 hours. Aloe vera cools the skin and helps decrease the burn's inflammation.

* Use a **Comfrey Ointment**. You can make your own from the leaves

and roots of this plant, or you can purchase ointments at the store. Comfrey ointment is a basic herbal treatment for all sorts of burns. Even in cases where blistering would be expected, comfrey heals the burn so that often blisters do not even appear. It also helps alleviate the pain and heat from the burn.

* **Drink lots of water**. Sunburn over large areas of your body can cause your body to become dehydrated, so extra fluid intake is important.

* Although I prefer natural remedies, if you feel your burn is severe, taking a dose of **ibuprofen** (Advil) immediately can help cut back on some of the redness, swelling, and pain that is going to occur.

* if your burn is mild, place **ice cubes** or a bag of frozen vegetables wrapped in a paper towel against the burn. Do not place the ice directly on the burn, always make sure to wrap it.

* if you have some available in your fridge, apply **yogurt** to the sunburned areas (Greek yogurt is best). Rinse the yogurt off in a cool shower and then pat dry.

* **eat extra fruits** such as watermelons, honeydew melons or cantaloupes which provide the body with additional hydration.

ACTION STEP:

On page 270 in Part II, write down 6 activities that are supportive of your health goals, as well as 6 activities that are unsupportive of your health goals.

"The only things that stand between a person and what they want in life are the will to try it, and the faith to believe it's possible." ~ Rich Devos

HEALTH TIP:

Colloidal silver, a suspension of microscopic particles of silver in water, is a superb natural antibiotic, and has been shown in studies to increase the effectiveness of antibiotics by up to 1000 times, even in low doses! It is the most powerful all-natural antibiotic and antiviral known (and without the health impairing side effects that modern antibiotics pose). In fact, silver was a common infection fighter dating all the way back to the days of Hippocrates in 400BC, but with the advent of Penicillin (and the F.D.A.), it has been shoved under the rug and forgotten in exchange for more profitable pharmaceuticals! Despite no pathogen being immune to silver, and hospitals once widely using silver, it's now dismissed as 'alternative medicine' and even 'quackery'. Still, scores of people swear by its ability to heal everything from pink eye to Staph infections, HIV, cancer and a host of other bacterial, fungal, and viral infections.

ACTION STEP:

The thyroid is a master gland that affects every organ in the body. With hypothyroid (the most common condition), everything slows down and symptoms can include weight gain, brain fog, hair loss, hormone imbalance, and lack of energy. In fact, thyroid problems can cause many recurring illnesses and fatigue. Conventional replacement of the thyroid hormone is not the answer, as while it might immediately make one feel better, it opens the door to a host of autoimmune diseases (lupus, rheumatoid arthritis, M.S., for example). If you want to heal the thyroid, begin by going off gluten. The gluten molecule mimics that of the thyroid, and when the body goes to attack the gluten is also inadvertently attacks the thyroid. (Note: While the following tips are important, so too is not discontinuing any thyroid medication without your doctor's consent).

TODAY'S INTENTION:

_____

_____

_____

POSITIVE OUTCOME(S):

_____

_____

_____

AFFIRMATION:

_____

_____

_____

GRATITUDE:

_____

_____

_____

_____

If hypothyroidism is a concern, then your action steps today (and going forward) include:

➤ going off gluten and avoiding all artificial and processed foods, HFCS, canola oil (which interferes with the production of thyroid hormones), table salt, hydrogenated oils and sugar.

➤ Check your mineral levels through HTMA (www.htmatest.com). Chances are you have a high calcium to potassium ratio, which indicates hypothyroidism. Since potassium is necessary in sufficient quantity to sensitize the tissues to the effects of thyroid hormone, while calcium blocks the absorption, a high Ca/K ratio strongly suggests reduced thyroid function and/or cellular response to thyroxine. Knowing your mineral levels, a mineral balancing protocol can then be designed to support these levels. There could also be connection with copper deficiency (either caused by true deficiency or copper toxicity where the copper is biounavailable). Low available copper decreases bioavailable iron which then decreases T4 production, increases rT3, thereby allowing mycotoxins to build up. Mycotoxins are one cause of Hashimoto's disease, which in turn is a primary cause of underactive thyroid. Copper toxicity also leads to an increase in tissue calcium...again...the high Ca/K.

➤ stay away from unfermented soy products (soy meat / soy milk / soy cheese). Soy phytoestrogens can lead to hypothyroidism and thyroid cancer. (Fermented, unprocessed soy is fine (ie: natto, miso, and tempeh)).

➤ Avoid fluoride (which suppresses the thyroid). Flouride (as well as chlorine) can block iodine receptors in the thyroid leading to hypothyroidism. Fluoride is found in toothpaste, drinking (tap) water, soft drinks, shower water...

➤ eating more seaweed (such as spirulina, hijiki, wakame, nori and kombu), and shellfish, all of which are good sources of iodine which the thyroid needs to produce the hormones that regulate body metabolism (however check first with your doctor as iodine rich foods, though beneficial, can interfere with the efficacy of thyroid drugs).

➤ Move toward a more alkaline diet (refer to page 240 for a list of alkaline foods).

➤ Eat organically (to reduce pesticide exposure).

➤ eat your carrots (people with hypothyroidism need a higher intake of beta-carotene).

➤ start cooking your broccoli, turnips, and cabbage. Cooking deactivates the goitrogens found in these foods. (Goitrogens block the effects of thyroid hormones).

➤ Reduce stress. Stress weakens your adrenals and increases cortisol, and cortisol negatively affects thyroid function. Remember that stress is caused not only by lifestyle, it is also caused by environmental toxins as well.

➤ Exercise

➤ Look into supplementing with L-Tyrosine and L-Arginine (both which help stimulate the thyroid and its hormones)

➤ (For women) balance estrogen levels as excess estrogen slows the thyroid gland. (Hint: dairy products and birth control pills both contribute to higher levels of estrogen!)

WEEK 9 / DAY 7 - DATE: _____

THIS WEEK'S REVIEW:

Today is your chance to go over the action steps of this past week, reincorporate any activities you may have forgotten, and complete any activities yet unfinished. Use today to catch up and take stock.

Check off the items you've completed below:

☐ I've completed my list of Dreams to Fulfill (knowing I can always add more as new dreams arise).

☐ I no longer drink diet soda, nor do I accept putting aspartame into my body.

☐ I've made a bottle of "Vinegar of the Four Thieves"

☐ I've written down what my ideal day looks like.

☐ I've made a list of activities that are unsupportive as well as supportive of my health goals.

☐ I've taken at least one step, from the list given yesterday, to improve the health of my thyroid.

☐ I completed all my daily journaling exercises, including today's which are on the pages that follow.

Of all the tips I've learned so far in this book, 11 action steps for my health that I fully **commit** to doing consistently from now on (the most important tips I'm taking forward with me) are:

1. _____

2. _____

3. _____

4. _____

5. _____

6. _____

7. _____

8. _____

9. _____

10. _____

11. _____

NOTES: Other Important Things I'd Like to Do or Remember:

HEALTH TIP:

One of the many tools we can use to heal ourselves and gain a more positive outlook is to release anger. Did you know that anger and poor liver health are connected, each contributing to the other? Everyone holds some anger or resentment inside them, some people more than others. Even if you find yourself to be a happy person, there is likely some anger hiding inside. When we keep anger inside it only poisons us, builds up, and eventually comes out in a way that potentially hurts others, or ourselves. Plus it saps away energy we could be using for healing. Writing out anger is a very powerful and cleansing process, both for the body and mind. It is also completely non-destructive in nature. It's important to examine your anger, is it toward someone else, or perhaps toward yourself even for triggering someone else to do something to you. Often it's someone else, but often too it's our own sensitivity and paranoia that stands in the way of emotional maturity. Either way, it's vital to release it, safely.

TODAY'S INTENTION:

_____

_____

_____

POSITIVE OUTCOME(S):

_____

_____

_____

AFFIRMATION:

_____

_____

_____

GRATITUDE:

_____

_____

_____

_____

ACTION STEP:

Turn to page 272 in Part II and follow the instructions to start releasing any anger that may be unnecessarily residing inside you.

"When I let go of what I am, I become what I might be."
~ Lao Tzu

WEEK 10 / DAY 2- DATE: _____

HEALTH TIP:

Vitamin D is known as the sunshine vitamin, and when it comes from the sun, it really does do us a lot of good. Oral Vitamin D however is not quite as shiny, despite all the claims made in the media and by doctors who extol its supposed benefits. For some people, supplementing Vitamin D can provide benefits, but certainly NOT for everyone! In fact, I would suggest for most people it's downright dangerous. Those promoting Vitamin D have simply not studied deep enough it's effects on the mineral system, nor do they understand that taking more Vitamin D is not the best way to actually raise your Vitamin D level. Understand what most don't and become Vitamin D 'smart' by reading this very important article starting on page 367. It should make you think twice before popping more of those little pills.

ACTION STEP:

Saying "I can handle it ALL BY MYSELF" is not only childish, but makes life a lot harder than it need be. If you need help, in any area, ASK FOR IT. Those who care about you are looking for ways in which they can help you. Step out of your comfort zone and ask someone today for help. In the box below record the names of people who you could approach for help. Beyond those immediately around you, you might also try including people in your life that might struggle with isolation (i.e. senior citizens, children, at-home moms, work-from-home friends). They want to help, be recognized, and be part of the community more than you know.

TODAY'S INTENTION:

_____

_____

POSITIVE OUTCOME(S):

_____

_____

AFFIRMATION:

_____

_____

_____

GRATITUDE:

_____

_____

_____

_____

"To the world you may be one person, but to one person you may be the world."
~Unknown.

154

WEEK 10 / DAY 3- DATE: _____

HEALTH TIP:

Today we look at one of the most important minerals in the body, yet it is a mineral that approximately 80% of the population is deficient in. The mineral is magnesium.

Magnesium is responsible for over 300 enzymatic processes in the body, It controls our ability to handle stress. We need it for the health of our bones and making calcium bioavailable, we need it to regulate blood pressure, to maintain the health of our liver and adrenals, for muscular strength, to properly assimilate Vitamin D, to prevent cancer, to enhance circulation, to create energy, to prevent calcification of organs and tissues, to give life to every single human cell. Most doctors don't test for it, and if they do, they'll typically use a blood test. Consider the irony therein since less than 1% of the body's magnesium supply is in the blood! Magnesium deficiency therefore goes widely unnoticed, and in many cases the symptoms of magnesium deficiency end up being treated with harmful drugs instead of a simple supplement.

TODAY'S INTENTION:

_____

_____

_____

POSITIVE OUTCOME(S):

_____

_____

AFFIRMATION:

_____

_____

_____

GRATITUDE:

_____

_____

_____

_____

"Magnesium is the most critical mineral required for electrical stability of every cell in the body. A magnesium deficiency may be responsible for more diseases than any other nutrient." ~ Dr. Norman Shealy

Signs of magnesium deficiency are numerous, and may include any of the following: leg cramps, muscle twitches and tightness, reduction in appetite, fatigue, weakness, tension headaches, eye twitches, tightness in chest (sensation of being unable to take a deep inhalation, or sighing a lot), mitral valve prolapse, constipation, kidney stones,

menstrual cramps, back pain, insulin resistance, high blood pressure, insomnia, headaches and migraines, angina, heart arrhythmias, numbness, constipation, and seizures. Beyond the physical, magnesium deficiency also affects the brain, leading to additional symptoms such as: clouded thinking, disorientation, depression, hallucinations, anxiety, irritability, panic attacks, agoraphobia, personality changes. Magnesium deficiency can also exacerbate osteoporosis (recall week 4), and plays a major role in diabetes and most if not all cardiovascular problems. Deficiency takes a toll on the adrenals as well, keeping the person in a constant state of fight or flight - all the while wearing down the adrenals.

"Magnesium deficiency appears to have caused 8 million sudden coronary deaths in America during the period 1940-1994"
~Paul Mason (magnesium researcher)

When one comes to understand the inter-relationship of minerals and how minerals affect both physical and psychological outcomes, we can better understand the role magnesium deficiency might play in conditions such as ADD, or in behavioral abnormalities. Let's look at an example. Many of our current lifestyle factors (as I'll discuss in the paragraph below) deplete magnesium, stress being one of the biggest factors. As magnesium drops, the calcium to magnesium ratio rises, and this leads various forms of addictive behavior (ranging from alcoholism to sugar cravings, even to sexual addictions). As magnesium (the calming mineral) drops, sodium (the stress mineral) rises. This rise in sodium creates a high sodium to potassium ratio (known as the stress ratio), and this in turn increases feelings of anger, fear, anxiety, depression. This high Na/K ratio further increases the loss of magnesium, and a vicious cycle is created. When stress becomes too intense, the person subconsciously feels a need to numb their emotions, and once again this is played out through addictive behavior. Magnesium deficiency supports denial, interferes with memory and concentration, and even increases the risk of violence.

So, why is magnesium deficiency so prevalent? In large part it's because naturally occurring magnesium has been removed from our drinking water (through treatment) and diet (food processing and soil nutrient depletion). But there are many more reasons too. Other factors include not eating enough greens (which are high in magnesium), copper retention/toxicity and stress in the body (which depletes magnesium), overconsumption of Vitamin D supplementation, consumption of coffee, alcohol, sugar, high phytic acid foods, glyphosate on our crops, prescription medications, diuretics, birth control pills, and stress...ALL of which deplete magnesium!!

For this reason, most people can benefit from magnesium supplementation. Ideally the best source is through diet (greens and nuts). Drinking magnesium bicarbonate water or doing transdermal magnesium therapy (magnesium oil, Epsom salt baths) are also effective

and provide higher absorption too. Be careful not to over-supplement though or take it 'blindly', as taking too much magnesium can cause problems by depleting antagonistic minerals. This is again why first having a HTMA test done is so important.

"There is a power and a force in magnesium that cannot be equaled anywhere else in the world of medicine. There is no substitute for magnesium in human physiology; nothing comes even close to it in terms of its effect on overall cell physiology. Without sufficient magnesium, the body accumulates toxins and acid residues, degenerates rapidly, and ages prematurely. It goes against a gale wind of medical science to ignore magnesium chloride used transdermally in the treatment of any chronic or acute disorder, especially cancer."

~ Sircus, M. "A Magnesium Deficiency Increases Cancer Risk Significantly." April, 2008

ACTION STEP:

Take a look at your diet, lifestyle, and symptoms and see if magnesium deficiency could be playing a role in your condition. Ultimately, testing one's magnesium level should be of prime importance. Unfortunately, as with other minerals, most doctors use serum blood testing which offer extremely misleading results and will most often come back showing 'normal', not showing magnesium deficiency until it's far too late.

"A serum test for magnesium is actually worse than ineffective, because a test result that is within normal limits lends a false sense of security about the status of the mineral in the body. It also explains why doctors don't recognize magnesium deficiency; they assume serum magnesium levels are an accurate measure of all the magnesium in the body."
Dr. Carolyn Dean

If you want to test your magnesium, a magnesium RBC (red blood cell) test may be somewhat more accurate, yet it too is lacking since it tests the red blood cells, and these cells don't have mitochondria which is where most magnesium should be. A properly interpreted HTMA (as you learned about in week 2) can paint a much better picture of magnesium status, including the rate of depletion and extent of deficiency. If you haven't already, read through the special article in Part V on HTMA which will offer you more insight into this area.

"Nutrients work synergistically and antogonistically in a complex dynamic system." ~ Roger Williams, PhD

HEALTH TIP:

Do you suffer from headaches or migraines? Since there are so many causes of headaches (stress, tension, allergies, coffee, eyestrain, hunger, sinus pressure, muscle tension, TMJ, alcohol, hormonal imbalance, weather, trauma, irritants...the list goes on), they are about as tricky to cure as the common cold. Below are a number of drug-free alternatives you can try the next time you feel one coming on (or as a preventative before they even start!).

➢ **Magnesium:** Magnesium is a big one as magnesium deficiency can cause headaches (and stress leaches magnesium). In addition to transdermal magnesium, some great natural sources include spinach, Swiss Chard, sweet potatoes, bananas, sesame seeds, and brown rice.

➢ **Vitamin B2:** Also known as riboflavin, this deficiency can also cause headaches.

➢ **Butterbur:** four months of supplementing with Butterbur has been shown to reduce migraine frequency by at least 50 percent in 2/3 of patients;

➢ **L-Tyrone and/or Guarana:** can help relieve cluster headaches

➢ **Kava kava:** can help relieve tension headaches

➢ **Make a salve** of ginger, peppermint oil and wintergreen oil. Rub on the neck and temples for tension headaches, or across the sinus area for sinus headaches.

TODAY'S INTENTION:

_____

_____

_____

POSITIVE OUTCOME(S):

_____

_____

_____

AFFIRMATION:

_____

_____

_____

GRATITUDE:

_____

_____

_____

_____

- ➤ **Lemon salt water:** Add the juice from half a lemon and a heaping teaspoon of Himalayan salt to a glass of water and drink. It may help in some cases.
- ➤ **Food sensitivities:** Gluten and eggs are two foods that a lot of people are sensitive to and that can cause headaches.
- ➤ **Dehydration:** hydrating your body can often help alleviate headaches (if you are dehydrated drink 1L of water for every 50lbs of body weight).
- ➤ **Ice Packs:** Place an ice pack on the back of the neck at the base of the skull. When using an ice pack there should be a barrier between the ice pack and the skin such as a wetted cloth or t-shirt that has had the water squeezed out of it. Ice therapy can lessen the flow of blood to the head resulting in less pressure in the head. It can often help relieve the throbbing pain of a migraine headache by decreasing the flow of blood to the head. It is often beneficial for a person to put their feet in a container of warm water at the same time. This can have the effect of attracting the blood to the feet instead of to the head.
- ➤ **Massage** – Apply gentle pressure to your scalp or temples, as well as alleviate muscle tension with a shoulder or neck massage.
- ➤ **Heat or a Hot Shower** – the heat can help relax tense muscles
- ➤ **Deep breathing** – here you can try lavender or peppermint oil as a topical solution or inhaler. These oils can be put in a vaporizer or on a washcloth.
- ➤ **Acupuncture** – helps calm the temporal artery and the sympathetic nerve system. Regular treatments over 3 to 4 months can help reduce the frequency.
- ➤ **Caffeine** – although I normally do not recommend caffeine in terms of being healthy for the body, it can however be used in the early stages of a migraine to enhance the pain-reducing effects of acetaminophen (Tylenol, others) and aspirin.
- ➤ **Proper Sleep** – Keep a regular sleep schedule. More than half of migraine episodes occur during sleep, and too much or too little sleep can trigger a migraine.
- ➤ **Regular Meals** – missed meals can cause fluctuations in blood sugar which can lead to migraines.

ACTION STEP:

Become aware today of how much hydrogenated soy bean oil you're consuming, and understand how dangerous it is. Sadly, hydrogenated soybean oil is in much of the processed food we eat (it's the highest source of fat in the human diet today according to food writer Nina Planck). According to Dr. Andrew Weil, it, together with high fructose corn syrup, are the two most dangerous government subsidized foods,

and are the major source of excess Omega 6 (which is one of the causes behind almost all inflammatory diseases).

In week 8 we looked at trans fats, and removing food with the Trans Fat label from your kitchen. The problem is that not all trans-fat containing foods need to be labeled as such. If an ingredient list contains partially hydrogenated soybean oil (about 70% of soybean oil we consume is partially hydrogenated), you can be sure there are at least trace amounts of trans fats. These trans fats interfere with the body's ability to fight cancer, interfere with insulin receptiveness, decrease immune function, and even affect the production of sex hormones.

The other problem with hydrogenated soybean oil is the soybean itself - most of which today in America are genetically modified to begin with!

Now, even though I'm ripping into soybean oil here (it is one of the worst), it's not the only unhealthy polyunsaturated fat oil that you should be avoiding. Some other processed vegetable oils that are high in inflammatory Omega 6 and through processing are degraded and likely rancid include canola oil, corn oil, cottonseed oil, sunflower oil, safflower oil, and grape seed oil.

What can you do? Choose healthier alternatives. Coconut oil is a great option. If you want to stick with soybean oil, at the very least make sure it's not hydrogenated (or partially hydrogenated - the worse of the two), and that's it's from a naturally grown and organic source.

"With the growing body of evidence linking environmental exposures to cancer, the public is becoming increasingly aware of the unacceptable burden of cancer resulting from environmental and occupational exposures that could have been prevented through appropriate national action."
~ President's Cancer Panel 2008-2009 National Report presented by the U.S. Department of Health and Human Services, National Institutes of Health and National Cancer Institute

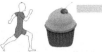

HEALTH TIP:

You're seeing a cupcake beside our running man icon above because today's tip also includes reducing a certain food: protein. What!? Protein is absolutely essential for growth and development. While athletes and body builders certainly need more protein than the average person (to build muscle), those with high protein diets are at risk of hyperacidity. (In fact, most Americans eat too much protein!) When the body is hyperacidic, the blood, lymph fluids and interstitial fluids thicken. This leads to a slowing of the immune response, sluggish cell metabolism, the collection of toxins, leaching of calcium and minerals from bones, aging, and many degenerative diseases. Long term hyperacidity from excess protein and sugar leads to high blood pressure, arterial sclerosis, osteoarthritis, osteoporosis, insomnia, disc problems in the back, various cancers, and intestinal problems. Too much protein without drinking enough water stresses the kidneys and can lead to urinary tract infections and kidney stones. When protein builds up in the body it produces free radicals and opens the door to disease – obesity, hypertension, coronary heart disease and the ones previously mentioned. So, while protein is good (and important), just be mindful not to have too much. For the average person, 50 - 60grams per day is

TODAY'S INTENTION:

_____

_____

_____

POSITIVE OUTCOME(S):

_____

_____

_____

AFFIRMATION:

_____

_____

_____

GRATITUDE:

_____

_____

_____

_____

ideal, with an allowance of 25% more for athletes and pregnant women. (For reference, an egg (the best source of protein) has about 6 grams, a skinless chicken breast about 45 grams).

ACTION STEP:

First, take a look at your protein consumption, and cut down if necessary. Secondly, you've probably heard that eating right before bed isn't good for you. Well, it really depends on WHAT you eat. Your metabolism slows at night, and so a stuffed gut is harder to digest and can also interfere with sleep. Small quickly-digested snacks, such as fruit or crackers, can be eaten close to bedtime; whereas a heavy, fatty dinner, like cheeseburgers and fries (which, well, you shouldn't be eating anyway if you've come this far, but if you were) should be eaten at least three hours earlier. So tonight, and going forward, remember to have dinner at least 3 hours before bedtime, and only light snacking after.

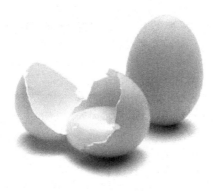

"Problems remain as problems because people are busy defending them rather than finding solutions. Stop wasting time defending your problems and work on addressing them instead."
- Celestine Chua

HEALTH TIP:

Try this recipe the next time you want to relieve a cough. Into a cup of boiled (hot) water steep the following for 3 minutes:

> ➢ Green tea bag
> ➢ ½ tsp cloves
> ➢ 3 –4 corns black pepper
> ➢ ½ tsp turmeric
> ➢ ½ tsp thyme
> ➢ 4 -5 basil leaves (optional)

Then straight out the ingredients (except the green tea bag) and add the juice of half a lemon and 2 tsp of Manuka honey.

Have a sore throat? Chop a ¼ garlic clove, let it sit for 10 minutes, then place it between your teeth for another 5 minutes. Not brave enough for that? Try this gargle solution. 6 drops oil of oregano, 1 dropper Echinacea tincture, 1 dropper Goldenseal, and a couple drops of bee propolis tincture – all mixed into about 2 tbsp of water. Sip, gargle, swallow, repeat every few hours. Whether you choose gargling or garlic, either way you'll be sending those throat germs packing!

ACTION STEP:

Spending time in nature has a number of health benefits. Some of these benefits include an increase in anti-cancer protein expression and natural killer cells to fight off infection and cancer growth, as well as decreased depression, anxiety, anger, confusion, and tension. It can help increase energy while helping reduce stress. Being in nature also helps us become centered, and fills our lungs with good, clean, oxygen.

Set a goal to spend time in nature today, reconnecting with Mother Earth, and the energy of the Universe from where we all came. Head to a local forest trail or park. Even if you have to drive a few miles to find a little green, it's worth it! Spend at least 10 minutes taking deep breaths of fresh air. Oxygenate yourself. Your body will thank you.

"Keep your face to the sunshine and you will not see the shadows."~Helen Keller

TODAY'S INTENTION:

_____
_____
_____

POSITIVE OUTCOME(S):

_____
_____
_____

AFFIRMATION:

_____
_____
_____

GRATITUDE:

_____
_____
_____
_____

THIS WEEK'S REVIEW:

Today is your chance to go over the action steps of this past week, reincorporate any activities you may have forgotten, and complete any activities yet unfinished. Use today to catch up and take stock.

Check off the items you've completed below:

☐ I've completed the Anger Journaling exercise.

☐ I've reached out to someone this week and have asked them for help (knowing my doing so helps them as well).

☐ I have taken a step to investigate my true magnesium level

☐ I've eliminated hydrogenated soy bean oil from my diet.

☐ I've spent time this week in nature, connecting with Universal energy, and practicing deep breathing.

☐ I completed all my daily journaling exercises, including today's which are on the pages that follow.

Of all the tips I've learned so far in this book, 12 action steps for my health that I fully **commit** to doing consistently from now on (the most important tips I'm taking forward with me) are:

1. _____

2. _____

3. _____

4. _____

5. _____

6. _____

7. _____

8. _____

9. _____

10. _____

11. _____

12. _____

NOTES: Other Important Things I'd Like to Do or Remember:

HEALTH TIP:

Silence... is a source of great strength and is an opportunity for self-reflection... and self-discovery.

ACTION STEP:

Spend at least 10 minutes today in complete silence. Turn off your phone and anything else that may disturb you. Sssshhhhhhh......quiet your environment... quiet your thoughts... sit in silence... just listen... listen not to the voice in your head which will eventually go away when you ignore it... but to the silence...and to your greater purpose.

TODAY'S INTENTION:

_____

_____

POSITIVE OUTCOME(S):

_____

_____

AFFIRMATION:

_____

_____

GRATITUDE:

_____

_____

_____

_____

"When the mind is still, tranquil, not seeking any answer or solution even, neither resisting nor avoiding, it is only then that there can be a regeneration. Because then the mind is capable of perceiving what is true and it is the truth that liberates, not your effort to be free."
~ Krishnamurti

HEALTH TIP:

While this is another controversial topic to some, today's news flash is that dairy is not good for you. In fact, adult humans were never meant to consume dairy (and we are the only adult mammal that does). For a hundred thousand generations dairy was never on the menu, and yet early man was lean, fit, and strong. You've been led to believe, through years of misleading advertising perpetuated by the dairy industry, that cow's milk is healthy when, in fact, it's probably hurting you, and your immune system, and is a hidden food allergy for large numbers of people. Dairy (including milk, cheese and ice cream) is a major contributor to allergies, and can even increase the risk of certain cancers. It can lead to congestion, inflammation, belly pain, bloating, gas, diarrhea, and a weaker immune system. The heating process of pasteurization also destroys 3 important enzymes that raw milk contains: lactase, lipase, and phosphatase. Lactase is needed to digest milk sugar (a.k.a. lactose). Lipase is needed to digest fats. Phosphatase is needed to absorb calcium which allows for lactose digestion. The lack of these enzymes in regular pasteurized milk is the reason why many people can't drink milk, or are milk intolerant. There is also an enzyme in cow's milk called 'xanthine oxidase' that, through the process of homogenization, comes unbound from the fat and can lead to cardiovascular disease in humans.

TODAY'S INTENTION:

_____

_____

_____

POSITIVE OUTCOME(S):

_____

_____

_____

AFFIRMATION:

_____

_____

_____

GRATITUDE:

_____

_____

_____

_____

Dairy (especially cheese) is also the most acid forming of all foods (and as you've already learned, for health we want to be increasing the alkalinity of our body, not the acidity). According to author, farmer and activist Howard Lyman, dairy is the number one thing to take out of the diet for optimal health – this coming from a fourth generation dairy farmer!!

"But, I need to drink milk to have healthy bones!" you say? No, that's just the message the media has fed us to believe. Dairy in fact can actually be bad for your bones. Cow milk has a substantially higher phosphorus to calcium ratio than human milk, and phosphorus inhibits calcium absorption. Not only that, but as you may recall from week 2, calcium can only be properly absorbed in bone with adequate magnesium, and the calcium to magnesium ratio of dairy has far too much calcium and far too little magnesium. As bad as the Ca/Mg ratio, it's actually become worse too over this past century. A 50 year study between 1940-1991 shows that while the calcium content of milk dropped around 4%, the magnesium content of milk dropped about 20%. In other words, it's less healthy for you today than it was for your grandparents. To get the calcium your bones need, there are much better sources – such as salmon, sardines, dark green leafy vegetables, sesame seeds, tofu, or fortified soy or rice milk. Almond milk and hemp milk are other tasty and healthy options. And remember...you need the balance with magnesium!

ACTION STEP:

You may have already eliminated dairy these past few weeks as part of your liver cleanse. For the remainder of this week, try to continue with that elimination (or reduction) of dairy. Opt for healthier alternatives (such as the calcium sources previously mentioned or, if you absolutely must have milk, then goat and sheep milk are better in terms of digestibility). You might be pleasantly surprised at the number of natural alternatives available in the stores, how your body feels, and that after a week or so, you might not even miss your 'regular' dairy.

"Every day do something that will inch you closer to a better tomorrow."
~ Doug Firebaugh

WEEK 11 / DAY 3- DATE: _____

HEALTH TIP:

In 1939, Duke University developed what was known as the Rice Diet Program. Known as a low sodium, good carb, detox diet, the Rice Diet has now for decades successfully treated high blood pressure and heart conditions, as well as weight and kidney problems. The diet's high fiber focus helps combat high blood cholesterol and reduces the risk of heart disease. The lower caloric intake of the program combined with moderate exercise makes the Rice Diet a proven short term weight loss solution.

ACTION STEP:

In week 4 I mentioned how collagen helps make bones flexible and lowers the risk of fracture. Well, collagen also has a number of other important benefits, a few of which include:

- ✓ Reduces cellulite
- ✓ Speeds up wound healing and skin regeneration
- ✓ Improves bone density
- ✓ Reduces gum recession
- ✓ Boosts joint health and reduces joint pain
- ✓ Reduces skin wrinkles
- ✓ Helps strengthen the intestinal gut lining (great for helping those with leaky gut or food sensitivities)

TODAY'S INTENTION:

_____

_____

_____

POSITIVE OUTCOME(S):

_____

_____

_____

AFFIRMATION:

_____

_____

_____

GRATITUDE:

_____

_____

_____

_____

If either this information on collagen or the aforementioned Rice Diet appear to offer help in your situation, spend some time today looking further into these options, either online, talking with your doctor, or visiting a health store and speaking with someone about collagen supplements.

"Embrace each challenge in your life as an opportunity for selftransformation."
~ Bernie S. Siegel

HEALTH TIP:

The proper vitamin and mineral supplementation is especially important for people with HIV. Low levels of vitamins A, B6, B12, and E along with the minerals zinc and selenium have all been linked to the progression of HIV to AIDS. Taking high potency formulations of these can help slow progression. Also of importance are Alpha-lipoic acid, glutamine, L-histidine, L-lysine, probiotics, and omega-3 fatty acids. The mushrooms maitake, resihi, and shiitake can enhance the activity of T-helper cells in people with AIDS, and in laboratory have been shown to kill HIV. One challenge is that symptoms of HIV might not even appear until 2 – 5 years after infection. During this time the immune system is becoming weakened, and the greater the degree of immune suppression, the greater the risk of contracting AIDS. Nutrient supplementation is very important as malabsorption is common with the disease. Even for the rest of us, the proper vitamin and mineral supplementation will help boost our immune systems.

TODAY'S INTENTION:

_____

_____

_____

POSITIVE OUTCOME(S):

_____

_____

_____

AFFIRMATION:

_____

_____

_____

GRATITUDE:

_____

_____

_____

_____

ACTION STEP:

People often forget the things someone else does, but people rarely forget how someone made them feel. Go ahead and make someone else feel great today! (You'll feel better in the process!)

"You never lose by loving. You always lose by holding back."

~ Barbara de Angelis

WEEK 11 / DAY 5- DATE: _____

HEALTH TIP:

Relationships can be empowering and healthy, or draining and toxic. If you're trying to get better and live healthy, yet people around you are negative, disbelieving, perhaps jealous, or even just not being helpful or supportive. you may need to move those relationships out of your life and make room for new, healthier ones. It's those healthy relationships that will inspire you, give you ideas and the confidence to keep going, and make life fun.

ACTION STEP:

Below, write down the names of any people you feel are toxic or negative. You may want to think twice about keeping those people in your life. Is their energy empowering or draining? Are they helping you move forward, or are they holding you back?

TODAY'S INTENTION:

_____

_____

_____

POSITIVE OUTCOME(S):

_____

_____

_____

AFFIRMATION:

_____

_____

_____

GRATITUDE:

_____

_____

_____

_____

"Keep away from people who try to belittle your ambitions. Small people always do that, but the really great make you feel that you, too, are great."
~Mark Twain

HEALTH TIP:

Brushing your teeth is more important than you might think. For most people, it's about being more attractive and reducing the risk of cavities. While this is important, good oral hygiene also has a direct link to your overall health. If you let food particles sit in your mouth, you are going to be building up bacteria. Usually, that bacteria is not at a harmful level. Without good oral health, however, things change. Bacteria continues to grow, and when bad bacteria build up in the mouth, they can easily travel to other parts of your body, leading to all sorts of infections and other diseases. Root canal treated teeth are especially susceptible to bacterial breeding, and these bacteria in turn produce toxins which systemically affect the body. Cavitations (common with root canals and pulled wisdom teeth, and not to be confused with 'cavities') can be breeding grounds for bacteria, even if one doesn't feel any pain in the area. A 'Cone Beam CT Scan' is far more effective than a standard xray at detecting cavitations.

TODAY'S INTENTION:

_____

_____

_____

POSITIVE OUTCOME(S):

_____

_____

_____

AFFIRMATION:

_____

_____

_____

GRATITUDE:

_____

_____

_____

_____

If you happen to have "silver" fillings, which about 75% of adults do, your risks of related health issues increase largely. There is approximately 400mg of mercury in a typical silver filling, which is several thousand times the amount found in contaminated seafood!! Your fillings are constantly releasing mercury vapor which makes its way into the bloodstream and causes oxidative problems in the tissues, especially impacting the nervous system. Mercury is an immune suppressant, and it the 2nd most toxic element on the planet...yet we put it into our mouths?! Heavy metal toxicity (as we've already looked at earlier in this book) is a major cause of a vast number of undiagnosed health

conditions. If you have a mercury filling, it's advisable to have it removed, however, it must be done cautiously. Not having it removed by a dentist properly trained in the removal of a mercury / amalgam filling can result in the release of significantly dangerous levels of mercury vapor into the body. Removal should ideally be done by a SMART (safe mercury amalgam removal technique) certified dentist following IAOMT (IAOMT.com) protocol).

If you have a systemic health issue where no other cause has been determined, it might be helpful to further investigate your oral health. When dead teeth are removed and the surrounding tissues cleaned of toxins, various elusive health concerns often seem to clear up.

Whether or not you have fillings, good oral hygiene is important. Your regimen should include:
✔ brushing after each meal, or at minimum twice a day.
✔ flossing
✔ eating a healthy, low sugar diet
✔ replacing your toothbrush as soon as the bristles become frayed, or after 3 or 4 months.
✔ having regular dental checkups at least once a year.

ACTION STEP:
Eight weeks ago you were introduced to the Personal Wellness Score. Have you used it yet? This tool that will accurately show exactly what changes you can make in your life that will have the biggest impact.

The Personal Wellness Score looks at the 12 areas of your life, which include: Healthy Habits, Spirituality, Romance/Love, Physical Environment, Personal Growth, Diet, Exercise/Fitness, Fun/Play, Friends/Social, Financial, Family, and Career/Work. They are all interconnected. To truly take your health to the next level, the other areas of your life also need to be 'healthy'. If you haven't yet, I encourage you to use this tool to bring greater balance into your overall life. Turn to page 226 to learn more.

"I wish I could show you, when you are lonely or in darkness,
the astonishing light of your own being."
~ Hafiz

THIS WEEK'S REVIEW:

Today is your chance to go over the action steps of this past week, reincorporate any activities you may have forgotten, and complete any activities yet unfinished. Use today to catch up and take stock.

Check off the items you've completed below:

☐ I've spent at least 10 minutes this week in complete silence, quieting my inner voice, and going within.

☐ I've reduced the amount of dairy I consume.

☐ I've looked further into how either collagen supplementation or the Rice Diet can benefit me.

☐ I have, or am going to, eliminate unsupportive toxic people and relationships from my life.

☐ I made someone else feel great this week. If I haven't yet, then for sure I will make someone feel great today! This world is about helping people, and making a difference in someone else's life.

☐ I am using the Personal Wellness Score to bring greater balance into my life.

☐ I completed all my daily journaling exercises, including today's which are on the pages that follow.

Of all the tips I've learned so far in this book, 13 action steps for my health that I fully **commit** to doing consistently from now on (the most important tips I'm taking forward with me) are:

1. _____

2. _____

3. _____

4. _____

5. _____

6. _____

7. _____

8. _____

9. _____

10. _____

11. _____

12. _____

13. _____

NOTES: Other Important Things I'd Like to Do or Remember:

HEALTH TIP:

As we begin the last week of this program, it's time to start planning where you'll be heading in the weeks, months, and years ahead. One of the ways to begin manifesting your vision of the future is to create a vision board. A vision board is a collage or images and words that represent the things you want in life. When you put these down on paper and place it somewhere where'll you constantly see it, it will keep you focused on where you're headed.

For some people vision boards work, and for others they don't. This brings up the question of 'why'. It's one thing to make a vision board and really want those 'things and experiences' in your future. It's another to believe you are deserving of it. The key to making your vision board come true therefore is to ensure your thoughts and belief systems are in alignment with what you create on the board. If there's a part of you that feels you're undeserving, not capable, etc, then you will be

TODAY'S INTENTION:

_____

_____

_____

POSITIVE OUTCOME(S):

_____

_____

_____

AFFIRMATION:

_____

_____

_____

GRATITUDE:

_____

_____

_____

_____

sabotaging your success. If this is the case, then go back and review the mindset exercises in weeks 2,3,4 and 8.

ACTION STEP:

Today you'll begin creating a vision board. It likely won't be (and shouldn't be) a one day process. Simply begin today, and over the next week or two, work toward completing it. You can use the list of dreams you created in week 9 as a foundation. Turn to page 278 for full instructions and to begin.

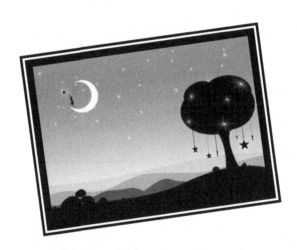

"First say to yourself what you would be; and then do what you have to do."
~ Epictetus

HEALTH TIP:

Rather than eliminating another food (I think I've already made you take enough things out of your diet for a while!), today's tip offers a few natural items that might not be on your radar to keep in your emergency kit for healing bruises, trauma and muscle soreness.

➢ **Arnica** (homeopathic pellets or spray): a premier remedy for trauma (falls, fractures, sprains, strains...) causing soreness, bruising, bleeding, as well as head injuries and concussions.

➢ **Aconite 30**: this is a homeopathic remedy great for sudden states of physical or emotional traumatic shock.

➢ **Calendula Tincture**: an important medical herb that reduces inflammation and promotes the healing of tissues while controlling bleeding and soothing pain.

➢ **Dit Da Jow:** A blend of Chinese herbs that helps treat impact injuries and is medically proven to increase circulation, disperse fluids, and speed healing

TODAY'S INTENTION:

_____

_____

_____

POSITIVE OUTCOME(S):

_____

_____

_____

AFFIRMATION:

_____

_____

GRATITUDE:

_____

_____

_____

_____

- ➢ **Magnesium**: helps with muscle pain and spasms by helping to relax the muscle. Transdermal magnesium chloride, in fact, offers an almost immediate effect on chronic and acute pain.
- ➢ **Hylands Cell Salts #8**: highly effective for the often quick relief of all kinds of cramps (leg, menstrual, abdominal...)
- ➢ **Traumeel Ointment**: a premade homeopathic ointment (containing arnica and aconite) to help reduce pain, inflammation and bruising in closed-wound injuries.
- ➢ **Zheng Gu Shui**: another Chinese herbal liniment great for broken bones, bruises, sprains and strains – it helps speed up healing time and reduces pain.

ACTION STEP:

Yesterday you began working on your vision board. Today you are going to write a personal vision statement for your life, to guide you towards the life you want, and give you strength to weather any storms along the way. Turn to page 280 in Part II to begin.

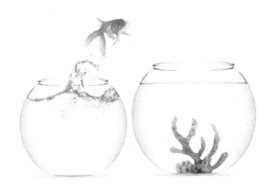

"Herbal medicine is older than human civilization – animals as diverse as primates, deer, rhinoceros, and wolves deliberately consume plants to deal with bacteria, viruses, parasites, or worms."
~(Engel.Veterinary Herbal Medicine.2007: 7-15).

WEEK 12 / DAY 3- DATE: _____

HEALTH TIP:

A few weeks ago you began incorporating some superfoods you're your diet. Today we'll get familiar with a few more to add to your healthy kitchen arsenal.

Sprouts are a super nutritious food that can easily be added to most any meal, salad, or even smoothie. They are a rich source of protein, anti-oxidants, and other vitamins. Research is finding that broccoli sprouts in particular offer many disease preventing benefits. A chemical compound called suforaphane shows promise in stopping the growth of malignant tumors, helping to treat or even prevent several cancers including prostate and breast. Interestingly, broccoli sprouts have 10 to 20 times as much suforaphane as does whole broccoli. Sprouts can also help with the prevention of ulcers, treatment of asthma, reducing blood cholesterol levels, and detoxifying blood.

Young Coconuts: have one of the highest sources of electrolytes found in nature. Coconut water, molecularly, is identical to human blood plasma – which means a cup (or coconut) full of coconut water is like an instant blood transfusion! It's great to add to smoothies, and much healthier than artificial sports drinks.

Raw Cacao: must be certified raw organic to offer the health benefits I'm talking about here (ie: this is NOT the cacao powder you buy in the store for hot chocolates nor is it that sugar laden chocolate bar!). It's high in both magnesium and iron, and is one of the world's most

TODAY'S INTENTION:

_____

_____

POSITIVE OUTCOME(S):

_____

_____

AFFIRMATION:

_____

_____

GRATITUDE:

_____

_____

_____

_____

antioxidant rich foods (14 times more flavonoids (antioxidants) than red wine and 21 times that of green tea).

Bee Pollen: is one of the most complete foods found in nature. It's an excellent source of protein (offering 5 to 7 times more protein than beef). Bee pollen has shown to be effective for fighting hayfever and sinusitis, countering the effects of aging, and helpful for recovering from illness.

Aloe Vera: contains numerous healing compounds (including natural steroids, antibiotic agents, amino acids, minerals and enzyme). It's excellent on skin irritations and injuries (nurns, cuts, eczema, etc). Aloe vera juiice is also beneficial for the digestive tract and can help reduce heartburn and ulcers.

Algae (including Spirulina, Chlorella, and AFA): Algae is a complete protein, high in beneficial chlorophyll, and great for detoxing and alkalizing the body.

Pasture-raised Beef Liver: While all the previous superfoods can easily be added to a healthy and tasty smoothie, this one you might want to leave out. But not out of your diet! Liver is fact is one of the most nutrient dense foods on the planet! Liver provides nature's most concentrated source of Vitamin A (retinol), abundant iron, high levels of copper, folic acid, purines, amino acids, phosphorus, Vitamin C, and Vitamin B12. While modern Western society has adopted a taste preference for muscle meats, organ meats such as liver provide a nutrient content 10 to 100 times higher!

ACTION STEP:

The next time you're at the store, pick up as many of these superfoods as you can and add them into your meals, salads, and smoothies whenever possible.

"The body is a self healing organism, but it needs the right fuel."
~Jessica Ess Marcus

WEEK 12 / DAY 4- DATE: _____

HEALTH TIP:

Alright, so today's topic is a big one, and one that everyone wants to have answers to. Today we take a look at remedies for those nasty colds and flus!

First, let's distinguish between cold and flu symptoms. The most common symptoms of a cold are runny stuffy nose, sneezing, and sore throat. The most common symptoms of flu are fever, headache and pain, tiredness, runny stuffy nose, sore throat, and chest discomfort. Colds typically last 7-9 days, although they can sometimes last up to 3 weeks. Flus tend to be shorter in duration, typically lasting 4 – 7 days.

So, you have a fever. Should you see a doctor? Not necessarily. A fever is your body's way of killing off the infection. Viruses have a harder time reproducing at higher body temperatures, and so a slightly raised body temperature is actually good in terms of your body acting effectively. This is why you want to avoid fever-reducing medications as, while they can provide short term relief, they can prolong your body's ability to fight off the infection. The time to see a doctor is when you have any of the following symptoms:

- fever above 102 degrees Fahrenheit
- greenish nasal discharge with possible pain around the eyes
- ear pain
- shortness of breath

TODAY'S INTENTION:

_____

_____

_____

POSITIVE OUTCOME(S):

_____

_____

_____

AFFIRMATION:

_____

_____

_____

GRATITUDE:

_____

_____

_____

_____

- uncontrollable cough
- coughing up green or yellow sputum persistently

Now let's look at a few things you can do to boost your immune system to fight off that nasty cold or flu!

➢ Avoid all sugars (this includes processed foods, artificial sweeteners, fruit juice, fructose, molasses, and grains (which break down as sugars). Sugars severely impair your immune system.

➢ Get lots of (extra) sleep and rest – that day or two of resting in bed that you think you can't afford may end up saving you a week of further sickness and even more time off work in the long run

➢ Diet: try to eat fermented foods such as miso, pickles or sauerkraut, coconuts or coconut oil, organic vegetables, and mushrooms (especially Reishi and Shiitake)

➢ Spice things up with garlic (remember the tip I gave back in the first week), turmeric, ginger, oregano, cinnamon, cloves, and cat's claw (unless pregnant in which case avoid).

➢ Drink lots (I repeat LOTS) of pure water – at least 8 to 10 glasses per day. This helps flush out the toxins.

➢ Supplement (as soon as symptoms first appear) with Vitamin C (up to 10,000mg per day for a couple of days (only) during the acute phase, although at these high levels it could cause bowel intolerance so ease in slowly and only take what your body can handle), Oregano Oil (contains carvacrol which is a strong antimicrobial agent), Bee Propolis (one of the most broad-spectrum antimicrobial compounds in the world as well as an immune booster), Andrographis, Goldenseal (hydrastis canadensis – a herb with strong antimicrobial properties), and Elderberry Syrup. Additionally, zinc (which is antimicrobial) and short term high dose Vitamin A (up to 5000IU) can be helpful. Vitamin D can also be helpful short term, but as it antagonizes (reduces) vitamin A, the two should be taken together to maintain a balance (such as through cod liver oil).

➢ Pocari Sweat, a Japanese sports drink available today in many countries (including Canada and the US), is an ion supply drink that helps effectively replenish water and electrolytes in the body that are lost through the perspiration that occurs during a fever.

➢ Try colloidal silver. With hundreds of studies there is today little doubt about silver's proven anti-bacterial properties – in fact it was commonly used as an anti-bacterial agent until the advent of antibiotics in the 1940s. For viruses however, evidence is growing that colloidal silver may also be effective. Studies have shown silver nanoparticles to inhibit the growth of HIV, small pox, SARS, hepatitis B, and many of the hundreds of flu-causing viruses. Available at

most health food stores, take a teaspoon under your tongue for 30 seconds, 4 – 6 times per day during the acute phase, or 1 – 2 times per day as a preventative.

➢ This natural antibiotic recipe should send those cold and flu germs packing. In a bowl with a half cup of lemon juice, mix a crushed garlic clove with 2 tbsp ginger powder, a pinch of chili powder, and a pinch of cinnamon. Store it in the fridge in a sealed container, and then take 1 tbsp daily (as a preventative) or several times a day (during an infection)

For your flu, you can also try some of these powerful formulas:

✓ Mix 1 oz of water with a dropper of goldenseal tincture, a dropper of bee propolis, and 5-8 drops of oil of oregano. Gargle with this mixture for 30 seconds and then swallow. Repeat this several times throughout the day to help kill any germs lurking in your throat.

✓ Brew a tea from elderflower, yarrow, boneset, linden, peppermint and ginger. Feel free to add echinacea root and schisandra berries to this tea if available. Drinking this tea hot will help you sweat, assisting your body to fight off the virus. Yes, I know making teas can be time consuming (not to mention shopping for all the ingredients). But if you're sick you've got time on your hands right? Joking aside, an advantage to drinking tea is that the liquid format thins congestion and helps flush out toxins. Try to drink several cups of tea throughout the day, followed up with a warm nap in bed – this keeps your body temperature high and slows down the virus.

✓ You can make another very powerful anti-flu drink using as many of these ingredients as you can find: boneset, cayenne, chamomile, echinacea, osha root, usnea lichen, ginger, and lomatium root.

✓ Load up on L-Lysine. L-Lysine is a natural amino acid that helps prevent the replication of flu viruses, regardless of strain. L-Lysine disrupts the virus's DNA replication cycle, thus putting the brakes on the next flu generation from being born, and subsequently, ending the flu. Taken with Vitamin C the efficacy of the L-Lysine is improved. In order for this treatment to be effective against the flu, your system needs to be flooded with L-Lysine right off the bat. Recommended dosage (always check with your medical professional first) is 4000mg for a first dose, then 2000mg every 3 hours (awake) while symptoms are present. Once symptoms are gone reduce the dosage to 2000mg twice a day for a week.

✓ Take a tablespoon of Vinegar of Four Thieves (remember that concoction you made back in week 9?) every few hours diluted in water.

What About the Flu Shot? A lot of people ask me about getting a flu vaccination as a preventative measure. After all, it's promoted almost

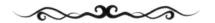

everywhere you look, almost to the point of instilling fear in the public that if one doesn't get it they'll be at risk of something horrible. In fact, some states are now enforcing a fear-based decision-making approach by making vaccinations mandatory, despite the fact that you can still get a horrible flu even after having receiving the vaccination, plus you're injecting a smorgasbord of known toxins into your body in the process. The decision to get a flu vaccination should be an individual one, based on choice and informed disclosure, especially when risk is shown. Aside from the shopping list of harmful ingredients found in vaccinations, you may want to consider these statements made by Dr. Michael T. Osterholm, et al, from the Center for Infectious Disease Research and Policy (2012) before running out to get your vaccine.

> *"We have over-promoted and overhyped this vaccine. It does not protect as promoted. It's all a sales job: it's all public relations."*

> *"The perception that current vaccines are already highly effective in preventing influenza is a major barrier to game-changing alternatives."*

If that isn't damning enough, here are the words of the former Chief Vaccine Control Officer at the FDA, Dr. J. Anthony Morris:

> *"There is no evidence that any influenza vaccine thus far developed is effective in preventing or mitigating any attack of influenza. The producers of these vaccines know that they are worthless, but they go on selling them, anyway."*

While we're at it, how about a few more quotes:

> **"Vaccines are highly dangerous, have never been adequately studied or proven to be effective, and have a poor risk/reward ratio."** – Dr. Allen Greenberg, MD

> **"There is no scientific evidence that vaccinations are of any benefit, but it is clear that they cause a great deal of harm."** – Dr. Gerhard Buchwald, MD

> **"The greatest lie ever told is that vaccines are safe and effective."** – Dr. Leonard G. Horowitz

So one then has to question, why do so many doctors still recommend the flu vaccine. The answer lays in education (and profits too of course), and is summed up nicely on the next page in a quote taken from the documentary film <u>The Greater Good</u> (www.greatergoodmovie.org) – a film definitely worth watching to understand in greater detail the dangers of vaccination. (The sites *www.learntherisk.org*, *www.nvic.org* and *www.vaccine-injury.info*

are three more great resources to educate yourself deeper regarding the benefits as well as substantial risks of vaccinations).

> *"They don't learn that no study exists comparing the medium or long term health outcomes of vaccinated to unvaccinated populations. They don't learn that vaccine safety studies don't use a true placebo, but instead use another vaccine or a solution containing mercury or aluminum as a placebo! They don't learn that vaccine safety studies often last a few days to a few weeks keeping hidden long term side effects. They don't learn that vaccines can overwhelm the immune system and cause autoimmune disease.*
>
> *They don't learn that the aluminum in vaccines is known to cause cognitive impairment, autoimmune disease, gut issues and a host of other damage to healthy adults – goodness knows what they do to tiny infants. They don't learn that the mercury in vaccines is documented in the medical literature as a potent neurotoxin and that it is still used in the manufacturing of some vaccines and as a preservative as well. They don't learn how the body processes the vaccine components because, well, no one has ever researched it."*

ACTION STEP:

People seek out coaches because they want to grow or become better. Perhaps they want to get healthier, be more fit, play a better game, grow their business, develop relationships or find more balance in their lives. Whatever the reason, having a coach is important for growing into the person you want to be. Even Tiger Woods has a coach for his golf game. Why? Not because the coach is better than Tiger at golf. Rather the coach can help Tiger see things that he himself can't. As Albert Einstein said, it takes a different kind of thinking to solve a problem than the kind of thinking which produced the problem. You've come a long way already and the guidance part of this program ends in a few days. Now it's time to take your life to the next level. Having a good coach (be it in life, health, business, relationships, etc) can help you get there. Today, consider working with a coach in one of those key areas of life – it could be the step that makes all the difference!

> *"The secret to success is not trying to avoid or get rid of or shrink your problems; the secret is to grow yourself so that you are bigger than any problem."* ~ T. Harv Eker

WEEK 12 / DAY 5- DATE: _____

HEALTH TIP:

If you're starting to get back into any form of an exercise routine, it's important to stretch beforehand in order to reduce the risk of injury. Some tips to keep in mind while stretching: never stretch cold muscles; ease into the stretch slowly and gently; never stretch to the point of unusual pain; don't bounce when you stretch; and hold each stretch for at least 30 – 45 seconds.

As your recovery improves you may want to get back into some sort of a healthy cardiovascular exercise activity. Whether fitness is your game or not, cardiovascular training is very important for your heart. If you haven't worked out for a while, you'll need to slowly reintroduce cardiovascular activity into your workouts. Knowing your target heart rate gives you a guideline for which to achieve an effective cardiovascular workout. Your target heart rate (THR) will be between 55% to 80% of your maximum heart rate (MHR). Your MHR can be measured roughly as 220 minus your age. Make sure to stay within your THR.

TODAY'S INTENTION:

_____

_____

_____

POSITIVE OUTCOME(S):

_____

_____

_____

AFFIRMATION:

_____

_____

_____

GRATITUDE:

_____

_____

_____

_____

ACTION STEP:

Begin today and make it a habit to always stretch before exercising. If you're not back into exercising, stretching is still good for your body. Do what you can, where you are, keeping the above points in mind.

In addition, for a little extra inspiration today as you persevere with your healing and health, visit https://vimeo.com/99080033 and watch the short 4 minute clip.

"The best preparation for tomorrow is to do today's work superbly well."

- William Osler

WEEK 12 / DAY 6- DATE: _____

HEALTH TIP:
Your body is in a constant state of replacing and renewing itself. While some cells (such as the nerve cells in your brain) do not replace themselves, the vast majority of the cells in your body will have replaced themselves several times throughout your lifetime. For example, your liver replaces itself approximately every half year, your heart every 20 years, your lungs every 2-3 weeks, your skin every 2-4 weeks, your intestines every 2-4 days, your bones approximately every 10 years, and red blood cells every 4 months. Think about that – since you've started this program nearly half your body has been completely replaced and renewed! A decade from now almost your entire body will have been reconstructed. With every cell replication comes another chance to change the state of your health.

ACTION STEP:
Congratulations. You have come a very long way over these past 3 months. You've been given another chance at health and life, and each day is a new chance to seize that opportunity. The future is now yours to pursue, and there's no time to waste in this lifetime. What legacy do you want to leave behind? Turn to page 283.

TODAY'S INTENTION:
_____

_____

_____

POSITIVE OUTCOME(S):
_____

_____

_____

AFFIRMATION:
_____

_____

_____

GRATITUDE:
_____

_____

_____

_____

"You are here to enable the divine purpose of the universe to unfold.
That is how important you are!"
~ Eckhart Tolle

THIS WEEK'S REVIEW:

Today is your chance to go over the action steps of this past week, reincorporate any activities you may have forgotten, and complete any activities yet unfinished. Use today to catch up and take stock.

Check off the items you've completed below:

☐ I've begin working on my Vision Board.

☐ I've written my Personal Vision Statement.

☐ I've purchased some superfoods this week and will incorporate them into my meals.

☐ I've watched the short movie at https://vimeo.com/99080033

☐ I'm in the process of finding a coach who can work with me for health and success as I go forward.

☐ I've completed all my daily journaling exercises, including today's which are on the pages that follow.

Of all the tips I've learned in this book, 15 of the key action steps for my health that I fully **commit** to doing consistently from now on (the most important tips I'm taking forward with me) are:

1. _____

2. _____

3. _____

4. _____

5. _____

6. _____

7. _____

8. _____

9. _____

10. _____

11. _____

12. _____

13. _____

14. _____

15. _____

NOTES: Other Important Things I'd Like to Do or Remember:

PART 2:

EXERCISES,

WORKSHEETS,

and

RESOURCES

MY COMMITMENT TO HEALING

I, (my name), hereby promise to commit 100% to my healing.
I purchased this workbook in order to heal myself. By doing so I am making a **12 week** commitment to myself. This commitment will not only affect my life, but also the lives of those people around me who care about me. I will not sell myself short by wasting this opportunity, or this information. This is no time for me to be lazy. This is my time to **follow through** 100% and place all of my focus and efforts into my healing. Feeling **GREAT** once again will be my reward.

I acknowledge there may be times when I won't feel like doing my exercises. I know I will need to make some changes to my diet, my lifestyle, even my thoughts, in order to optimally heal. However the alternative to not healing is unacceptable and therefore **I will do what's necessary**! I refuse to be a victim of my injury or illness. Others before me have healed from equal or greater adversity, and I know within me **I have the power** to do the same. I have powers within me greater than I am aware – I will discover them, and I will prevail. This is not about 'trying'. 'Trying' something leaves open the possibility of failing. Instead, I will **DO**, leaving upon the table **no other alternative** except for success. My health and my life deserve nothing less.

Practitioners and various treatments will help me. However I acknowledge that the key to my healing begins with my

mindset. Even if I don't fully understand the 'how' to my healing, I will focus on the 'why' (the reasons for my healing) and **I am committed to finding a way**, no matter what it takes. It all begins inside **ME**.

More than any other person, I know what is best for me. I am in control and take **responsibility** for my own healing. I do not let things happen to me. Rather I am the destiny of my ship, and chart my course. I am willing to do whatever it takes for me to get better. **TODAY I commit** to beginning. And tomorrow I commit to **following through**. Quitting will not produce winning, and therefore I will not quit, nor be lazy. Nor will I criticize myself. I will remain **positive**, and **focussed on my goal** of being healed. I **love** myself, and make my own healing my number 1 priority.

TODAY – and for the next 12 weeks, I make these commitments to myself.

F.O.D.M.A.P. FOODS

Incorporate less of the High FODMAP and more of the Low FODMAP.

	HIGH FODMAP ☹		LOW FODMAP ☺	
FRUIT	Apple	Nectarine	Banana	Lemon
	Apricot	Peach	Blueberry	Lime
	Avocado	Pear	Cantaloupe	Orange
	Blackberry	Prune	Grapefruit	Passion Fruit
	Cherry	Persimmon	Grapes	Pineapple
	Lychee	Watermelon	Honeydew	Raspberry
	Mango	Canned Fruit	Kiwi	Strawberry
VEGETABLES	Artichoke	Leek	Alfalfa	Eggplant
	Asparagus	Mushroom	Bamboo Shoot	Ginger
	Beets	Okra	Bean Sprouts	Lettuce
	Brussel	Onion(!!)	Bok Choy	Olives
	Cabbage	Peas	Carrots	Potato
	Cauliflower	Shallots	Celery	Spinach
	Fennel	Snow Peas	Chives	Sweet
	Garlic		Cucumber	Tomato
DAIRY	Cottage Cheese	Cow's Milk	Lactose Free Milk	
	Ice Cream	Goat Milk	Coconut Milk	Rice Milk
	Yogurt	Sheep's Milk	Cheeses (cheddar, Swiss,	
	Sherbet	Sour Cream	parmesan, feta,	
	Margarine	Whip Cream		
	Evaporated Milk			
GRAINS	Rye	Spelt	Oats	Quinoa
	Wheat (includes wheat-based		Rice	Polenta
	pastas, cereals, bread, pastries)		Gluten-free pasta	
OTHER	Baked Beans	Lentils	Beef	Chicken
	Kidney Beans	Chickpeas	Egg	Tofu
	Soy Beans		Fish	
	Corn Syrup	Fructose	Nuts (Walnuts, Almonds,	
	Honey	Molasses	Seeds (chia, flax, pumpkin,	
	Sorbitol	Xylitol	sesame, sunflower)	

MY H.E.A.L.T.H. GOALS

Today you are going to begin setting your own 'H.E.A.L.T.H goals, using the My HEALTH Goals Worksheet. Before embarking on setting those goals however, it would be prudent to first review the importance of why and how to properly set goals.

In health, as in life, we need to know where we're going. If we don't, we'll be blown around by whichever direction the wind takes us, and detoured by whatever distraction pulls our fancy. Having a set of goals becomes your roadmap to getting to where you want to be. How can you possibly know where to go if you don't know what your destination is.

Knowing where you are going is what helps drive you forward to achieving what you want. There will certainly be challenges along every journey, but with a goal you'll be motivated to keep going even when the going gets tough.

By setting goals, you are placing the focus of your mind on improving yourself, or your life, in some way. Goals help us strive for new heights, and in turn help us reach our highest potential.

In terms of healing and health, it's easy to get lazy. Some days you may not feel like doing your recommended treatment, therapy, or action step. Some days a greasy hamburger in bed is all you feel like! Remembering and being committed to your health goals will help you make the right decisions, the healthy decisions.

Believe it or not, there is a worse place to be than being in pain with sickness or injury. When we are in pain, it is very clear that we want to be 'out of pain', and we are thus naturally motivated to take action to get there. However, once our healing begins and the pain starts to subside, we fall into the 'comfort zone' where "Oh well, I'm good enough now" invades our thoughts. The motivation for getting out of pain is now gone, and it's easy to settle for 'good enough'. Is just 'good enough' acceptable to you though? Or do you want to be fully healthy and living your dreams? Do you want to be once again at your best?

Keith Cunningham (the original 'Rich Dad from Robert Kiyosaki's book 'Rich Dad Poor Dad'), once said that "hell on earth would be meeting, on the last day you have to live, the 'you' you could have been". Imagine all those unfulfilled dreams that would just die along with you. This is why you need goals – to remind you of what it is you truly want, to motivate you, to guide you through challenges with unwavering focus, and to get you there, step by step.

Properly Setting Goals

There is a right and a wrong way to set goals. If the only goal you set for yourself is to "be pain free and healthy" and you add no further specifics to the goal, you are setting yourself up for failure. A properly thought out goal has several elements to it. Applying these essential elements of goal setting will greatly increase your chances of achieving your goal(s) and dream(s). This information can be used in all aspects of your life whenever you set goals, be it health, weight loss, career, dating, adventure, etc.

The 3 Essential Rules to Setting Goals

1. Goals must be behavioural in nature. In other words, they must represent your planned action as opposed to an outcome. After all, the outcome only occurs after a well-executed plan of action. Additionally, many external influences beyond your control can affect an outcome whereas you and only you are fully in charge and in control of your actions.

Example, "I'm going to lose 10 pounds" is not a behavioural goal, rather, it is an outcome. A better worded goal would be "I'm going to work out 4 days a week and stop eating cheesecake".

2. Goals must be measureable. The behaviour itself needs to be measureable, and there must be a time element attached (either a rate of repetition or a completion date). Without these elements how will you know if you're on the right track, or have achieved the goal.

Example: "I'm going to exercise" is not a measureable goal. However, by saying "I'm going to do core exercises 4 days a week for 30 minutes for the next 3 months" is measureable. It is very easy to tell if you are achieving your goal or not.

3. You must create accountability. To create true accountability, there must be communication of the goal combined with a reward or consequence.

If you're like most people, it's easier to be held accountable to someone else than to be accountable to yourself. We can always give ourselves excuses, but it's harder to give excuses to someone else. By communicating your goal to others you are therefore more likely to achieve your goal. Make sure that those you share your goals with are supportive of you as naysayers and doubters will only suck away at your motivation and belief.

The second part to creating accountability is include a consequence for failure. There are two motivators in life, pain and pleasure. Pleasure can be a powerful motivator, yet the desire to avoid pain is even more so. Therefore, both a reward (pleasure) for achieving your goal as well as a consequence (pain) for failing to achieve your goal should be communicated to those you share your goal with.

When choosing a reward, make sure it is something that excites you. For smaller goals your reward may be something such as a nice evening out or a day at the spa. For larger goals your reward may be a trip to some dream destination, buying a new car, etc. Make sure that you can afford whatever your reward is (both in time and money), and make sure to follow through on your reward upon successful completion of your goal. In life we tend to beat ourselves up at failures yet downplay our successes. It's important to celebrate when we achieve something. This is your reward for the effort and commitment you've put in toward achieving your goal.

When choosing a consequence, make sure it is something that you will dread doing. The consequence needs to be painful, yet in no way should it be physically harmful. The consequence needs to be able to be carried out in a day or less, and is to be done the day after failing to

achieve your goal. In other words, a consequence such as 'No vacation time for me until I'm able to achieve my initial goal' does not work as it is not immediately fulfill-able nor can it be performed in a day or less. Some possible consequences may include: leaving a day's pay on the street for someone to find, publicly admitting your failure and reasons why, walking down the block in your underwear (granted you need a good sense of humor for that!), offering a paid-for plane ticket to your ex for a trip to Hawaii, spending a night on the street, etc. Some of these consequences seem harsh, and they are. Their sole purpose is to drive you to achieving your goal and to motivate you to do whatever it takes to avoid having to carry out the consequence.

A Word of Caution

Some goals are controllable where the time to achievement is based directly upon the effort you put in, and this time can be estimated. Healing is a little different. Absolutely it is true that the more effort (properly applied) you put in to your healing the quicker your healing will take place. However everyone heals at a different pace dependant on a variety of factors (physical condition, extent of the injury or illness, age, lifestyle, mindset, determination, etc). It is therefore very important that you:

1. Do not create a timeline for your healing based on how someone else has healed. Perhaps you know someone with a similar injury or illness who has healed in 'x' amount of time. That time is irrelevant to you. Perhaps (unknown to you) their injury or illness was less severe than yours and therefore they healed sooner, leading you to feel disappointment if you haven't reached their level of healing by 'x' time. Alternatively, who says that you aren't able to heal faster than that other person? Perhaps their injury or illness was more serious than yours, or maybe they were not as ambitious in their rehabilitation. Why therefore slow your progress down by thinking it will take 'x' amount of time when you might achieve success even sooner. Remember, this is your journey, and there is no one else in the race but you.

2. Do not create goals with consequences based on being 'healed' by a certain date. As I've discussed above, everyone heals at different speeds. There is no harm placing a timeline in your mind as doing so

gives you something to strive for. However an exact date for 'being healed' should not be written in stone as there are too many variables beyond your control that influence the outcome. As a result, if you place a consequence for not being healed by a certain date, you are in danger of unnecessarily punishing yourself.

Create your goals, rewards, and consequences based only upon behavioural actions that you control.

Using the "My H.E.A.L.T.H. Goals Worksheet"

The My H.E.A.L.T.H. Goals Worksheet (on the pages that follow – with additional printable worksheets available at www.TheHealingWorkbook.com) should be filled in at the beginning of each month, reviewed weekly, and scored at the end of each month.

Begin by filling in the start and end date of the month (your month begins today).

Next, write down your 2 biggest health goals for the coming year. Writing down your health goals reinforces in your mind what you are working toward.

Under each of the 6 (H.E.A.L.T.H.) sections, complete the initial sentence by writing your intention for that area. These intentions should all be supportive of your two main health goals that you wrote at the top of the page.

In the HABITS section (which is a different format from the rest), you'll continue by writing a supportive habit goal to replace your unsupportive habit. It is more difficult to break an old habit if there is nothing to replace it with. Therefore, when choosing your new supportive habit, make sure it can directly replace the old habit. For example, if your old habit is watching TV an hour each night, this could be replaced by substituting that time with doing exercises. If your old habit is eating potato chips, this could be replaced with eating fresh veggies.

For the remaining sections, break the intentions you've written in the first sentence down even further into two stages. The first stage ("At Least") should be an easy first step toward the attainment of your intention (at minimum you will 'at least do this'). The second stage should be a loftier yet still achievable goal (achieving that goal will feel great). For both the 'At Least' and the 'Goal', include the date by which you will have accomplished each stage.

As you achieve your 'At Least', circle the corresponding single star to the right. As you achieve your 'Goal', circle the corresponding two stars to the right.

At the end of the month, total up your stars. A total of 18 points is possible if you achieve ALL your 'At Leasts' and 'Goals'. It's up to you how you choose to score yourself and carry out rewards or consequences. My suggestion is to place rewards and consequences for the overall number of stars each month as follows:

12 - 18 Stars: Excellently done! Reward yourself!

8 - 11 Stars: Not a bad effort, room for improvement though. No reward or consequence.

1-7 Stars: Lack of commitment. Time for a consequence, and then start with renewed vigor and determination next month.

MY **H.E.A.L.T.H.** GOALS WORKSHEET

MY 2 BIGGEST HEALTH GOALS ARE:

1. _____
2. _____

Today's Date
(Start of Month)

HABITS

H This month I will stop doing the unsupportive habit of _____

by _____ and I'll replace it with the supportive habit of

_____ by _____.

EXERCISE

E This month my exercise goal is to _____:

ATLEAST: _____ By: _____

GOAL: _____ By: _____

ACKNOWLEDGE

A This month I will acknowledge _____ for _____:

ATLEAST: _____ By: _____

GOAL: _____ By: _____

LEARN

L This month I'll improve my overall health & vitality by learning more about _____:

ATLEAST: _____ By: _____

GOAL: _____ By: _____

TRANSFORM

T This month I will positively transform my life by :

ATLEAST: _____ By: _____

GOAL: _____ By: _____

HAPPINESS

H This month I will do the following for my own fulfillment and happiness:

ATLEAST: _____ By: _____

GOAL: _____ By: _____

/18

MY **H.E.A.L.T.H.** GOALS WORKSHEET

MY 2 BIGGEST HEALTH GOALS ARE:	Today's Date (Start of Month)
1.	
2.	

HABITS

H This month I will stop doing the unsupportive habit of _____

by _____ and I'll replace it with the supportive habit of

_____ by _____.

EXERCISE

E This month my exercise goal is to _____:

ATLEAST: _____ By: _____

GOAL: _____ By: _____

ACKNOWLEDGE

A This month I will acknowledge _____ for _____:

ATLEAST: _____ By: _____

GOAL: _____ By: _____

LEARN

L This month I'll improve my overall health & vitality by learning more about _____:

ATLEAST: _____ By: _____

GOAL: _____ By: _____

TRANSFORM

T This month I will positively transform my life by :

ATLEAST: _____ By: _____

GOAL: _____ By: _____

HAPPINESS

H This month I will do the following for my own fulfillment and happiness:

ATLEAST: _____ By: _____

GOAL: _____ By: _____

/18

HEALTHIER SNACK IDEAS

For those who are always looking to nibble, often we turn to unhealthy snacks because we don't know what a healthy alternative might be. If this sounds like you, use the list below for a few healthier snack ideas you can just grab and go.

Handful of nuts (walnuts, almonds, pistachios, cashews)
½ sliced apple with natural peanut butter
½ cup blueberries with a bit of yogurt
1 cup of raspberries
Handful of raisins
Fresh veggie mix (broccoli, cauliflower, etc)
Celery sticks with natural peanut butter or hummus
½ cup egg salad on lettuce
1 hardboiled egg chopped & mixed with avocado
½ cup edamame
½ sliced cucumber
Bean and chickpea salad
Fruit and/or green smoothie
½ cup non-fat frozen yogurt
½ cup beet chips with Greek yogurt
2 squares of dark (70%+) chocolate
1 cup of soup
1 cup of grapes
½ cup Greek yogurt with granola
1 slice Wasa bread with apple slices
1 cup kale chips
Half an avocado
Cherry tomatoes topped with goat cheese
Handful of pumpkin seeds

MY FOOD JOURNAL

	MONDAY		TUESDAY		WEDNESDAY		THURSDAY		FRIDAY		SATURDAY		SUNDAY	
	Food	How I feel	Food	How I feel	Food	How I feel	Food	How I feel	Food	How I feel	Food	How I feel	Food	How I feel
BREAKFAST (and Late Morning)														
LUNCH (and mid Afternoon)														
DINNER (and Evening)														
Glasses of Water														
Other Comments														

SCHEDULING PRIORITIES

There is a story of a professor who one day brought in to his class a large jar filled to the top with rocks. He asked his students, "Is the jar filled?". The students responded "Yes.".

He then took out from his desk a small bowl of pebbles, and dropped them into the big jar. The small pebbles filtered themselves into the spaces between the big rocks. He then asked the class, "Is the jar full?", to which they again responded "Yes".

He then took out from his desk a small bowl of sand, and sprinkled it into the big jar. All the sand filled in the remaining gaps between the rocks and pebbles. He then asked the class once again, "Is the jar full?", to which they once again responded "Yes!".

To the student's surprise, the professor then took out from his desk a cup of water. He slowly poured the cup of water into the big jar. He was able to empty the entire cup of water into the jar that was 'already full'. The water filled in all remaining spaces between the rocks, pebbles, and sand.

The jar was now full.

He then asked his class, "What would have happened if I had reversed the order, putting in the water first, then the sand, then the pebbles, and then the large rocks?". The answer was unanimous – the large rocks wouldn't fit.

The lesson he taught his class that day was that, in life, your priorities are the large rocks, while the pebbles, sand and water represent all the other distractions, errands, chores, appointments, etc that inevitably

come up and we fill our time with. In this case priorities are the things that are most important to you, the things that mean the most to you, the things that, if you accomplished nothing else, would still fulfill you. When you fill your jar (representing your life) with your priorities first, there still somehow seems to be enough time to work in everything else as well. However, if you always fill your life with the sand, water, and pebbles first, you'll never have enough space in your life for what really matters the most to you.

The exercise that follows will help ensure you keep enough space for your 'large rocks'.

Step 1:

On the following page make a list of all the things and activities that are most important to you in life. (Although your list may be completely different, some examples might be: spending time with children, going to the gym, Sunday night family dinners, meditating, volunteer work, travel, weekly nature walk, reading, doing a favorite sport or hobby, etc.) Write them all down below, and then in the column to the right, mark down how often ('Frequency') you ideally want to allot time for this activity (D= daily, W= weekly, M= monthly, Y= yearly).

My Big Rocks (Priorities in Life) Are: Frequency:

_____   _____

_____   _____

_____   _____

_____   _____

_____   _____

_____   _____

_____   _____

_____   _____

_____   _____

_____   _____

_____   _____

_____   _____

_____   _____

_____   _____

_____   _____

_____   _____

_____   _____

_____   _____

_____   _____

_____   _____

_____   _____

_____   _____

_____   _____

Step 2:

Now that you're clear on your priorities, it's time to start scheduling them in. After all, why would you only schedule medical appointments, oil changes and business meetings, and yet never schedule in the things that really matter most? Use the calendar on the next page as practice to begin. Afterward, you will surely want to use your own calendar system to schedule your priorities. For now, fill in the calendar with all your big rocks from the previous page that apply to the coming month. Once you've done so, grab a highlighter and **highlight** each of these activities. The key is that, **once you schedule a big rock, it MUST NOT be altered**!! This is what happens in life – we plan something fun or important, and then a meeting comes up and we postpone or forfeit our big rock – and this is why we are left feeling unfulfilled – the things that matter most to us often get pushed aside for the things that really don't matter in the grand scheme of things. It's time to change that habit. Once you write in your big rock, you are committing to keeping that appointment with yourself, ensuring you achieve what really matters most to you. Go ahead, and do that now.

Step 3:

Once you've filled in your big rocks, schedule in all upcoming appointments around those big rocks. Your appointments and meetings are the pebbles. You will find a way to fit them in around your big rocks. **Remember, your big rocks should never be moved** (except of course in an extreme emergency). The sand and water are everything else that happens from day to day, and they will naturally filter in between your pebbles and rocks.

Sunday	Monday	Tuesday	Wednesday	Thursday	Friday	Saturday

VICTIM VS VICTOR

Holding on to a victim mentality makes it very difficult to ever recover fully. We cannot heal ourselves when we are blaming someone or something else for our misery. We have no control over those external influences, and by blaming we send all our energy towards that negative person or event that caused our distress.

We have only control over ourselves. When we take responsibility for all outcomes, we shift from a victim to a victor mentality. We accept responsibility for the event (good or bad), and we acknowledge that whatever happens next is ultimately in our hands. Our energy can now be directed fully toward victory, or in this case, healing.

A victor mentality is also important to eliminating those negative patterns that keep showing up in life. When life throws you those hard curveballs, so long as you keep viewing it with victim mentality, that pattern will repeat over and over, leading to a lot of suffering. By looking at the situation the eyes of a victor, asking the question 'what am I here to learn from this', the outcome becomes positive.

Do the following simple exercise to discover which mentality dominates you. On the following page are 2 columns of words. Go down each column and circle every word which resonates with how you feel. You are not comparing words across from each other, rather you are looking at each column independently and circling all words that resonate. When you're done, count how many words you've circled in each column. The column with the most counts will show whether you have a victim or a victor mindset. If you tend more towards the victim, follow the instruction on the page that follows to shift yourself more towards that of a victor.

VICTIM	or	VICTOR
Frustration		Happiness
Defeated		Healthy
Weak		Strong
Obese		Free
Sickness		Accepted
Conflict Avoidance		Responsible
Failure		Peaceful
Empty		Abundance
Tortured		Loved
Scarcity		Triumph
Deceitful		Faith
Fearful		Courageous
Loneliness		Truth
Pessimistic		Creative
Overwhelmed		Powerful
Abandoned		Open
Trash		Treasure
Stress		Excited
Blaming		Self-Respect
Life is Hard		Worthy
Stuck		Fulfilled
Misery		Honor
Broke		Rewarded
Pain		Brightness / Light
Doubtful		Diligent

Here are some steps you can take to help you shift from victim to victor mentality.

1. Acknowledge that this is where you are right now, and that now does not need to represent the future.

2. Choose today to take responsibility for where you are now, and where you want to get to.

3. Whenever you blame, complain, or rationalize why you can't do something, interrupt yourself. For example, after a negative thought about your limitations, you might say something such as "Cancel. Cancel. That's not true. I *can* do it!"

4. Love yourself, and avoid self-judgment and criticism.

5. Trust and be confident in your abilities. Declare to yourself that "I can and will succeed!"

6. Live with integrity and honor and choose actions that serve the well-being of everyone.

7. Forgive yourself when you fail to live up to your new standards, especially at the beginning. Be kind to yourself.

8. View life's challenges as happening "through you" to help you grow, rather than "to you" to make you suffer. Really let this concept sink in for it is key.

9. Work with the affirmations (page 243), choosing the one each day you feel you need the most.

10. Make a conscious effort each day to adopt at least 1 new victor quality into your actions and persona.

EMOTIONAL CLEARING

"By listening to the story in our mind, we come to understand
the movie of our life. To change the picture on the screen,
we must first adjust the programming within ourselves.
And to be able to see it, we need to first be willing to look."
~ Rick Fischer

We are all running on 'programs' – messages and patterns we picked up early in life that control us, for good or for bad, as adults. Holding on to hidden negative emotions and patterns can affect us in various aspects of life, from repeated disappointments in relationships and career to serious health concerns. In fact, almost all health concerns can be traced back to some energetic or emotional imbalance. This is why, in order to heal, we must be introspective and work on our inner selves. As you'll notice more and more in the coming weeks, this book deals heavily with our inner world and mindset – this is because all healing begins within.

As Louise Hay addresses in detail in her bestselling book <u>You Can Heal Your Life</u>, many negative physical health conditions can be traced back to specific unresolved emotional issues. Drawing from her book in this regard, a few common ailments are listed below along with a very simplistic look at some potential underlying emotional issues.

ADDICTIONS: not loving oneself, running away from self.

AIDS: feeling defenseless, denial of true self, sexual guilt

ALCOHOLISM: guilt, inadequacy, self-rejection

ANOREXIA: denying the self, fear of rejection.

ANXIETY: distrusting the natural flow of life.

ARTHRITIS: feeling unloved, resentful

BACK (upper):   lack of emotional support, feeling unloved

BACK (lower):   financial woes and concerns.

BULIMIA: getting rid of self-hatred.

CANCER: deep hurt, grief

CATARACTS (eyes): not being able to see the joy ahead

DIABETES: longing for what might have been

HEADACHES: self-criticism

LARYNGITIS: fear of speaking up.

LIVER PROBLEMS: fear, anger, hatred

LUNG PROBLEMS: Depression, grief, not feeling worthy

MIGRAINES: sexual or intimacy fears, feeling pressured

OBESITY: feeling need for emotional protection, insecurity

OSTEOPOROSIS: feeling there is no support left in life.

SHOULDER PROBLEMS: carrying a heavy burden

SLIPPED DISK: feeling unsupported in life.

THYROID PROBLEMS: humiliation, repression

ULCERS: feeling unworthy or not good enough

The above causes may or may not resonate with you, at least on the surface. It may however warrant a closer look to see if there might be truth in this or not for you. Regardless of how you view Louise Hay's findings, there is a definite connection between emotional pain and the manifestation of physical symptoms. Let me give you an example.

Suppose you grew up in a home where mom and dad were always fighting, and the tension in the air was high. Arguments would always come up at the dinner table. Years later you go from doctor to doctor trying to understand why your digestive system is messed up – perhaps you've been diagnosed with Irritable Bowel Syndrome. Could there be a connection to your childhood? Quite possibly. A relaxing environment during meal time allows for proper digestion. The child in this example grew up in an environment where meal times were never

calm, and this began impairing their digestion at an early age. Medically, the diagnosis may be I.B.S., and while diet will certainly be part of the treatment, the issue also needs to be healed emotionally.

We finally have hard scientifically proven evidence of this connection between emotional pain / childhood trauma and physical symptoms, as laid out in the highly praised (and recommended) book "The Impact of Early Life Trauma of Health and Disease: The Hidden Epidemic" by Lanius, Vermetten, and Pain. As excerpted from this book:

> *"Traumatic events of the earliest years of infancy and childhood are not lost but, like a child's footprints in wet cement, are often preserved life-long. Time does not heal the wounds that occur in those earliest years; time conceals them. They are not lost; they are embodied."*

> *"...we contribute to the problem by authenticating as biomedical disease that which is actually the somatic inscription of life experience on the human body and brain."*

In other words, the trauma, the abuse, the abandonment in childhood, these events show up in our diet, in our addictions, the way we treat ourselves as adults. So ask yourself, "Are you willing to look inside at your truth?", because that is where healing begins.

Very often when the emotional side is properly addressed and cleared, so too will the symptoms resolve themselves. The two exercises on the following pages can help you begin working through this.

Exercise #1

Step 1:

Are there any people in your life that bring out the emotion of anger in you? Write down their names:

_____

_____

How about frustration? Who contributes to your feelings of frustration?

_____

_____

How about hurt? Who contributes to your feelings of hurt?

_____

_____

Step 2:

Think of the people you wrote down above, write 2 things that come to mind when completing each sentence below:

I feel most angry when:

_____

_____

I feel most frustrated when:

_____

_____

I feel most hurt when:

_____

_____

<u>Step 3:</u>

Write 2 things that come to mind when completing each sentence below: What things do I do to myself that make me feel angry?

_____

_____

What things do I do to myself that make me feel frustrated?

_____

_____

What things have I done to myself to hurt myself?

_____

_____

<u>Step 4:</u>

Using the above instances to help intensify the emotions, for each emotion (anger, frustration, hurt, etc), close your eyes and try to discover where that emotion resides within your body. Focus your mind inward and let it travel through all the parts of your body. You may discover for example a feeling of pressure in your chest, or warmth in your leg. As you discover where these emotions reside, place your hand on that area and express the emotion out loud by saying "I feel pressure here", or "It hurts here".

<u>Step 5:</u>

Next, while keeping your attention focused on the area of negative emotion, for the next 30 seconds on each exhale visualize expelling that emotion.

Step 6:

Finally, imagine you could speak to that person who caused you to feel that negative emotion. What would you say to him or her? It is important to remember that they were not the cause of your negative emotion, but rather it was your response to what they did. If the case involved them intentionally trying to hurt you, then consider viewing that incident as you unintentionally allowing them to do so, and recognize that you will no longer fall into that trap. Speak to them. Release the emotion. Forgive.

Exercise #2

This exercise is especially powerful for releasing emotions (perhaps unconscious) that have been haunting us throughout our lives and have been sabotaging our greater potential, and especially relationships. A simple traumatic event in childhood can have long reaching effects in adulthood. There is a child within all of us (our 'inner child') that carries with us some of our deepest wounds. As we go through life as adults, we project those wounds (drama) onto the people we bring into our life, hoping to 'get it right this time' and to make up for what happened in our past.

A baby for example, who may have been distraught with the fear of abandonment when mommy left for 3 days on a business trip and grandma was left to take care for the baby, may be left with deep seated fears of abandonment as an adult. The mother did nothing wrong, she made sure the baby was in good care. But to the baby, who has no sense of time, watching mommy leave meant that mommy would never come back. Thirty years later this plays out in a relationship when a well-meaning partner walks away from a small argument but unknowingly triggers the fear of abandonment in the now grown baby, causing tension in the relationship.

Another example is that of a one year old, still very close to mommy, who sees mommy distraught after she found out daddy cheated on her. Mommy and daddy still love baby very much, but baby just sees mommy's crying and sadness not understanding why. Baby begins to

think that she is the cause, leading to a lifelong pattern of guilt and unworthiness.

These are just a couple of examples of patterns developed by events in childhood. We also inherit patterns from our parents, and their parents. Let's say your grandfather was a high school dropout, and your dad was a high school dropout. Chances are you might be (or were on the path to be) a high school dropout as well. Do you think that dad and grandfather led an easy life? Do you think they wished the pain and hardship they went through on their children? Of course not. But despite their intentions and wishes the child grows up to repeat the cycle, which then gets passed down to their children, and their children's children. Only YOU can break the cycle. Only you can change the history of your family that your children will inherit.

In relationships it's common for a partner to seek out in their partner what they didn't receive as children from their parents. This is often seen in women who look for men that resemble their father, either in physical attributes or in the type of person the father was. As explained in Neo-Freudian psychology and as proposed by Carl Jung, the 'Electra complex' explains why these women will often look to acquire, in a partner, the father they never had in childhood. In this endeavor however they are subconsciously seeking the 'emotionally unavailable man' in the hopes that she can somehow 'fix' him. A loving and healthy partner may come along for her, but eventually if she is being subconsciously driven by her Electra complex, she'll sabotage the relationship because he does not fit who her father was. The same is true for men and women alike. Beginning at birth, the person forms an unconscious image of the opposite sex based on the inputs around the child at the time. As the person grows up, they may subconsciously be seeking out that unconscious image, even if consciously they say that's not what they want. As explained brilliantly in the book Getting The Love You Want by Harville Hendrix, Ph.D, both sexes are seeking to heal in their partner a wound they acquired in childhood. The wound created by a parent will unintentionally be repeated by the partner which then unconsciously triggers old emotions, causing the wounded partner to in some way withdraw. This pattern can often be seen when looking back through one's history of relationships.

Whether we inherited a pattern directly from our parents or developed one in childhood, we all have patterns in our lives... and it's time – and your duty – to break the cycle! If there is a repeating pattern going on in your life that is causing you pain, or holding you back from what you deserve, it's your duty to figure out why, and learn the lesson from it, in order for it to stop. Healing can only begin when we bring our hurt out of the shadows, shedding loving light on it.

My repeating pattern (or family cycle) that I want to stop is:

_____

_____

_____

Seeing the pattern is the first step towards learning the lesson from it, and subsequently healing. For example, it could be you have a pattern of bombs that fall out of the blue onto relationships that end painfully. To figure out why, you need to go back in time and find the source of that bomb. Using the example of the baby above who's mommy was distraught after daddy cheated, in this case that event was the first bomb for the baby. It was a traumatic event for that baby, as the baby assumed it was all because of her.

In meditation, try to go back into your early life and figure out when this negative pattern first might have appeared. What emotions did you take on from someone else at that time? In the second example we used earlier, mommy was sad, feeling guilty of not being good enough, and alone. Being a one year old baby who's still very attached to mommy at that time, the baby took on these same emotions. Once you discover the emotions or feelings you took on at this first experience, chances are you'll recognize that these are still prevalent in your life today.

The first time this pattern may have emerged was

_____

_____

_____

I was about _____ year(s) old.

The emotions that I felt around me and took on were

_____

_____

_____

_____

What is this pattern or cycle within me or my family costing me? What is it costing my children? What will it cost my children's children? How is it hurting me, or those people around me who love me?

_____

_____

_____

_____

_____

_____

_____

_____

_____

The key to healing from this is to now ensure you replace these negative emotions with what was missing at the time. The baby did nothing wrong, and has nothing to be guilty about, and so she should focus now on being proud of who she is, not allowing guilt in. The baby was always good enough in the eyes of mommy and daddy, and that grown person now needs to focus on feeling worthy. And if loneliness is still being felt, with or without friends around, focus on being your own best friend. All these positive emotions can be programmed into the subconscious mind by repeatedly saying them to yourself, and giving yourself positive affirmations.

The emotions I need to focus on giving myself to heal are:

_____

_____

_____

_____

I can help myself do this by incorporating those positive thoughts in these affirmations which I will repeat to myself daily:

_____

_____

_____

_____

_____

_____

_____

_____

Additional Resources for Emotional Clearing Work

Over the next few weeks you'll be introduced to additional methods for accessing the subconscious and healing yourself of emotional, mental, and spiritual hurts and patterns that can manifest themselves physically. A few of these techniques, if you're interested in jumping ahead in this area, include the Dalian Method as mentioned on page 81 as well as the Ho'oponopono exercise on page 241 and The Emotional Freedom Technique (page 259).

In addition to techniques I specifically cover in this book, additional tools and processes that I also recommend for emotional clearing include:

1. If you are dealing with cancer, the book "The Journey" written by Brandon Bays offers a remarkable story of her own healing and walks you step by step through the 'Journey process'. The Journey Process will help you access and clear out deeply hidden emotions that may be blocking your healing.

2. 'The Work' by Byron Katie is a powerful and well respected way of identifying and questioning the thoughts that cause anger, fear, depression, addiction, etc. So much disease, and unnecessary suffering, is caused by holding on to unhealthy thoughts. You can begin doing the work by asking yourself the 4 foundational questions:

   i. Is the thought true?
   ii. Can you absolutely know that it's true?
   iii. How do you react, what happens, when you believe that thought?
   iv. Who would you be without the thought?

   To learn more about The Work and to go deeper, visit www.thework.com

3. The charitable foundation 'Choose Again' offers a variety of intensive, mindfulness programs to enable clients to heal anxiety, addictions, depressions, dysfunctional relationships and other issues.

4. Personal development seminar companies such as Peak Potentials Training, Tony Robbins, and PSI Seminars among others offer not only courses to help you grow both personally and professionally, they also offer in many of their courses the chance to do powerful emotional clearing exercises.

5. Imago Relationship Therapy (as developed by Harville Hendrix and explained in his book Getting The Love You Want) is very helpful for relationships and uncovering self-sabotaging relationship patterns.

6. Processes such as Breathwork, Rebirthing, and Past Life Regression can also help you access and clear deeply hidden emotions.

TOP FOODS TO BUY ORGANICALLY

The U.S. alone uses 1.2 BILLION pounds of pesticides a year, leading to a wide range of health risks including skin, eye and lung irritation, hormone disruption, brain and nervous system toxicity, cancer, blood disorders, and birth defects. When you regularly eat foods grown with pesticides, you're putting yourself at risk. However, not all foods need to be purchased organically, especially is price is a factor. Some foods contain more pesticides than others. At the same time, even some produce sprayed with large amounts of pesticides might still be okay if they have a thick skin (such as bananas or watermelons). The chart below shows the 'cleanest' foods (lowest in pesticides and insecticides) and the 'dirtiest' foods (highest in pesticides and insecticides). As much as possible, the 'dirty' foods should be purchased organically, while you can probably get away with buying the clean foods non-organically.

CLEANEST FOODS	DIRTIEST FOODS
Avocados	Apples
Sweet Corn	Strawberries
Pineapples	Grapes
Cabbage	Celery
Sweet Peas (frozen)	Peaches
Onions	Spinach
Asparagus	Sweet Bell Peppers
Mangoes	Imported Nectarines
Papayas	Cucumbers
Kiwi	Cherry Tomatoes
Eggplant	Imported Snap Peas
Grapefruit	Potatoes
Cantaloupe	Hot Peppers
Cauliflower	Domestic Blueberries
Sweet Potatoes	Lettuce

NON-ORGANIC IS OK

BUY ORGANIC!

Source: http://www.ewg.org/foodnews/list.php (April 2014)

MY INSPIRATION LIST

When we think of people who have come before us, who have achieved something we aspire to be, we become inspired to do and be better. Whatever your challenge is right now, think of 9 people who inspire you, whether they are living or not. They might be a movie or TV idol, a sports figure, a parent or family member, a person from history, a person you know who overcame disability, or even a fictitious character. Write their names in the left column below. Then, once you have completed that, beside each name write out how you think they would handle your situation. What would they do? Think of their attitude, their actions, their advice. Place them in your shoes, or you in theirs. What strength, knowledge, and guidance can you gain from them?

1. _____ _____

2. _____ _____

3. _____ _____

4. _____ _____

5. _____ _____

6. _____ _____

7. _____ _____

8. _____ _____

9. _____ _____

PERSONAL WELLNESS SCORE

The "wellness wheel" concept is often used in various counseling practices to visually display how balanced one's life is in various areas. The Personal Wellness Score™ takes this concept a step further through a very comprehensive series of questions, the answers of which are then calculated using a specific mathematical formula and plotted visually on a modified wellness wheel displaying both one's current situation as well as one's "ideal". As everyone's "ideal" is different, the Personal Wellness Score gives a much truer reading of the areas in which improvement would make the most impactful difference in one's life.

While this book is about health and healing, these concepts are not independent of other areas of your life. Stress in career or relationships, or a negative environment, can lead to poor health. Likewise poor health can affect finances and 'play'. Even if you eat the healthiest food every day, if other areas of your life are 'empty' or stressful, your health will continue to be sub-par.   By using the Personal Wellness Score, one can quickly see which areas of life might be adversely affecting health, and what changes can have the biggest impact.

The exercise you'll do on the following page will give you a quick glimpse of the wellness wheel concept, using the same 12 areas that are represented on the Personal Wellness Score. The center of the circle represents '0', meaning completely non-existent, horrible, or unfulfilled. The outer edge of the circle represents '10', meaning amazing, wonderful, perfect. To begin, in each of the 12 areas, draw a line that represents how you currently feel about that aspect of your life. When you're finished, you'll have a wheel, and usually a rather crooked one at that. When we imagine a wheel turning smoothly, we see a nicely inflated, perfectly round, balanced wheel. Likewise, for our lives to go as smoothly as possible, we want the wellness wheel to also be balanced. If even one segment falls dramatically short, it's going to give our life a bumpy ride. The great news is that a person's wellness is constantly changing. Simple everyday choices in our lifestyle can raise our wellness score and lead to a smoother wheel.

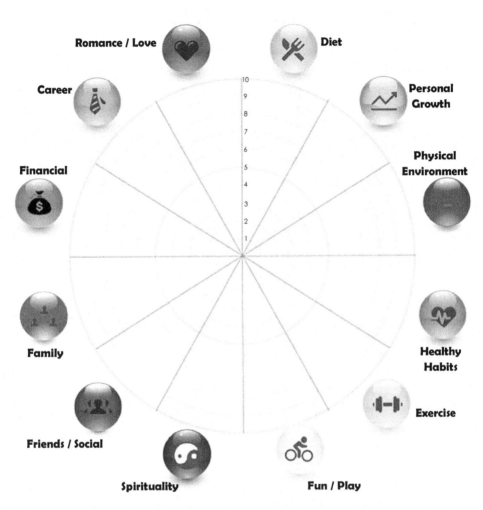

Keep in mind that this is simply an introduction to the wellness wheel concept. If you'd like your actual Personal Wellness Score created and calculated, together with a complete personalized report that will help you create better balance in your life, I offer this at http://www.integrativehealthcoaching.ca/wellness-score.html

SPECIAL OFFER TO ALL READERS

After filling out your Personal Wellness Score Questionnaire, email it back to me and mention Promo Code PWS30 to receive a complimentary 30 minute phone consultation with me to go over your Personal Wellness Score results together.

ASKING THE RIGHT QUESTIONS

On this and the following two pages are a number of powerful questions that can help you discover not only your inner self, but can also help inspire creativity, self-empowerment, and guidance toward the right answers that will serve you in your healing and life. Do not rush this exercise. For each question, spend at least 5 to 10 minutes in quiet contemplation reflecting on the question itself, and the answers that come up.

The questions are presented in no particular order. Simply choose the ones that resonate most with you.

~ Who do I need to forgive?

_____

_____

_____

_____

~ What is my body trying to tell me?

_____

_____

_____

_____

~ Is it *possible* for me to heal fully? If so, what is holding me back?

_____

_____

_____

_____

~ What things am I assuming? Are they really true?

_____

_____

_____

_____

_____

~ Is there something else I can be doing to heal myself in addition to what I'm already doing?

_____

_____

_____

_____

~ What am I holding on to that needs to be let go?

_____

_____

_____

_____

~ Who am I?

_____

_____

_____

_____

~Who am I listening to?

_____

_____

_____

_____

~ Am I being pulled by hope or pushed by fear?

_____

_____

_____

_____

~ What am I not doing that I could be?

_____

_____

_____

_____

~ Who can I draw strength from?

_____

_____

_____

_____

~ What am I resisting?

_____

_____

_____

_____

~ What story am I telling myself (and others)? Is it really true?

_____

_____

_____

_____

~ What habits/actions/thoughts do I need to change?

_____

_____

_____

_____

~ Am I able to see any linkage between emotional pain (or unfulfilled needs) I might have experienced as a child and struggles I've seen in my (health, relationships, work) as an adult?

_____

_____

_____

_____

~What feelings and emotions am I feeling? Why am I feeling this way? In there an inner emotional conflict going on inside me? Am I willing to explore this further (why these feelings resonate within me)?

_____

_____

_____

_____

~ What is this experience teaching me?

_____

_____

_____

_____

~ What must I do to overcome the obstacle(s) holding me back
from reaching my fullest potential in life?

_____

_____

_____

_____

_____

_____

_____

_____

_____

_____

UNSUPPORTIVE THOUGHTS

<u>Step 1:</u>

In the circle below write down all the unsupportive thoughts that run through your mind repeatedly. What is that negative little voice inside your head always telling you?

(continue on the following page...)

Step 2:

Think of what colors represent healing to you. Using that color or colors, draw a thick line around the circle, imagining that that 'healing line' will contain all those negative thoughts within the circle and will protect you from those thoughts escaping the circle. Imagine all those thoughts being trapped within the circle, and you being outside of it, free.

Step 3:

Commit to releasing those thoughts. They no longer serve you. Let them go. You may do this through a meditation. Or you may choose to tear out this page and ceremoniously burn it in a fire (carefully of course!).

NEGATIVE PATTERNS

"If you don't acknowledge your history, you're doomed to repeat it."

When we objectively look at our lives, we can often see patterns. Some of these serve us well, while others sabotage us from leading the life we would like to. You've already begun looking at a few of these earlier in this workbook. Negative patterns cause unnecessary suffering emotionally, adding to stress and further affecting the health of our body. Patterns are those life events that over time keep coming up. They might be in business (for example failures), in relationships (for example repeated similar endings), health (for example frequent injuries or illness), or in any other area of life. When patterns are repeated over time, it's the universe's way of telling us we have a lesson to learn. Until we learn this lesson, these patterns are destined to be repeated. Becoming aware of and acknowledging these patterns is the first step in the journey towards uncovering what our lesson(s) may be. You've already done a lot of work in this area. Today, begin by looking at what other patterns may exist in your life. You might then want to refer back to the exercises on pages 220 and 221 to work through and eliminate these negative patterns.

Patterns I've seen over time in my relationships are:

_____

_____

_____

_____

_____

Continued on next page...

Patterns I've seen over time in my business or career are:

_____

_____

_____

_____

_____

Patterns I've seen over time in my health are:

_____

_____

_____

_____

_____

Patterns I've seen over time in some other area of my life are:

_____

_____

_____

_____

_____

_____

_____

_____

pH TESTING & FOOD GUIDE

There is a simple test you can do at home to check your pH balance and determine how acidic or alkaline your body is. Ideally, your body's saliva should be between 6.7 – 7.2 (slightly higher up to 8.4 immediately after meals). Urine (a slightly less accurate measure) should be between 6.3 – 6.9 (again slightly higher up to 8.4 immediately after meals). (Note that these numbers are for saliva and urine which have a different pH range from that of blood).

To test your pH, get some pHydrion paper (pH paper strips) at your local pharmacy. You'll need about 60 strips. On day 1, do your first test immediately upon waking and before drinking, eating or brushing your teeth. Wet the end of a strip with your saliva and record the pH number. Next, test your first urine of the morning by urinating on a new strip and recording the pH number. If you can, hold off on breakfast until you've urinated and tested your urine a second time. Then, eat breakfast. Wait five minutes and check both your urine and saliva again. The next urine and saliva test should be done a couple of hours after breakfast, and then again 2 – 3 hours after lunch.

Use the table on the next page to conveniently record your pH numbers.

Make sure your numbers are in the ideal pH range. If your numbers show below this range a couple of hours after meals, you need to lower the acidity in your body. The same is true if your numbers decrease between your 1st and 3rd A.M. tests.

My pH Levels:

My pH Numbers	Day 1	Day 2	Day 3	Day 4	Day 5	Day 6
Saliva Test #1						
Urine Test #1						
Saliva Test #2						
Urine Test #2						
Saliva Test #3						
Urine Test #3						
Saliva Test #4						
Urine Test #4						
Saliva Test #5						
Urine Test #5						

The pH Level Effect of Various Foods on the Body

EAT MORE OF THESE FOODS ⬆

10 — Raw Spinach, Raw Kale, Raw Broccoli, Raw Asparagus, Cauliflower, Cucumber, Seaweed, Lemon, Lime, Alfalfa Grass, Wheat Grass, Chia Sprouts, Collard Greens, Raw Onions, Celery

9 — Avocado, Lettuce, Raw Zucchini, Red Beets, Raw Tomato, Parsley, Raw Eggplant, Green Beans, Garlic, Lemon Grass, Cayenne Pepper, Green Tea, Red Radish, Raw Peas, Chives

8 — Brussel Sprouts, Green Cabbage, Cooked Broccoli & Spinach, Cooked Asparagus, Cooked Peas, Cooked Eggplant, Millet, Raw Almonds, Wild Rice, Quinoa, Coconut Water, Olives, Flax Seed Oil

7 — Tap Water (most), Olive Oil, Coconut Oil, Pumpkin Seeds, Sesame Seeds, Sunflower Seeds, Fennel Seeds, Raw Goat Milk, Barley

EAT LESS OF THESE FOODS ⬇

6 — Brazil Nuts, Macadamia Nuts, Hazelnuts, Walnuts, Lentils, Wheat, Brown Rice, Spelt, Grapes, Papaya, Blueberries, Raspberries, Peach, Plum, Pineapple, Banana, Watermelon, Fresh Water Fish

5 — Honey, Cocoa, Soy Milk, White Rice, Whole Grains, Cooked Corn, Potato, Sweet Potato, Bread, Fruit Juice, Oysters, Mayonnaise, Ketchup, Most Bottled & Reverse Osmosis Water (on average)

4 — Ocean Fish, Turkey, Chicken, Eggs, Beer, Wine, Cream Cheese, Hard Cheese, Popcorn, Peanuts, Pistachios, Coffee, Chocolate, Cranberries, White Sugar, Canned Fruit, Tomato Sauce

3 — Pork, Beef, Lamb, Veal, Black Tea, Tobacco Products, Artificial Sweeteners, Soda, Mocha Frappuccinos, Hard Liquor, Soy Sauce, Processed Foods, Vinegar, Pickles, Sweetened Fruit Juices

NOTE: The alkaline / acidic values shown here are average values and reflect the affect the foods have on the body, not necessarily the actual pH level of the food itself. For example, lemons are very acidic, however they have a high alkalizing affect when digested and assimilated in the body, thus they are shown here with a high alkaline pH. Another example is meat which usually tests as alkaline but is acid-forming in the body.

HO'OPONOPONO

If you need additional help forgiving someone or getting unstuck from a pattern of negative thoughts, the ancient Hawaiian practice of Ho'oponopono can really help. In its common form it is a meditation comprising of the words "I'm sorry, please forgive me, thank you, I love you". While the words are simple, the healing behind the chant is profound. The technique is based around the premise that everything we see in someone else (good or bad) we first create within ourselves. To heal or 'change' someone else, we must first heal ourselves, taking full and complete responsibility for everything. We can set the intention, but then we must let go, step back and have faith in allowing the universe to unfold whatever is meant to happen in the best interest of ourselves and those around us. There are many versions of the musical meditation available on YouTube. Choose one you like, and then, as you listen to it, focus on the person that needs to be forgiven – this could even be yourself which, in all cases, you should always begin with. For a deeper study of Ho'oponopono and its powerful effects, Dr. Joe Vitale's book 'At Zero' is an excellent resource.

Use the following steps to practice basic Ho'oponopono, anywhere, anytime.

1. Think of the person you need to forgive or wish to heal (you or someone else).

2. If your answer to the first question was 'someone else, then what is it within YOU that needs to be forgiven or healed (relating to the frustration you have or issue with that person)?

3. Begin repeating the mantra, either silently or aloud, of "I'm sorry, please forgive me, thank you, I love you."

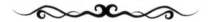

With "I'm sorry", you are simply opening a door to taking responsibility, acknowledging that you (or your ancestors) are sorry for whatever has caused this adverse circumstance.

With "Please Forgive Me", you are asking for forgiveness for having forgot how much the universe loves you, and forgiving yourself as all wrongdoings by someone else is first created by thought or memory within yourself.

With "Thank You" you are simply acknowledging that your request has been heard and is being acted upon.

With "I love You" you are tuning your mind to the energy of love, for with it comes great healing power.

AFFIRMATIONS

Affirmations are positive declarations said to oneself stating that something is true. The more you tell yourself positive, supportive, and expansive thoughts, the more positive your outer reality will become. *"What you dream, what you feel, and what you really are, will all be manifested through the word."*[1] However simply saying the words is not enough; you must also 'feel' them. When thoughts are mixed with any of the feelings of emotions, a magnetic force is created around that thought which then attracts similar thoughts. Adding emotion to the affirmation gives it greater strength and meaning. The more conviction with which you express the affirmation, the better it will transform into reality. *"Remember, therefore, when reading aloud the statement of your desire... that the mere reading of the words is of no consequence – unless you mix emotion, or feeling with your words. Your subconscious mind recognizes and acts only upon thoughts which have been well-mixed with emotion or feeling."*[2] It is the repeated thoughts and words you think and say in absolute faith that transform positive thought into positive focus and create the orders your subconscious mind acts upon. Therefore, as you go through the following affirmations and meditations, make the subconscious mind believe (because you believe it) that you are healthy, that you must have the good health you're visualizing and that this good health is just waiting for you to claim, and that the subconscious mind must guide you to the best practitioners and treatments available, and guide the cellular functions of your body towards this good health. (It must be reiterated that the words are only as good as the underlying belief. If you need to work further on your underlying beliefs, the Dalian Method as mentioned in Week 4 is a powerful place to start).

[1] Ruiz, D. M. (1997). The Four Agreements. San Rafael: Amber-Allen Publishing
[2] Hill, N. (1960). Think & Grow Rich. U.S.A.: Fawcett Books.

On the following pages is a list of healing affirmations. You may also wish to come up with your own affirmations. In doing so, keep the following rules in mind. Affirmations should always be:

- ✓ Written in the present tense
- ✓ Written in a positive way (stating what you want rather than what you don't want).
- ✓ As short and simple as possible
- ✓ Written in a way and with words that feel right to you. If the wording of a particular affirmation sounds silly to you, say it in a way that you feel comfortable with. You can also try saying it in an E.F.T. type manner using "Even though". For example, "Even though I'm still hard on myself, I'm moving toward treating my body and my mind with love and respect."
- ✓ Written in a way that allows you to create a feeling of belief as you say it, allowing you to say it with conviction.

Affirmations can be used in a variety of ways. The most common would be reading them aloud to yourself. You may wish to copy the affirmation pages that follow and post them on your wall, and then each morning and evening read through all the affirmations once. Alternatively, you may wish to choose one or two affirmations that really hit home with you and bring them with you into meditation.

Some other techniques for using affirmations include:

- ✓ Read through the list silently to yourself
- ✓ Re-write the affirmations several times while focusing on the meaning and the feeling of the affirmation as you write.
- ✓ Post a few affirmations in various locations around your home / car / office. Each time you pass by one of the locations you'll be reminded to say those affirmations to yourself.

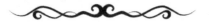

- ✓ Pay attention to your conversations and try to include affirmations whenever possible (and of course appropriate) while speaking with others.
- ✓ Record yourself saying the affirmations, and then play back the recording each night as you fall asleep.
- ✓ Compose a song to a tune you know well and use the affirmations as lyrics. Songs are memorable, allowing the affirmations to 'stick' much easier.

The following pages offer you a list of powerful healing affirmations for you to begin with.

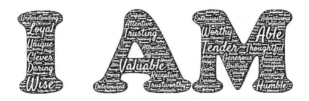

** I trust and believe in my body's innate ability to heal

** I treat my body and my mind with love and respect

** I am good to my body and my body is good to me

** I am disciplined in my exercises

** I eat nutritionally

** I sleep soundly

** I am supported and loved

** I take time to relax and rejuvenate

** I breathe deeply to oxygenate my cells

** My subconscious mind is my partner in healing

** I let go of all negative ideas about my body.

** I let go of all limiting concepts about myself.

** Healing energy is flowing freely and abundantly through my body

** I understand that my thoughts, positive or negative, create my reality and I therefore observe my thoughts and choose my words wisely

** I trust in the process of life. I am safe and taken care of.

** I now let go of all fears, guilt, frustration and anger

** I allow my life to unfold effortlessly and easily

** I am centered and in control

** I live with purpose and passion

** I am willing to do whatever it takes

** I accept this challenge as an opportunity to grow

** I am grateful for the new doors that are currently opening
for me

** I realize that everything happens for a reason and that that
reason is there to serve me in a positive manner

** I allow myself to stay focused on receiving healing energy,
even in the presence of painful symptoms.

** I let go of all sickness in my body. I don't need it anymore.

** I am willing to ask for help and to receive it

** I choose to be happy right now

** I am bigger than any obstacle

** I love and accept my body completely

** I am worthy and deserving of good health and happiness

** I maintain good posture in all my movements

** I fully let go of old, negative patterns for my physical body.

** I am strong and healthy, full of energy and vitality

** My back is completely healed and strong

** I forgive myself.

** I focus on positive outcomes

** I am in perfect health

** I love myself

LOVING ONESELF

Whether it's a physical or a mental state being healed, both involve opening oneself up to love - loving oneself, loving those around us who care (and even those who don't), and loving the part of us that is ill or hurts. To love that part of us that is causing pain can be scary, because it often means looking at it (how did **I** in some way cause this?), and then move on to acceptance, rather than resistance. Resistance only increases suffering. Acceptance allows us to understand, learn, and move through the pain.

When a child or loved one hurts, we instinctively want to do everything we can to make them feel better. The loving we give them during their hurt helps them in their healing. So if we know that this loving helps others, and it is what we naturally do for others, then why don't we do it for ourselves?

As children, when things went wrong, even if it had nothing to do with us, we perceived it as there was something wrong with us. These thoughts grow into 'I'm not good enough', and we learn to reject ourselves, instead of loving ourselves. Our inner dialogue as adults, if we listen carefully, is often that of us as a parent scolding our own inner child (negative self-talk). We instead need to nurture that child within, accept every part of him or her. Every one of us, no matter how young, old, man, woman, or self-reliant we are, needs love and acceptance. In every woman there's a tender little girl that needs help, and in every man is a little boy who needs warmth and affection.

> *"It is through healing our inner child, our inner children, by grieving the wounds that we suffered, that we can change our behavior patterns and clear our emotional process... The one who betrayed us and abandoned and abused us the most was ourselves... It is necessary to own and honor the child who we were in order to Love the person we are."*
>
> ~ Robert Burney

We are all born with love inside us. Self-love is our nature, and our birth right. As we've seen, somewhere between infancy and adulthood, many of us lose this connection to loving ourselves. We pick up messages as children that we're not good enough, we compare ourselves to societal standards that further that message, we've been wronged and hurt by people, and before we know it, our minds are full of negative self-talk, and feelings of unworthiness, guilt and inadequacy, and self-punishment pervade. This makes life harder than it needs to be, and it shows up with negative consequences in our health, relationships, and work life. Self-hatred, or being frustrated with oneself in any way, is not conducive to the positive energy required for healing. We need to be forgiving, not just of others, but of ourselves (including our inner child), and learn how to love ourselves again.

Learning to truly love oneself again isn't easy, but with awareness and effort we can get back to that place, and by doing so, we allow great inner healing to take place. The following are some ways for you to practice that rediscovery of self-love.

1. Begin your day with gratitude. Using either the daily journaling pages in this book or a separate gratitude journal, write down 5 to 10 things each morning that you are grateful for. There is so much to give thanks for – where you live, your health, your friends, sacrifices people have made for you in the past, your opportunities, etc. Beginning your day by giving thanks creates a positive vibration that opens the door to more positivity entering your life throughout the day.

2. Avoid negative distractions such as the news, gossip, and trash TV. As interesting as these may be they are not serving you in loving yourself. You don't need negative news every day. You don't need to live your life vicariously through people on TV. This is *your* life, not someone else's! Create your own positive and inspiring story – one that you can be proud of.

3. Meditate daily, and open your heart chakra. Spend even 5 minutes a day just sitting at peace, quieting your mind. You may choose to focus on one empowering thought (such as peace, love, gratitude, forgiveness, your accomplishments and successes, etc), or just sit with no thoughts at all. Chakra work is also beneficial - meditate on opening the back of your heart chakra and allowing pink loving light to enter and flow through your body as you accept yourself exactly as you are.

4. Use positive affirmations and self-talk. Allow yourself happy and loving messages throughout the day. *"I am perfect, complete and whole, just as I am"*.

5. Act with integrity. When we make a promise and don't keep it, or act not in integrity, we let ourselves down, our words lose their meaning, and our worth takes a hit. To truly reach self-love, we must have honor and keep our word.

6. Create a life of fun. Rediscover what excites you in life; what moments you enjoy most; your passions. Consciously add those moments and experiences into your life as best you can. When you build a life that you truly enjoy – one that fulfills you – that fulfillment helps with loving oneself.

7. Add meaning and purpose to your life. Find a way to contribute more – to others, to community, to a greater cause. With that sense of contribution and purpose comes a renewed sense of worth and love.

8. Even when things don't work out the way you would like, trust your intuition and keep having faith. Trust that things are happening the way they are meant to in order to serve a higher purpose. By fighting what we cannot change, we are only increasing our own suffering. Instead, accept, learn, and trust that whatever is happening is happening for a reason. When we find acceptance and peace so too do we find self-love.

9. Be patient with yourself. So things haven't happened for you as quickly as you had hoped. Again, things happen for a reason. Rather than fight the timing of events, accept it, and trust that everything is happening for a reason. Take a deep breath, smile, and know that everything will unfold at the time it is meant to unfold. In the meantime, you can love yourself.

10. Live in the present, and love what is. Living in the past takes away from the love you can be experiencing today. And worry and fear are emotions that only exist in the future. Those things haven't even happened, and they too take away from the love we can feel right here, right now.

11. Forgive. Holding on to resentment or regret only poisons our body and mind, while at the same time giving power to that which we resent. So let it go. Even if someone has done you wrong, forgive them, and love them. Keep practicing Ho'oponopono and the other forgiveness exercises presented in this book. And forgive yourself. Honor and be good to your inner child.

12. Believe in your worth. If someone doesn't believe in you , it doesn't matter – you are not what someone else's opinion is of you. If finances are rough, it doesn't matter – your net worth should not equal your self-worth. Your worth is only controlled by your thoughts. Believe you are worthy. Feel it and remind yourself daily. You are worthy of success, love, and abundance. When you embrace your own worthiness, you embrace self-love.

MY IDEAL HEALTH

If I were to describe my ideal health, including how I look, feel, and act, it would look like this:

_____

_____

_____

_____

_____

_____

_____

_____

_____

_____

_____

_____

_____

EGO vs SPIRIT

Our 'Ego' mind is the part of us that runs off pride, that needs to be right, that says "Once everything falls into place I will find peace". It is constantly striving for perfection, thereby exacerbating unhealthy levels of stress.

Our 'Spirit' mind on the other hand has no need for pride or for being right, as it is connected to a higher universal power. Knowing that everything happens perfectly as it should, it comes from a place of love and acceptance, and says "Find peace and everything will fall into place". By shifting our thoughts from ego to spirit we automatically become more at peace with ourselves, eliminating stress, and allowing for a healthier flow of energy.

Are you living in your ego or your spirit? Take the test on the next page. Comparing phrases in each column (left and right) on the following page, put a check mark beside the phrase that best describes your outlook. The total number of checkmarks in each column will show you how weighted you are in ego versus spirit. Following each category are questions to ask yourself to help you elevate your thinking away from ego and into that of spirit.

EGO

SPIRIT

GENERAL

____ I dwell on mistakes

____ I learn from mistakes

____ I complain about life

____ I am amazed by life

____ "You can't do that"

____ "How can I do that?"

What is the universe trying to teach me?

How can I be more flexible?

What is distracting me?

How can I be more accepting of what is?

MONEY

____ In business only to make money

____ In business to help people

____ Brag of success to elevate self

____Talk of success to inspire others

____"I can't afford that"

____ "How can I afford that?"

____Riches allow for self-gratification

____ Riches allow me to do more good

How can I serve the greatest number of people?

How can I give people what they want?

What's holding me back?

EGO

SPIRIT

RELATIONSHIPS

____ The other person is the problem   ____ By changing myself I influence others

____ My relationships are reactionary   ____ I sustain relationships with gratitude

____ Measure people by their mistakes   ___Measure people by their character

What can I learn and change about myself to make this relationship better?

What is this other person really feeling right now?

What am I grateful for in this relationship?

Why is this person perfect for me / how have they been the perfect guide for me in life?

HEALTH

____ I will do it tomorrow   ____ My daily actions create strength & health

____ I do it if it feels good   ____ Health comes from planning & commitment

____ Health & success are separate   ____ Health is key to my success

What can I do right NOW?

What can I do to eat/live better today?

How often do I tell myself 'Everything I need to heal is within me now?"

What is my body trying to tell me, and how can I use this to make me stronger?

VAKS Instructions

1. Think of a goal or affirmation. Allow 2 to 3 minutes to complete this activity. Begin by standing up and stating your goal or affirmation aloud one time.

2. **Visual**: Stretch your arms out in front of you and clasp your hands together, keeping your thumbs pointed upward. Imagine a sideways figure 8 in front of you. Starting in the middle, move your hands (together) to the top left of the 8 and continue the motion in the shape of the sideways 8, always moving your hands up through the middle of the 8. Without moving your head, have your eyes stare constantly at your moving thumbs while stating your affirmation once out loud on each rotation. Repeat this process for 30 seconds.

3. **Auditory**: Using your index finger and thumb, gently squeeze and massage the outer rim of both your ears simultaneously. Starting at the top of the ear, massage your way to the bottom, while keeping your eyes closed and repeating your affirmation. Repeat for 30 seconds.

4. **Kinesthetic**: Begin standing, arms raised and bent at the elbows. Slowly raise your left leg off the ground as you twist your body to bring your right elbow to your left knee. Alternate in a slow flowing motion for 30 seconds while continually saying your affirmation aloud. Warning: If this movement is difficult or uncomfortable, you may do this instead lying down. With your hands by your head and knees bent, lift one knee up while bring the opposite hand (not elbow) to meet it.

5. **Spirit**: With one hand on top of the other placed over your heart, close your eyes and repeat your affirmation aloud for 30 seconds while feeling the vibration of your voice and envisioning your affirmation being true.

SHIFTING FROM FEAR TO POSITIVITY

The human mind is programmed to feel fear – instinctively it serves to protect us from harm. However, when we let our fears run wild, they crowd out positive advancements, hinder achievement, and lure us toward the very thing we fear. We must learn to acknowledge that fears exist, and then turn them around to create positive outcomes. To begin, complete the sentences below. Write your answers quickly without putting too much thinking into them. Write the first thing that comes to mind.

I am afraid that

_____

_____

The thing I fear most about my health is that

_____

_____

I have been sabotaging the full extent of my healing progress because I am afraid that

_____

_____

Next, to shift those fears to create positive results, for each sentence above rewrite a positive intention on the following page as if the fear didn't exist. How would you think? What would you be feeling if that fear didn't exist?

For example:

I am afraid that *I will never be able to do XYZ again.*

Turn it around to:

I wake up feeling overjoyed every morning because I am once again doing XYZ and doing it better than I ever have.

Take control of your fears now by turning them around below:

_____

_____

_____

_____

_____

_____

_____

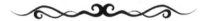

EMOTIONAL FREEDOM TECHNIQUE

EFT (Emotional Freedom Technique), also referred to as acu-tapping, is another method of releasing dysfunctional beliefs that hold us back from the health and life we deserve. EFT is a meridian based energy healing system working on the premise that "the cause of all negative emotions and beliefs is a disturbance in our body's energy system." Negative emotions cause disruptions in our flow of energy along these meridians, leading to the development of pain or disease. By tapping on specific areas along the meridian channels while making a specific statement, negative memories, emotions, and beliefs which block the natural flow of energy can be released. Acu-tapping can be done to you by someone else, or you can do it to yourself as well. A basic instruction is included below.

1. Bring to mind the problem you are facing at this time (the negative thought, fear, frustration, etc).

2. State the problem in an easy to remember phrase (think of it as creating a title for a movie). For example:
     * I felt alone & unloved when my father abandoned me.
     * I have a nagging pain in my right shoulder

3. On a scale of 1 to 10 how would you rate the intensity of this feeling, in other words, how much is it bothering you (10 being the greatest intensity).

4. Create a Self-Acceptance affirmation phrase using the format: "Even though (insert the phrase you created in step #2), I deeply and profoundly accept myself."

5. Locate the point at the side of your hand just below your pinky finger where you would hit if you were to do a karate chop. Rapidly tap this point using 2 or 3 fingers from your other hand while stating three times the Self-Acceptance Affirmation Phrase.

6.   Next, you will go through a series of tapping each of the points shown on the diagram below while stating the Problem Phrase (from step #2). Simply tap quickly with 2 or 3 fingers on each point as you say the problem phrase once, and then move on to the next point. It does not matter the order of points, nor which side of the body you choose to work on (there is no need to repeat actions on the other side of the body). There is also a point on your wrist, the width of 3 fingers below the inside crease formed between your arm and hand, that should be tapped as well (in this case patting the point with your whole hand). Once you've tapped all 9 points, this is considered one complete pass. Then do another complete pass, beginning with the Self-Acceptance Affirmation Phrase on your karate chop point (Step #5).

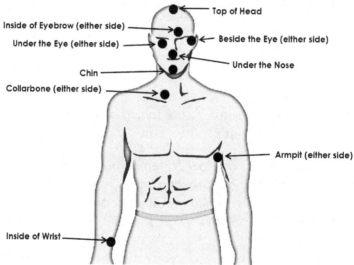

7.   After 2 complete passes, reassess the intensity of your feelings. Has it gone down at all? If you notice a drop by 1 or 2 points, then the EFT is working for you. Continue with steps 4 through 6 until you bring the intensity down to zero or as low as you can. If you are noticing improvement, it's important to adjust your phrases to acknowledge your progress.   Adjust your Self-Acceptance Affirmation to "Even though I still have some (insert problem phrase), I deeply and completely accept myself". Adjust the Problem Phrase during the tapping to incorporate the word 'Remaining', for example "I have remaining pain in my right shoulder."

This is not presented as a complete study on EFT as that is beyond the scope of this book. However these basic steps can certainly get you started on the road to emotional healing through the benefits of acutapping.

PRAYER

A few healing prayers are presented on the following pages. Choose the ones that resonate most with you. Depending on your religious beliefs, feel free to substitute the word 'Universe' with 'Lord' or vice versa, or any other name to which a higher power is represented to you.

(1) [The Footprints Prayer]: One night I had a dream... I dreamed I was walking along the beach with the Lord, and Across the sky flashed scenes from my life. For each scene I noticed two sets of footprints in the sand; One belonged to me, and the other to the Lord. When the last scene of my life flashed before us, I looked back at the footprints in the sand. I noticed that many times along the path of my life, There was only one set of footprints. I also noticed that it happened at the very lowest and saddest times in my life This really bothered me, and I questioned the Lord about it. "Lord, you said that once I decided to follow you, You would walk with me all the way; But I have noticed that during the most troublesome times in my life, There is only one set of footprints. I don't understand why in times when I needed you the most, you should leave me. The Lord replied, "My precious, precious child. I love you, and I would never, never leave you during your times of trial and suffering. When you saw only one set of footprints, It was then that I carried you.

~

(2) Lord, I come before you today in need of your healing hand. In you all things are possible. Hold my heart within yours, and renew my mind, body, and soul. I am lost, but I am singing. You gave us life, and you also give us the gift of infinite joy. Give me the strength to move forward on

the path you've laid out for me. Guide me towards better health, and give me the wisdom to identify those you've placed around me to help me get better. In your name I pray, Amen.

~

(3) Universe, I hurt, my body isn't functioning as it needs to function. I am in pain. But you already know all that. I'm not coming to tell you what is wrong, but to ask you to do what is right and best for me. As it fits your plan, heal me, mend my body and my mind, and grant me days of better health and renewed strength. As I wait, give me an extra measure of patience, endurance, and perseverance. When my energy to press forward is lacking, pour your power into me like a fresh mountain stream flowing into a beautiful lake. Universe I know you are able to heal, I know it with utmost confidence. Grant me now the wisdom to understand your timing and the courage to accept your healing as sufficient for the moment.

~

(4) Lord, heal me. Heal me in whatever You see needs healing. Heal me of whatever might separate me from You. Heal my memory, heal my heart, heal my emotions, heal my spirit, heal my body, heal my soul. Lay Your hands gently upon me and heal me through Your love for me. Amen.

HABITS

UNHEALTHY HABITS	HEALTHY HABITS
Going to bed late or at odd hours	
Sleeping in late	
Smoking	
Watching TV excessively	
Overworking	
Road rage	
Losing one's temper in general	
Aimlessly surfing the Internet	
Addicted to watching the news	
Using drugs or alcohol	
Negative self talk	
Not taking time to reflect or meditate	
Eating an unhealthy diet	
Getting distracted easily	
Living or working in mess / clutter	
Obsessing over worries and problems	
Telling lies to yourself or others	

Skipping breakfast	
Nail biting	
Staying in an unhealthy relationship or social circle	
Not feeling good enough or feeling worthy (not loving yourself)	
Seeing things only as black or white	
Not being able to say 'no'	
Small mindedness	
Taking negative comments personally	
Blaming others or ignoring personal responsibility	
Having to be 'perfect'	
Holding on to anger or resentment (not forgiving)	
Refusing to look at (or work on) one's weaknesses	
Being resentment of people who are richer / healthier / 'better' than you	
Exposing yourself to harmful chemicals and toxins	
Poor hygiene (oral or otherwise)	
Not exercising (being physically lazy)	
Greed	
Constantly feeling stressed	
Physically hurting yourself	

DREAMS TO FULFILL

It often takes our comfortable life as we've known it being taken away from us before we realize how precious every day is, and for that matter our lives. Having a serious injury or illness gives us a chance to reflect on our lives, and quite often during these times we find ourselves begging for a second chance. If you're given that second chance are you going to take it? Are you going to do all those things you've always dreamed of doing? Without a clear direction or goal the winds of change will continue to blow you around and you may never get to realize your dreams or, worse yet, you'll even forget what they were. View this experience as a blessing, for this is your chance to get clear again on your life, your dreams, the things that inspire you, those things which wake you up in the morning looking forward to a new day and the future. Focusing on these dreams will build up a kinetic energy inside of you that will explode into potential and momentum once you're given that second chance and 'released' back into health.

Begin by taking some time to reflect on and answer the questions on the following pages. They will give you an idea of why you are here, and what you are all about. Then, on the subsequent page, begin recording all those things you want in your life, the activities you enjoy doing or would like to do, places you'd like to see, lives you'd like to touch, legacies you'd like to leave....

When you were a child, what did you want to be once you grew up?

_____

_____

_____

Who are the 3 people who've had the biggest influence on your life, and why?

_____

_____

_____

Think of a moment when you are the happiest you can ever be in your life. What are you doing that is making you so happy?

_____

_____

_____

What do you think are your greatest strengths?

_____

_____

_____

_____

What more can you do in life to maximize your strengths?

_____

_____

_____

If there is a piece of wisdom that you have learned from your life to date and could pass on to the world, what would it be?

_____

_____

_____

What do you value the most in your life?

_____

_____

_____

What is it that you would really like to do with your life?

_____

_____

_____

Given a second chance, dreams I want to fulfill are:

_____

_____

_____

_____

_____

_____

_____

_____

(continue onto the next page...)

Record all the dreams and things you want in your life, the activities you would like to do, places you'd like to see, lives you'd like to touch, legacies you'd like to leave....

DREAM   **ACHIEVE BY**

_____

_____

_____

_____

_____

_____

_____

_____

_____

_____

_____

_____

_____

_____

_____

_____

_____

_____

_____

My IDEAL DAY

Describe your ideal day being healthy. What would you be doing, with whom, and when? How do you spend your morning? Your afternoon? Your evening? Who is part of your life, and who do you connect with? What are your accomplishments for the day? Have fun with this, use your imagination, and dream big.

_____

_____

_____

_____

_____

_____

_____

_____

_____

_____

_____

_____

_____

_____

_____

_____

SUPPORTIVE vs UNSUPPORTIVE ACTIVITIES

Every day we do things that support us as well as things that don't support us. This is true for all areas of our life – business, relationships, and health. So many of these activities have become so habitual it's easy to not even recognize the benefit or detriment they bring. It's therefore important to reflect from time to time on just what supportive and unsupportive activities we do daily.

A few weeks ago you did the exercise on habits. Have you reduced your unhealthy habits? Have you added in new healthy habits? Today, write down 6 activities you do regularly that support you in your health goals. Are you able to do any of these more often? What are 3 more positive activities you could do but currently aren't that would support you in your health goals?

1. _____

2. _____

3. _____

4. _____

5. _____

6. _____

(one more): _____

(one more): _____

(one more): _____

(continued on next page)....

Next, write down 6 activities you are still doing regularly that are NOT supporting you in your health goals. For this exercise set aside any beliefs about food or excuses you may have. You know the right answers inside of you. Which of these activities, starting today, will you vow to stop doing, or at least do less of. Remember, it's your health we're talking about.

1. _____

2. _____

3. _____

4. _____

5. _____

6. _____

ANGER JOURNALING

Although this process may seem like a stretch to some, it can be a powerfully positive experience. I am going to ask you to commit 100% to this exercise for the next 3 days. If after that time you have not felt the benefits, you are free to stop. If you find it useful, then you may continue on your own as often as you wish. You may use either the space provided here or a separate sheet of paper, perhaps even a private journal. For at least 3 full minutes you will write non-stop whatever anger comes out. Allow yourself to write whatever comes to mind without any analyzing or thinking (also known as stream of consciousness writing). Do not edit spelling or grammar, and do not censor words or thoughts just because they shock you. If it's in your mind it needs to come out, and there is no safer place than your sheet of paper. You may find that your handwriting changes; or that much of what you write is illegible. This doesn't matter. Just continue writing without stopping.

Once you are done, you may choose to review what you've written, or not. You may choose to keep it stored somewhere private, or shred or burn it. This is for no one else to ever read but yourself. Therefore it does not matter what you write or if you choose to dispose of it after.

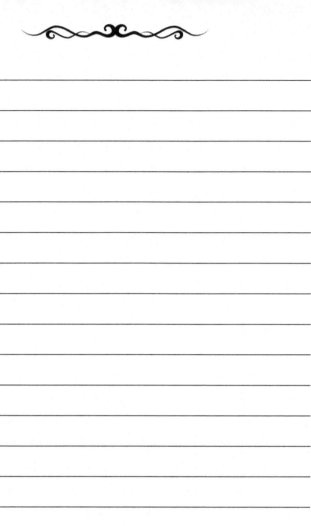

BASIC LIVER CLEANSE

This is a basic 1 week liver cleanse (as outlined in Week 3) that can help rejuvenate your liver, one of the most important organs for the overall health of your body.

The Program

For the course of each of the next 7 days:

1. AVOID ALL of the following: Meat, Sugar, Gluten, Alcohol, Dairy (probiotic yogurt is ok), Salt (sea salt or Himalayan salt is ok), Nuts, Caffeine, Wheat, and Processed Foods.

2. Drink an amount equal to half of your body weight (in ounces) of water and apple juice. Half to 1L should be unsweetened apple juice. The balance should be pure, room temperature water. (In other words, if your weight is 150lbs, then you'll be drinking 75oz of these liquids. 1L is about 33oz. In this case you might drink 3/4L unsweetened apple juice and about 1.5L of water. This high liquid consumption is imperative. Start the day with a glass of lemon water.

3. In addition, you'll drink 1 to 2 glasses of beet juice per day. Use a juicer (ideally, if you have one), or otherwise a blender with extra water as a base. The basic recipe will use 1-2 peeled beets (start with 1, work up to 2), 1 cored apple, and ½ squeezed lemon. In addition, you can also experiment adding any of the following for extra flavor: freshly squeezed orange juice, ginger, nutmeg, cinnamon, stevia. (Drinking this beet juice is essential as it helps stimulate the genesis of new liver cells).

4. Also in addition, have a cup or two of any of these teas throughout the day: dandelion root, peppermint, fennel, green or wormwood.

5. Drinking a daily cup of nettle infusion is also a good idea. Into an empty bottle or large canning jar pour a quart of boiling water over 1 cup of dried nettles. Allow to stand for at least four hours before drinking, storing the remainder for drinking on subsequent days.

6. Your meals for this week will be limited to greens (smoothies or salads). Specifically, any combination of broccoli, sprouts, cabbage, avocado, asparagus, artichoke, Spirulina, blue-green algae, kale, and any other dark green leafy vegetable. Fermented foods (such as organic sauerkraut) as also fine. Yes, you'll be eating less than usual,

but that's the idea. Not stuffing yourself with so much food allows the liver a chance to rest a bit and catch up on the important work it has to do.

7. Take a teaspoon of apple cider vinegar mixed with water before meals.

8. Supplement with either psyllium husk or flaxseed (these could be added to your beet juice is desired). Additional beneficial supplements can include turmeric, food grade diatomaceous earth, garlic, desiccated liver, and milk thistle. If you're able to source some He Shou We (from your local Chinatown), it's a great liver tonic – boil it in a bit of water for about 45 minutes and then add the resulting water to your tea.

9. Take a good probiotic daily. Yogurt with active bacteria culture is also acceptable.

Note: As your liver cleans out you may feel worse before you feel better. The first few days might be hard, and you might be hungry, but stick with it for as long as you can – at minimum for 5 days if you can't do 7.

VISION BOARD

Creating a vision board will give you inspiration, a clear direction, greater energy, and will further amplify your reasons to heal. You've already learned that the bigger your 'why' the smaller the 'how' becomes. The vision board is another tool to make your 'why' even bigger.

Having a dream in the back of your mind is one thing, but visually seeing it on paper every day in front of you helps bring it closer to reality. Making your own vision board is not only a powerful tool for manifesting the things you want in your life, but it's also a lot of fun in the process. Before beginning your vision board, it's recommended that you spend at least a week or so filling in your 'Dreams to Fulfill' in the previous section. Now you're ready. On page 279, begin drawing an image of what you want your life to look like. It doesn't matter if you can draw or not, there are no prizes for best picture, no one needs to see this but you. Draw in the objects / feelings / people / achievements etc you'd like to have in your life, even if they are just representations. How do you see yourself? Be as creative as possible. The images can all be separate, or you can make them flow together into a unified scene. It doesn't matter. Draw what speaks to you. Go back to the child inside you and color in the picture with markers or crayons. You don't need to get it perfect right away, you can always come back and add to it.

Once you're satisfied with your Vision Board reflecting how you'd love your life to be, rip it out of this workbook and post it on your fridge, bedroom wall, desk, or wherever you'll see it on a daily basis. Then spend a few moments each day reflecting on your Vision Board, seeing the amazing life that lies ahead of you, see what it looks like, feel how it feels, smell how it smells. The more real you can make it the more your inner mind will help manifest it.

Down the road you can take this a step further by purchasing magazines of topics that inspire you and cutting out images from these magazines. Buy a large piece of construction paper (Bristol board) and glue these images on top.

PERSONAL VISION STATEMENT

Your personal vision statement concisely represents what you want to be, do, feel, associate with and accomplish at some future date. The statement may be one sentence, or it may be 3 or 4, and can include several areas of your life (physical, mental, social, spiritual, emotional, recreational, career, etc). The statement, although it is occurring at a future date, is written in the present tense. As you begin to write it, answering the following questions first will help give you some guidance.

What are some of your favorite activities (things you could do all day long every day and never get tired of)?

_____

_____

_____

What do you need to do every day to feel fulfilled?

_____

_____

What are 4 or 5 of your core values?

_____

_____

If you never had to work another day in your life, how would you spend your time?

_____

_____

_____

_____

What must you do in this lifetime to not feel regret when it comes to an end?

_____

_____

_____

_____

What strengths do you see in yourself? And what strengths have others seen in you?

_____

_____

_____

_____

Excellent. Now you're ready to start combining all this information into your vision statement. The following is an example only, simply to give you an idea of what one looks like.

> I wake up each morning to the sound of the ocean outside and our children playing. After my successful financial career I now spend my time helping others through philanthropy. My wife and I travel regularly, and when we're home we enjoy playing golf and hosting dinner parties for our friends. I am grateful and proud of all my accomplishments, and the adventures I have fully lived.

Now it's your turn. Write your personal vision statement on the following page:

My Personal Vision Statement

_____

_____

_____

_____

_____

_____

_____

_____

_____

_____

_____

_____

_____

_____

_____

_____

_____

_____

_____

_____

_____

_____

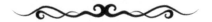

MY LEGACY

There are many forms of writing legacy letters out there, most of which have more to do with passing on a message to a future generation as part of a will or departure letter. This is not what we are going to create here. While others in the future will feel its influence, the purpose of writing your legacy here is more to serve as a life-guide for you.

This is about you getting clarity, as you go forward from here, on what legacy you want to leave behind. As you write it, think about the following:

> What have you done already, and what do you still want to create and achieve in this life?

> Who have you, and who do you still want to, touch / inspire / help?

> What important dreams lay dormant inside you that will simply die with you if you don't act on them?

> How do you want to be remembered?

Imagine, today was your last day alive, and just before you depart you meet the YOU you could have been. How does that feel? If it feels painful, there is no better time to start than today. And yes, today! Every day we have the same excuses, and they will be there tomorrow as well. Why is starting tomorrow any better than starting today? This is your opportunity, in the here and now, to begin creating your future, your life, your legacy.

On the following page, write your legacy.

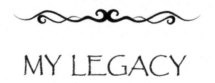

MY LEGACY

DOCTOR / THERAPIST LOG

During this time you may be introduced to various doctors and therapists, some better than others. Use this page to record the names of those people who stand out as unique or exceptional in their ability to heal in case one day you'd like to refer back to them.

Name	Therapy	Phone or Email	Notes

PART 3:

GUT HEALING

and

ELIMINATION

DIET

RECIPES

By Aga Postawska

THE ELIMINATION DIET

What is an elimination diet? Well, it's all in the title: you eliminate certain foods for a period of time, usually three or four weeks, then slowly reintroduce those specific foods and monitor your symptoms for adverse reactions. If you observe a negative response, congratulations, you've just identified a food sensitivity, food that is silently damaging your gut and robbing you of your health and vitality.

When choosing to do an elimination diet you have plenty of options of how you can go about doing it. Either removing 1 specific food, such as bread, an entire group of food such as gluten containing grains, or removing multiple groups of foods at once such as the most popular allergens and irritants: sugar, gluten, dairy, soy, corn, and eggs.

You can refer to the list below to see what foods are typically included and removed during an intense elimination diet. Once you've chosen what you'd like to remove, completely cut that food out of your diet for 21 days. The more diligent you are the better, and louder, of a response you'll get back from your body when you re-introduce that food again in 3 weeks.

ELIMINATION DIET FOOD LIST

Foods	Include	Exclude
Grains	whole gluten free grains like: buckwheat, millet, brown rice, amaranth	Wheat, corn, barley, spelt, kamut, rye, oats, white rice, all gluten-containing products
Nuts		*Peanuts, all nuts
Dairy	coconut milk	Milk, cheese, cream, yoghurt, butter, ice cream,
Legumes		Soybeans, tofu, tempeh, soy milk, all beans, peas, lentils
Fats	olive oil, flaxseed oil, coconut oil	margarine, butter, processed and hydrogenated oils, mayonnaise
Meat and fish	fish, turkey, lamb, wild game	beef, chicken, pork, eggs, cold cuts, bacon, hotdogs, canned meat, sausage, shellfish, meat subtitles made from soy

Vegetables		night shades: tomatoes, eggplant, potatoes, peppers (sweet potato, yams are okay)
Fruit		citrus fruits: orange, pineapple, lemon, lime
Sweeteners	Stevia	white or brown sugar, honey, make syrup, agave nectar, high fructose corn syrup, desserts
Spices/ Condiments	sea salt, fresh ground pepper, fresh herbs and spices: garlic, dill, oregano, rosemary, thyme, turmeric, ginger, parsley, cilantro	ketchup, mustard, relish, chutney, soy sauces, BBQ sauce, vinegar
Beverages	filtered water, loose leaf herbal teas(caffeine free): peppermint, chamomile, rooibos,	alcohol, caffeine (coffee, black and green tea, soda, tonic water, sparkling water, carbonated drinks)

RE-INTRODUCTION

After the 21 days is up, to reintroduce a food, continue following the elimination diet, but add in one food you eliminated 3 times a day for 3 days.

For example, after 3 weeks of cutting out gluten, eat a piece of toast for breakfast, a sandwich at lunch time and then maybe a little bit of pasta with dinner. During those 3 days it's important to be food journaling. Write down what you ate and how you feel: physically, emotionally, and mentally.

Pay careful attention to any symptoms experienced such as joint pain, headaches, sinus issues, foggy thinking, fatigue, nausea, skin issues, poor sleep, mood swings, and anxiety.

If you experience any symptoms of discomfort or dis-ease this means that this food is creating an inflammatory and immune response. Your body has a sensitivity or intolerance to it and your digestive tract isn't in a healthy state to properly and safely digest it at this moment. Avoid your identified food sensitivities for 3-6 months.

Now, you don't necessarily have to avoid this food forever. Just wait a complete of months, give yourself the time for your gut to heal, and then reintroduce it at a later time to see how you react then.

BUILDING A STRONG NUTRITIONAL FOUNDATION

The elimination diet still remains the gold standard for identifying food sensitivities in the alternative medicine fields of nutritionists, health coaches, naturopaths, functional medicines doctors, and even acupuncturists.

Why not just get food allergy testing done? Well, it's often expensive and unreliable. On the other hand an elimination diet is easy to do and empowering because you do it, not someone in a laboratory. Plus, you experience the results first-hand, which is a powerful motivator for future dietary changes. It's a lot more empowering to feel the difference food is making in your life rather than a written diagnoses of do's and don'ts from some complete stranger.

Following fad diets, dogmatic views on nutrition, and bias dietary advice from health professionals can sometimes do you more harm than good because 'every body' has a unique biological and metabolic make-up, each needing different forms of nutrition. An elimination diet allows you to see and feel what really works for you, what's nourishing your body and what's causing you harm. By using this method, you can build a strong nutritional foundation that is tailored to your individual needs.

Try an easy round of an elimination diet for yourself, remove just one food item, and see how it goes. Play detective, be curious, listen to what your body has to say, and most importantly have fun!

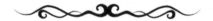

The Elimination Diet Recipe Plan

Sometimes the elimination diet can seem a bit overwhelming, especially as you are first transitioning from an unbalanced SAD diet to a healthier way of eating. With so many things that you can't eat, sometimes you may wonder what you can eat. The good news is that the elimination diet is not only better for your health, it can be delicious, too! To help get you started, here you can find a whole week's worth of recipes for breakfast, lunch and dinner – and even tasty snacks and desserts! These recipes assume you are trying the basic elimination of the five most common allergens from your diet – wheat, dairy, soy, corn and sugar.

Bon appetit!

BREAKFAST

FLAXSEED PORRIDGE

<u>Base ingredients</u>
2 tbsp. ground flax
2 tbsp. chia seeds
2 tbsp. of hemp hearts
1 tbsp. ground almonds
1 tbsp. coconut oil

OPTIONAL ADDITIONS	SUPERFOOD ADDITIONS	SWEETENERS
coconut milk	maca	fruits
almond milk	ashwaganda	stevia
nuts and nut butters	cacao powder	raw unpasteurized
banana	vanilla bean powder	honey
berries	spirulina (added when	molasses
cinnamon	porridge is cooled)	
cardamom		

<u>Method</u>
Mix base ingredients with your choice of additions and hot water to desired consistency. This recipe is great for an on-the-go breakfast, as you can pre-mix in a container and just add water.

TROPICAL COCO-QUINOA "OATMEAL"

Ingredients

1/2 cup cooked quinoa	1/4 cup chia seeds
1/2 cup coconut milk	1/2 sliced banana
2 tbsp. chopped walnuts	1 mango
Handful of pumpkin seeds	Pinch of Himalayan sea salt
1/4 cup ground flax	Cinnamon to taste

Method

Prepare the quinoa the night before. Bring 1 cup of water to a boil and then add quinoa. Cook for 10-15 minutes, until all the water has been absorbed and the quinoa has released its rings. It is a good idea to make extra when preparing quinoa, as it is delicious in salads and added to the side of any dinner dish.

In the morning, heat up the coconut milk and pour in the quinoa, cook until warm and the quinoa is tender again.

Preheat the oven to 350 degrees F (180 degrees C) and roast the walnuts and pumpkin seeds on a baking sheet for about 5 minutes, until they are golden brown.

Once the quinoa and coconut milk mixture is warmed, pour it into a bowl and top with the reminding ingredients. You can sweeten it with unpasteurized organic honey, maple syrup or molasses.

GREEN MONKEY PANCAKES

Ingredients

1 green plantain	Pinch of salt
5-6 kale leaves	1 tbsp. ground flaxseed
Handful of walnuts	Stevia or honey to sweeten
2 organic free range eggs	Coconut oil

Method

Combine all ingredients in a food processor to make a thick dough and fry on low heat with coconut oil.

You can enjoy your green monkey pancakes with some coconut milk kefir, lemon or lime, cinnamon or cardamom.

EGGS IN AVOCADO "TOAST"

Ingredients
2 organic free range eggs
1 avocado
Salt & pepper

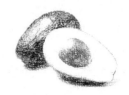

Optional additions
Nutritional yeast
Spices such as cayenne, paprika, thyme, rosemary or whatever you like
    with your eggs
Fresh herbs like basil, cilantro or green onion

Method
Slice an avocado in half and remove the pit. Scoop out a few tablespoons of avocado flesh from each side, to make enough room for an egg.

Crack an egg into the hole in each half of the avocado. Top with salt, pepper and your choice of optional additions, then place in a preheated oven at 250 degrees F (120 C) for 3-5 minutes, depending on how cooked you like your eggs.

You can serve with slices of tomato, cucumber and bell pepper if you wish. You can also fry up some organic humanely raised bacon in ghee with a handful of crimini mushrooms.

TORTANG TALONG (EGGPLANT OMELETTE)

Tortang Talong is a traditional breakfast dish from the Philippines. The eggplant adds an impressive spectrum of nutrients to your morning meal: vitamins C, K and B6, fiber, folate, potassium, manganese, phosphorus, copper, thiamin, niacin, magnesium and pantothenic acid.

Ingredients
2 or 3 baby or Japanese eggplants
3 organic free range eggs
1 tbsp. coconut oil
Salt and pepper

Optional additions
Diced onion and tomato
Nutritional yeast

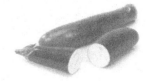

Method

Place 1 eggplant, skin still on, in a fry pan over a medium-high heat. Cook one side for 1-2 minutes, until slightly softened and the skin is evenly charred. Rotate and repeat for the other sides. The whole process should take about 4-5 minutes per eggplant. Remove from the heat and repeat with the remaining eggplants. When they've cooled, use a knife to peel off the skin.

Next, beat the eggs in a shallow bowl. Season with salt and pepper. Place 1 eggplant in the mix, and using a fork to gently squash the flesh so the eggplant is flat but still remains attached to the stalk. This is key – the stalk adds to the visual aesthetics of the dish.

Scoop the egg mixture onto the eggplant, ensuring it is coated, and place your additional toppings. Allow to soak for about a minute.

Meanwhile, heat the oil in a frying pan over medium-high heat. Once hot, gently slide the eggplant into the pan. Cook for about 1-2 minutes on each side until golden. Repeat with remaining eggplants, soaking them in the egg mixture, adding toppings and frying until golden.

MEXI-VEGGIE SCRAMBLE

Ingredients

2 tbsp. chopped red or white onion
Handful of your favorite mushrooms, chopped
1/2 bell pepper
1 tomato
1 clove of garlic

2 organic free range eggs
coconut oil or ghee
1 tbsp. cumin
1 teaspoon paprika
Cilantro to garnish
Nutritional yeast (optional)

Method

Chop the mushrooms and vegetables into bite-sized pieces. Heat the oil or ghee in a fry pan, then add the onions and cook for 3-5 minutes. Add the mushrooms, bell pepper, tomato and garlic. Cook for 3-5 minutes until the vegetables are tender. In a separate bowl, beat the eggs with the cumin and paprika and then pour into the frying pan. Cook to your desired consistency of egg scramble. Serve hot with fresh cilantro garnish.

GREEN SMOOTHIE

Ingredients

1 cup coconut or almond milk
Handful of your favorite nuts, such as almonds, cashews or walnuts
Handful of spinach
2 kale leaves, stems removed

1 banana
Half an avocado
Handful of frozen berries of your choice
1/2 inch cube of ginger

Optional superfood additions

chia seeds
hemp hearts
ground flaxseed

spirulina
maca
matcha

Method

Combine all the ingredients in a blender and blend until smooth.

You can use frozen banana to give the smoothie a cooler and creamier texture, or adjust the amount of coconut or nut milk to achieve your preferred consistency.

LUNCH

Cream of Mushroom Soup

This recipe has 3 parts because we are making it from scratch.

Vegetable Soup Stock

To make about 4 cups of veggie stock you'll need:

1 big onion	1 bunch of parsley
6-8 cloves of garlic	A few bay leaves
3 carrots	Sea salt
5 celery sticks	10 peppercorns

Roughly chop the vegetables and cover with water in a pot. Bring to a boil, then reduce heat and simmer for 30 minutes to an hour. Strain and enjoy your homemade vegetable stock. It is a good idea to make a big batch that you can use in many different recipes.

Cashew Cream

Ingredient: 1 cup raw cashews

Soak 1 cup of raw cashews in hot water for 30 minutes. Drain and add to a blender. Blend slowly, adding just enough water to get the blades moving and create a thick cream-like consistency.

Main Recipe

Ingredients

1 medium onion	2-3 tbsp. ghee or olive oil
6-8 cloves of garlic	Salt and pepper
2-3 big handfuls of brown button mushrooms	Your choice of spices, such as thyme, cayenne, paprika,
4-5 cups vegetable stock	cumin,
1 cup cauliflower, finely chopped or pulsed in a food processor	pepper

Method

Chop the onion and fry for 10 minutes in olive oil or ghee. When the onions start to become transparent, add the garlic and mushrooms with a 1/2 cup of veggie stock. Cook for another 10 minutes.

Add the cauliflower. Food-processed cauliflower can add to the creamy consistency of the soup. Add the remaining veggie stock, salt, pepper and your choice of spices, experimenting to achieve a flavor that you love. Bring to boil, then reduce the heat to a simmer.

If you like a creamy consistency in your soup, put half of the soup into a blender and blend until smooth. Then return it to the pot with the rest of the soup. Simmer for an additional 10 minutes.

Serve with a spoonful of delicious cashew cream. You can also garnish with fresh herbs such as fennel or dill.

Focaccia Flatbread Sandwich

Bread ingredients
 1 cup almond flour
 3/4 cup arrow root flour
 1/4 cup ground flaxseed
 1 tsp. baking soda
 2 organic free range eggs

1/3 cup almond milk
Herbs such as rosemary and thyme
 (you can use oregano for a great pizza base)
Salt and pepper to taste

Method
Combine all the ingredients except the herbs in a bowl. The mix will be more watery than your typical bread batter. Pour onto a baking sheet lined with parchment paper and spread evenly. Top with your desired herbs and spices. Bake for 15 minutes in an oven preheated to 350F (180C).

Remove from oven and cool. Cut into slices as desired for sandwiches, flatbread or panini.

Add your favorite vegetables or sandwich ingredients, such as tomato slices, cucumbers, avocado, olives, lettuce, hard boiled eggs, bell peppers, jalapenos, crispy chicken left overs (see recipe under dinners).

Tabouli Twist Summer Salad
Ingredients
 1 1/2 cup water
 1/2 tsp. sea salt
 1 cup of quinoa
 4 large tomatoes or 1 pint of cherry
  tomatoes
 2 Persian cucumbers or 1 long English cucumber

1 stalk of celery
1 bunch of cilantro
2 handfuls of red grapes
5 tbsp. olive oil
Juice of 2 lemons
1/2 tsp. ground black pepper

Method

In a medium saucepan, bring the water to a boil. Then add the quinoa and reduce heat to medium-low. Cover and simmer until the quinoa is tender, about 10 minutes. The quinoa is done when the rings begin to loosen from the seed. Remove from heat, cover and stand for 5 minutes. Let cool.

Finely chop the tomatoes, cucumbers, celery, cilantro and grapes and place them in salad bowl.

Combine the olive oil, freshly squeezed lemon juice, salt and pepper, then pour over the salad. Stir in the cooled quinoa and serve.

You can make this the night before, at it tastes better the longer it sits. You can serve with hardboiled eggs or avocado on the side. Try using parsley instead of cilantro and adding some fresh mint.

Turkey Taco Wraps

Ingredients

1/2 onion, finely chopped
1 tbsp. ghee or olive oil
500grams organic ground turkey
1 tsp. garlic powder
1 tsp. cumin
1 tsp. paprika
1 tsp. chili powder
1/2 tsp. oregano

1/2 bell pepper
1/2 cup water
4 oz. can of tomato sauce (gluten free)
A few large romaine or iceberg lettuce leaves to use as 'taco shells'
Cilantro & nutritional yeast to garnish

Method

Heat the oil or ghee in a large skillet and fry the onion for 5-10 minutes until it becomes transparent. Add the turkey, breaking it up as it cooks. When it is no longer pink, add the spices including garlic powder, cumin, paprika, chili powder and oregano.

Add the pepper, water and tomato sauce (or fermented ketchup) and cover. Simmer on low for about 20 minutes.

Wash and dry the lettuce of your choice. Create little taco shells with the leaves and add the meat in the center. Garnish with nutritional yeast and cilantro. Great to serve with salsa and guacamole.

Zucchini Boats

Ingredients

1 zucchini
1 small onion, chopped
4 cloves of garlic, minced
1/2 bunch of cilantro, finely chopped
3-4 crimini mushrooms, chopped
2 kale leaves, stems removed and chopped

1/2 orange bell pepper
2 tsp. cumin
1 tsp. paprika
1 tsp. coriander
Salt and pepper to taste
2 tbsp. nutritional yeast
2 tbsp. of ghee or olive oil

Method

Preheat the oven to 400 degrees F (200C).

Cut the zucchini in half lengthwise and scoop out the flesh. Set aside the zucchini boats.

Chop the scooped zucchini flesh, onion, garlic, cilantro, mushrooms, kale and pepper, then sauté in a frying pan over medium-high heat in 1 tbsp. olive oil for 5-8 until tender. While cooking, season the veggies with cumin, paprika, coriander, salt and pepper.

Place the zucchini boats in a greased pan, flesh side up. Fill the boats with the cooked vegetable mixture and drizzle with remaining olive oil. Bake for about 25 minutes or until the zucchinis is tender.

Garnish with nutritional yeast and serve.

Black Bean Quinoa Burgers

Ingredients

1 (12 oz.) can of black beans, drained and rinsed
1/2 cup cooked quinoa
1/2 onion, chopped
3 cloves garlic, chopped
1 tsp. cumin

1 tsp. paprika
1/2 tsp. coriander
1/2 tsp. Himalayan salt
1/2 tsp. freshly ground pepper
1 tablespoon nutritional yeast
1 tbsp. olive oil

Method

Preheat the oven to 400 degrees F (200C).

Combine all the ingredients except for oil in a bowl and mash to make a dough-like mixture. Shape the dough into 4 equal patties no more than 1/2 an inch thick.

In an oven-safe saucepan, cook the patties on high heat in olive oil to brown each side.

Transfer them to the oven. If you don't have an oven-safe saucepan, transfer them into a glass casserole dish with additional oil. Bake for 15-20 minutes.

Serve over fresh greens and avocado slices.

Veggie Frittata

Ingredients

7 large organic free ranges eggs
1 packed cup of kale, stems removed and finely shredded
1 packed cup baby spinach, finely shredded
2 medium-sized carrots, grated
1 large zucchini, grated
1 small bell pepper (red, orange or yellow), diced

1/2 onion, finely chopped
4 cloves garlic, minced
2 tbsp. of dried herbs, such as basil, rosemary, thyme or oregano
1 tbsp. olive oil
5 tbsp. coconut flour
Pinch of sea salt or pink Himalayan salt
Pinch black pepper

Method

Pre-heat a fan-forced oven to 150°F (65C).

In a bowl, whisk the eggs and then add the vegetables, garlic, herbs and olive oil. Mix well.

Add coconut flour, salt and pepper. Mix and let stand for 5 minutes to allow the coconut flour to absorb any excess liquid.

Spoon the mixture into a lined or greased baking dish or casserole dish. Bake for 35-45 minutes or until cooked through and golden on top.

Serve warm or chilled with salad greens or steamed veggies.

DINNER

Crockpot Curry

Ingredients

1 onion
5 cloves of garlic
1/2 inch cube of ginger
1 tbsp. coconut oil or ghee
A large handful of crimini
  mushrooms
1 parsnip
1 carrot
1/2 zucchini
1 large or 2 small yams
1 tomato
1 (7 oz.) can of organic tomato
  paste (gluten-free)
400-500 grams of ground
humanely
  raised turkey, lamb or beef (or
  omit meat for vegetarian
option)

2 bay leaves
1 tsp. fenugreek seed
2 tbsp. coriander
1.5 tbsp. paprika
1 tsp. cinnamon
3 tsp. cumin
2 tsp. chili powder
2 tbsp. turmeric
1/2 tsp. nutmeg
3 pods of cardamom
1 tbsp. garam masala
Salt and pepper to taste
1/3 cup water
1/2 bunch of cilantro (to garnish)

Method

Dice the onion and garlic, and grate the ginger. Add to the bottom of a crock pot with the coconut oil (or ghee).

Chop the mushrooms, parsnip, carrot, zucchini, yams and tomato into small cubes so they all cook evenly, and add to the pot. Add the tomato paste and ground meat (if using).

Add all the spices and mix with a spoon, then add the water. Cover and cook on low for 5-7 hours. You can prepare the curry in the morning around 10am and then dinner is ready for 5pm.

Serve garnished with cilantro and accompany with quinoa instead of rice.

Crispy Chicken

The amount of batter that you need will vary, depending on the size and quantity of chicken breasts you're preparing. Fortunately it is quick and easy to make more batter if you need it. If you make too much, you can store it in the fridge for a week or so.

Ingredients

1 organic free range egg
5 tbsp. ground flaxseed
4 tbsp. almond meal
2 tbsp. arrowroot powder (optional)
Organic free range chicken breasts

1 tsp. each of cayenne, paprika, cumin, sea salt and pepper
Add whatever spices you love, such as turmeric, thyme, rosemary, garlic, oregano, etc.

Method

Beat the egg in a bowl and set aside. Mix the dry ingredients and spices on a large plate.

You can cut your chicken breast into strips or leave it large. Dip it into the egg, then the spice mix, then onto a greased baking pan or glass casserole dish.

Place into a preheated oven at 300F (150C). Bake for 10 minutes, then turn and bake for 5-10 minutes more. Check that the chicken is not pink in the center before removing from the oven. Thinner strips will cook faster than whole breasts.

Serve on top of a salad, sandwiched between romaine lettuce leaves for a chicken burger, with stir fry veggies, a baked yam and steamed vegetables or with curried cauliflower rice.

Not Your "Mac and Cheese"

While this recipe contains neither macaroni nor cheese, it is a healthy alternative that will satisfy your craving.

Ingredients

1-2 tbsp. of ghee or coconut oil
Half an onion, sliced or diced
3-5 cloves of garlic
Half a head of green cabbage, sliced or chopped
Handful of brown button mushrooms, chopped

2-3 tbsp. turmeric
Salt and pepper to taste
Water, a small amount
Nutritional yeast to taste
Organic humanely raised bacon (optional)

Method

In a large saucepan, heat the oil or ghee. Add the onion and cook for about 5 minutes. Add the garlic and cook for another minute. If you're using bacon, add it in now.

Add the cabbage and mushrooms with a splash of water and the generous amount of turmeric. Season to taste with salt and pepper. Cover and cook for about 5 minutes until the cabbage is soft. When the cabbage has reached your desired tenderness, remove from the heat. Add nutritional yeast, stir and serve.

Rosemary Orange Baked Salmon

Ingredients

Wild sockeye salmon fillet
1 tbsp. rosemary
1 tsp. thyme
1 tsp. turmeric
1 tsp. coriander
1/2 inch of ginger
4-5 cloves of garlic

1/2 an orange
Juice of 1/2 a lemon
1 tbsp. of red wine vinegar
3-4 tbsp. of olive oil (until desired consistency)
Dash of salt and pepper
1 tbsp. of honey

Method

Preheat oven to 300F (150C).

Combine all the ingredients except for the salmon in a blender.

Place salmon in casserole dish or in tin foil. Pour the sauce from the blender on top, sprinkle with some additional rosemary and garnish with some lemon slices. If using tin foil, seal the salmon into a tight package, then place on baking tray in the oven.

Bake for 15-20 minutes to cook the fish as desired, whether slightly pink or cooked through. A shorter bake time will leave the salmon moist, while a longer cooking time can dry it out.

Any leftover sauce makes a delicious salad dressing.

Portobello Burgers

Ingredients
1 medium white onion
2-4 gloves garlic
1 organic free range egg
1 pound of organic humanely
   raised ground beef, lamb or
pork
Olive oil or ghee
2 Portobello mushrooms for each
   burger, stems removed

Spices, such as chili powder,
   paprika, salt, pepper
Burger toppings such as sautéed
   onions, tomatoes, bell peppers,
   fried egg, romaine lettuce,
   fermented ketchup, humanely
   raised bacon

Method
Chop onion and garlic. Combine with the egg and meat in a bowl. Roll
the mix into burger sized balls. Fry the burgers in a pan with plenty of olive
oil or ghee for 5-7 minutes each side or until cooked all the way through.

In a casserole dish, drizzle olive oil (or spread ghee) on top of the
mushrooms and then sprinkle with spices. Roast them in a preheated oven
at 300F (150C) for 10-15 minutes until the mushrooms browned and cooked
through.

Place your meat patty between two mushrooms to form a burger. If you
can't find Portobello mushrooms, wrap your burger patty in lettuce leaves.
You can top your burger with sautéed onions, tomatoes, bell peppers,
lettuce, fried egg or even humanly raised organic bacon. Add healthy
homemade condiments like fermented ketchup, horseradish or mustard. If
you want to enjoy fries with your burger, use parsnip fries or roasted
asparagus instead of potato fries.

Pizza

Ingredients
3-4 tbsp. of fermented ketchup
(see
   bonus recipes)
Oregano
Crimini mushrooms
Bell pepper
Spinach
Onion
Olives
Nutritional yeast

Optional additions
Pine nuts
Apple
Ginger
Pineapple
Organic humanely raised bacon
Garlic
Kale

Method

Using the same bread ingredients as the Focaccia recipe in the lunch section, add oregano, and spread it thin in a pizza crust pan. Bake for ten minutes in a preheated oven at 350F (180C).

Remove from the oven and brush with olive oil. Spread with fermented ketchup. Chop up the mushrooms and vegetables and top the pizza. You can use our suggested vegetables or choose your favorites.

Sprinkle a generous amount of nutritional yeast on the pizza. Pop it back in the oven for another 10-15 minutes, until the veggies are cooked as desired.

You can add leftovers from the crispy chicken recipe if you desire.

Triple Mushroom Cabbage Rolls

Filling and wrap Ingredients
1 small cabbage, using 8-10 full
leaves
Olive oil
1 medium onion, chopped
3 cloves of garlic, minced
1 cup brown and white mushrooms,
    chopped
1 cup Portobello mushroom,
chopped
1 tbsp. rosemary
1 tbsp. thyme
1 tbsp. sage
Salt and pepper to taste

Sauce Ingredients
1 tbsp. olive oil
2 cloves of garlic, minced
1 cup tomato paste or
    fermented ketchup
1/2 cup almond milk

Method

Gently remove 8-10 large outer leaves from the cabbage. Make sure to keep the leaves fully intact. This may take some practice and patience.

Bring a large pot of water to a boil and add the cabbage leaves. Reduce the heat to a low simmer and let the leaves cook for about 3 to 5 minutes, until they are soft, but not falling apart. Drain the leaves and set them aside to cool. These are the wraps for the filling.

In a saucepan, warm the olive oil over medium heat. Add the onion and sauté until it begins to soften and become transparent. Then add the

minced garlic, chopped mushrooms, herbs, salt and pepper. Cook over medium heat for about 8-10 minutes.

Set the pan aside to cool. Once the mushroom mixture has cooled, place it in a food processor and mix it until blended. If you don't have a food processor, use a blender or just try to chop up the mixture a bit more. This is your filling.

To make the sauce, use a separate saucepan. Heat the olive oil over medium heat and add the minced garlic. Then add the tomato sauce or ketchup and almond milk and stir. Reduce the heat to low and let it simmer for about 10 minutes.

Lay one cabbage leave out flat and place about 1 tablespoon of the mushroom mixture about 1-2 inches from one edge of the leaf. Fold in the sides and roll up the leaf as you would a burrito, making a tightly stuffed cabbage leaf. This can get a bit tricky if your leaves aren't fully intact, but wrapping it tight will do the trick. Continue with the rest of the leaves or until the mushroom mixture runs out.

Place each roll, seam-side down, into the saucepan with the sauce. Use a spoon to drizzle some of the sauce over the top of the rolls. Cover, and let them simmer in the tomato sauce for about 10 minutes.

CONDIMENTS

Baconnaise

Ingredients

2 egg yolks from organic free range eggs
1/4 tsp. sea salt
1/4 tsp. mustard seed powder
½ cup of bacon grease from organic and
    humanely raised bacon

Juice of half a lemon
1 tsp. white wine vinegar
1/8 cup olive oil

Method

Whenever you cook with bacon, save the grease in a glass container to make delicious baconnaise. Place all the ingredients (except olive oil) in a food processor. Mix well, then very slowly (very, very slowly) add the oil while blending. It will soon emulsify into a delicious mayonnaise that you can drizzle on top of just about everything.

Fermented Horseradish

Ingredients

1 cup peeled horseradish root
1 tsp. sea salt

1 cup of brine from sauerkraut or kvass
½ cup turnip (optional)

Method

Blend the ingredients in a food processor until smooth. If the ingredients aren't blending well, add a little more brine.

Place in a mason glass jar and seal. Make sure it is airtight. Leave it on your counter or in a cupboard for 2-3 days, allowing the dish to ferment.

Once opened, store in the fridge.

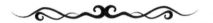

Mustard

There are two ways to make mustard and both ways are quite simple. Either use mustard seeds or mustard powder.

Mustard powder version

1/2 cup water
1/2 cup of mustard powder
Salt to taste

<u>Optional additions</u>
1-2 tbsp. vinegar (apple cider or balsamic)
Lemon or lime juice
1 tsp. arrowroot powder to thicken if desired
1/4 tsp. of turmeric
Dash of garlic powder
Paprika
Cayenne

<u>Method</u>
Add all the ingredients together and mix. Store in a glass jar in the fridge.

Mustard seed version

1/2 cup dark mustard seeds
1/2 cup light mustard seeds
1/2 cup water

1/2 tbsp. apple cider vinegar or
Balsamic vinegar

<u>Method</u>
Combine the ingredients and let stand overnight, until the seeds have absorbed all the water and vinegar. Blend in a food processor with any optional additions. Place in glass jar and store in fridge.

At first, this mustard will be spicier. Allow to rest for a few days and the flavors will infuse and the taste will improve.

SNACKS

Parsnip Fries

Ingredients
3 or 4 parsnips, cut into French fries
3-4 tbsp. olive oil
Spices to taste, such as paprika, cumin, cayenne, salt, pepper, chili powder
[**You can also use yams or beets in this recipe to make yam or beet fries. Or use them all for colorful mix!]

Method
Preheat the oven to 350F (180C).

Place the slices of parsnips into a bowl. Add spices, usually about half a teaspoon or so of each. Drizzle with olive oil, enough to cover the parsnips and stick the spices to the fries.

Spread the fries in a single layer on a baking sheet and bake for 15-20 minutes, depending on their thickness. Turn halfway through cooking. They are finished when they are toasted, slightly darker than golden brown. They taste better slightly overcooked than undercooked.

Serve with fermented ketchup.

Flaxseed Crackers

Ingredients
Any mixture of leafy greens with stalks, such as parsley, kale, spinach, chard or cilantro
1 small white onion
6 cloves of garlic
1 cup walnuts, soaked

1 cup sunflower seeds, soaked
1 cup pumpkin seeds, soaked
Ground flaxseed
Sea salt and pepper
Spices such as cumin and cayenne
Sesame seeds, to garnish

Method
In a food processor, combine the greens with onion, garlic, walnuts, sunflower seeds and pumpkin seeds. You may have to do this a couple times as you dump the mixed ingredients into a larger bowl.

Once all the ingredients are finely chopped, add just enough water to make it slightly watery and ground flaxseed to create a thick paste/dough. Add spices generously to taste.

Spread the paste evenly onto a dehydrator sheet. Score with a butter knife or spatula into desired shapes and sprinkle with sesame seeds.

Dehydrate overnight or to desired crispness, making sure to flip the crackers half way through.

If you don't have a dehydrator, you can spread the mixture on a cookie dough sheet and bake in the oven at the lowest temperature with the oven door ajar until desired crispness.

Serve with hummus or guacamole, or use them to make little mini sandwich bites. If you make them thinner and softer, you can use them to make mini wraps.

If you use a juicer, you can use apple and carrot pulp with some cinnamon to make sweet crackers. You can also use fruits like banana and mango with ground flax to make something similar to crepes, just be sure to take them out of the dehydrator when they are still soft.

Sprouted Chickpea Hummus

Seeds, grains and legumes are like little treasure chests filled with nutrients. Each one contains a little plant embryo, packed with all the nutrition that the plant needs to sprout. To get inside this magic box and access these nutrients, you need the right key to get in. These foods are protected by anti-nutrients such as phytic acid and enzyme inhibitors that prevent you from absorbing their full nutrition and can even steal nutrients from you! These compounds make it very difficult for your body to digest the food and to absorb its nutrients. It is a defense mechanism that protects the seed from being eaten. After all, this tiny little seedling longs to one day grow into a big adult plant.

This is why legumes and grains can aggravate the digestive system, so anyone with digestive distress such as bloating, constipation, gas or cramps should stick with easy-to-digest foods that allow the digestive tract to heal.

By soaking and sprouting legumes, grains, seeds and some nuts, you neutralize the phytic acid and enzyme inhibitors. This transforms the dormant protective seed into a living baby plant. The complex and super

dense vegetable proteins transform into more simple amino acids which are easier for your body to digest and absorb.

You can do this with almost any seed, grain, legume or nut, including rice, mung beans, chickpeas, lentils, lima beans, kidney beans, almonds, walnuts or broccoli seeds.

Sprouting Method
Soak the seed of your choice in water. To make hummus, use chickpeas. Always use dried beans, not canned. Cover them in plenty of water and let them sit overnight.

In the morning drain and rinse the chickpeas. Once drained, place in a colander covered with a dish towel. Several times throughout the day, rinse and drain again. You can do this every 2-3 hours, or even just 2-3 times a day.

When they are ready, visible sprouts, which look like white tails, will appear. Many seeds, grains and legumes take 2-3 days. Some foods, such as rice, can take up to 5 days.

Ingredients for hummus

6 cups sprouted chickpeas	4 tsp. turmeric
Juice of 2 lemons	6 tsp. cumin
5 cloves of garlic	2 tsp. paprika
1 tomato	1 tsp. cayenne
Handful of sun-dried tomatoes, soaked in water for 5 minutes	1 tsp. chili powder
	1/3 cup nutritional yeast
1/2 red pepper	Salt and pepper to taste
1/2 cup olive oil	

Method
Combine all the ingredients, except the spices, in a food processor and blend until smooth. Then add the spices. Taste as you go to get the balance right. When in doubt, add more olive oil, nutritional yeast or salt.

Serve with cucumber, carrots, celery, orange pepper slices or flaxseed crackers.

Cinnamon Plantain Bites

These plantain bites are a healthy way to satisfy your sweet tooth. They are sweet, tasty and super easy to make. A sprinkle of cinnamon even helps control the mini-sugar spike after you've devoured this scrumptious treat. Plantains are similar to bananas, but generally larger and they contain more starch. They must be cooked before eating. When still green they are boiled and a bit similar potatoes, generally served mashed or as part of a veggie burger. They ripen to yellow and are then used in sweet dishes like this one.

Ingredients
1 yellow plantain
1 tbsp. of coconut oil
cinnamon

Method
Peel the plantain and cut it into long strips.

Melt the coconut oil in a frying pan at medium to low heat. Fry the plantain slices until cooked all the way through and golden brown. Sprinkle with cinnamon to serve.

Spicy Chickpea Popcorn

Ingredients
1 (15 oz.) can of chickpeas
2 tbsp. olive oil
1 tsp. paprika
1 tsp. cumin
1/2 tsp. cayenne
Sea salt to taste

Method
Preheat the oven to 400F (200C).

Drain and rinse the beans, then dry them with a kitchen towel.

Add the oil and spices to a bowl, and toss the chickpeas in the bowl to coat them.

Pour the beans onto a baking sheet and bake for 35-40 minutes, shaking the pan halfway through.

Serve warm and store in an air tight container once fully cooled.

Guacamole

Ingredients

2 avocados, peeled and pitted	1 tsp. garlic, minced
1-2 tomatoes, diced	1 tsp. salt
1/2 cup onion, finely diced	1 tsp. cumin
1/2 cup cilantro, finely chopped	1/2 tsp. cayenne
Juice of 1 lime	Salt and pepper to taste

Method

Mash the avocado with a fork, then mix in the remaining ingredients. Allow to sit for 30 minutes in the fridge to enhance the flavor.

Serve with veggie sticks, flaxseed crackers or focaccia slices. It is also great as a side dish to a main meal.

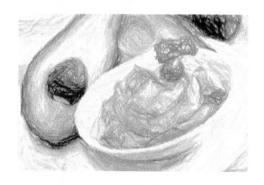

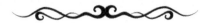

DESSERT

Cashew Cream

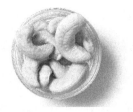

Ingredients
1 cup cashews
water

Method
Add boiling water to cashews and soak for 20 minutes. Drain, then add to a blender. Slowly add water to make it blend and to reach your desired consistency.

You can use this in soups or smoothies, or add lemon juice and serve it with frozen blueberries.

Coconut Ice Cream

Ingredients
1 cup cashews
2 cups young coconut flesh
coconut water
vanilla extract
pinch of salt

Method
Soak the cashews in hot water for 20 minutes, or in room temperature water overnight (for a raw vegan option).

Crack open fresh young coconuts. Reserve the water and collect about two cups of flesh. Blend the coconut meat with the soaked cashews, adding coconut water to create your desired consistency. Add vanilla extract to taste and a pinch of salt.

Eat immediately or place in the fridge or freezer, depending on what you'd like cream or ice cream.

Raspberry Lemon Sorbet

Ingredients
Handful of frozen raspberries
1 cup coconut milk kefir
Dash of almond milk

Juice of half a lemon
Few of drops of vanilla extract
1/2 tbsp. of raw honey

Method
Blend all ingredients and enjoy, or you can freeze and enjoy later.

Chia Seed Pudding

Base Ingredients
chia seeds
water

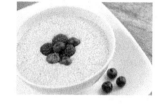

Method
Soak 1 part chia seeds in 10 parts of water. After about 20 minutes, the chia seeds will release a tasteless jelly. This is your pudding base. You can then add whatever flavors you like to create a pudding.

Blueberry Flavor Optional Ingredients
1 cup soaked chia seeds
1/4 cup almond milk
Juice of 1 lemon
1 cup blueberries (fresh or frozen)
Stevia or honey for sweetener

Blend almond milk, blueberries, lemon juice and sweetener of choice in a blender. Once smooth, add this to 1 cup of the chia seed pudding. Serve fresh or chill and serve later.

Chocolate Flavor Optional Ingredients
2 tbsp. cacao powder
2-3 tbsp. honey
1/2 cup almond milk
1/2 frozen banana (or 1/2 an avocado)

Blend ingredients in blender and add to a cup of chia pudding base.

PART 4:

CANCER

AND

DIABETES

(A special section for holistically treating these two diseases)

CANCER

This section is provided not as a 'cure' for cancer as that would be making light of a very complex and devastating disease; rather this information is given to use as a supplementary resource that can improve your chances of cancer prevention and successful treatment. There are over 100 types of cancer, and more than 1/3 of Americans will get cancer in their lives. In fact everyone has cancer cells in their body, but for most people their immune system is able to prevent those cells from growing out of control. Each cancer treatment protocol will be slightly different depending on the type of cancer and stage. For this reason, it is imperative that you work with a health care professional who understands your particular condition. Like the rest of this book, this information is not to replace the advice or treatment given to you by your doctor, it is only to open doors to further treatment and prevention options you might not be aware of that may hold answers for you. The truth is that, despite the cancer industry's alleged and never ending 'search for the cure', current mainstream cancer treatments are toxic to the body, marginally successful, and fail to look at the underlying cause(s).

"Everyone should know that the "war on cancer" is largely a fraud."
~ Dr. Linus Pauling (two time winner of the Nobel Prize for Medicine)

I would like to propose a more holistic restorative and preventative approach.

FOODS TO CONSUME MORE OF

✓ Salvestrols are naturally occurring nutritional compounds that seek out cancer cells, and literally destroy them. How do they do this? Over 98% of all cancer cells have an enzyme called CYP1B1, something not present in almost any normal cells. Salvestrols are able to 'seek out' these enzymes, and when contact is made, a chemical reaction is activated which kills the cancer cell. This all happens in as quickly as 30-60 minutes after ingestion. Salvestrols are found in many fruits and vegetables (and herbs too). However, through the use of fungicides which are sprayed on produce and modern food processing, salvestrols are lost. For salvestrols to effectively fight cancer, they need to come from organic sources, which contain 30% higher levels than non-organic. Here are a few organic sources high is salvestrols:

Fruits: apples, grapes, blueberries, cranberries, oranges, strawberries, tangerines

Vegetables: avocados, bell peppers, broccoli, brussel sprouts, cabbage, cauliflower, olives

Herbs: basil, parsley, dandelion, milk thistle, mint, rosemary, sage, thyme

✓ A Ketogenic diet is beneficial. This high fat, adequate protein, low carb diet starves cancer (cancer cells cannot metabolize ketones (from fats)) yet gives fuel to normal healthy cells. Such a diet is contrary of course to conventional cancer treatment protocol which emphasizes carbs. However, this excerpt from an article written by the Weston A Price foundation explains the reasoning well:

> *"The reason the cancer patient starves while the cancer cells grow is because they [cancer cells] are much better at taking up the sugar than are normal cells. If we understand this selective metabolism of cancer well enough to diagnose its growth, then the next step is to withhold sugar and see what happens. The trouble is we need a backup fuel source. And there is a backup fuel source: ketones from fats. Cancer cells cannot metabolize ketones. Normal cells do fine on ketones; we know this from fifty years of successfully utilizing a therapeutic very high-fat ketogenic diet. Cancer patients on a ketogenic diet will often have their tumors shrink and will halt their cachexia—their physical wasting and weight loss. The cancer cells starve on a ketogenic diet, but normal cells thrive... Our whole notion of the right diet for cancer patients today is backwards. The knee-jerk dietary prescription for cancer patients is a low fat, high-carbohydrate diet."*

✓ Chaga mushrooms (powerful anticancer substance that also contains properties that help remove radiation). Of the 150 species of medicinal mushrooms that are able to inhibit the growth of tumors (especially of the stomach, esophagus, and lungs), chaga is the most powerful.

✓ Reishi mushrooms (especially good for prostate cancer, and recognized as a cancer treatment in Japan)

✓ Maitake mushrooms (activate T-cells which defend against viruses and cancer cells. Maitake can limit and even reverse tumor growth).

- ✓ White button mushrooms (beneficial especially against breast cancer)

- ✓ Brussel sprouts, broccoli and broccoli sprouts (all contain suforaphane which may help stop the growth of malignant tumors). Also, cruciferous vegetables such as broccoli contain large amounts of the nutrient indole-3-carbinol which is powerful against breast cancer by reducing cancerous development from hormones and blocking cancer cell progression.

- ✓ Garlic and onions

- ✓ Green vegetables and organic plant foods - the key here though is cutting, blending, or chewing those vegetables well. (There is a chemical in the plant cell that attacks cancer but that chemical only comes out with chewing).

  "Phenols have been found to modulate distinct cell receptors and signal transduction pathways that suppress the carcinogenic process both in vivo, in vitro, and to a lesser extent in humans. And even during chemotherapy, plant phenols can potentially reduce side effects, decrease tumor resistance, and increase the effectiveness of cytotoxic drugs."
  ~ Pamela Yee, MD

  The importance of green vegetables is further underscored by a massive 1996 review of hundreds of studies and published in the Journal of the American Dietetic Association that clearly showed greater vegetable and fruit consumption offers a protective effect against many types of cancer including stomach, esophagus, lung, oral cavity and pharynx, endometrium, pancreas, and colon. The types of vegetables that offer the greatest protection against cancer are raw vegetables, allium vegetables, carrots, green vegetables, cruciferous vegetables, and tomatoes.[1]

- ✓ Alkaline foods (recall Dr. Warburg's Nobel Prize winning discovery back in the 1930s that cancer cannot survive in an alkaline environment)

---

[1] J Am Diet Assoc 1996 Oct;96 (10):1027-39.

✓ Curcumin. There is an enormous amount of evidence based literature that exists supporting curcumin as a cancer fighter. Effective against almost all cancers, it has the ability to destroy cancer cells and promote healthy cell function. Research has also shown that it can work together with certain chemotherapy drugs to enhance the elimination of cancer cells, while also reducing the adverse effects of chemotherapy on healthy cells..

✓ Beets or beet juice, daily. The betacyanin in beets helps prevent the formation of cancerous tumors while also detoxifying the body.

✓ Green tea (which contains EGCG, a powerful anticancer compound)

✓ Goji berries

✓ Flax seeds and chia seeds (both of which help fight estrogen fueled cancers)

✓ Artichokes (contains enzyme that stop the replication of cancer cells)

✓ Yew tip oil

✓ Iodine. The work of Dr. B.A. Eskin who published 80 papers over 3 decades investigating iodine and breast cancer showed that iodine deficiency is a cause of breast and thyroid cancer.

✓ Magnesium chloride (used transdermally, as most cancer patients are magnesium deficient)

✓ other foods not already mentioned above but that are antiangiogenic (see below under Treatments & Processes) include: blackberries, blueberries, grapefruit, lemons, apples, pineapple, red grapes, red wine, bok choy, ginseng, licorice, nutmeg, tuna, olive oil, grape seed oil, dark chocolate

✓ in summary, think of the acronym GOMBBS as your anti-cancer menu. It stands for Greens, Onions, Mushrooms, Beans, Berries, Seeds...the highest cancer reducing foods.

THINGS TO AVOID / USE LESS OF

➢ sugar (cancer feeds and thrives off of it!)

➢ high fructose corn syrup

➢ nicotine (stop smoking, and avoid smoke-filled environments)

➢ acidic foods (which create an environment in which cancer can flourish)

➢ high protein (recall from week 10 that diets high in protein lead to hyperacidity which helps foster a cancer-friendly environment).

➢ trans fats (interfere with the body's ability to fight cancer)

➢ charred foods (these are carcinogenic)

➢ processed meats (especially bacon, sausage, and ham which have been declared as cancer causes by the World Health Organization) and rotisserie chicken

➢ sunscreens (and skin creams) that contains parabens

➢ Avoid BPA, phthalates and other xenoestrogens.

➢ Prolonged use of the birth control pill and estrogen replacement therapy

➢ Dairy, especially from cows injected with genetically engineered growth hormone.

➢ Aspartame

➢ Folic acid (excessive folic acid has been shown to fuel tumor growth, whereas folate has been shown to prevent certain cancers)

➢ pesticide-laden foods (an important reason to buy organic instead). (Did you know that a regular head of lettuce can contain over 50 types of pesticides!)

➢ Over the counter sleeping pills. Studies show a direct link between increased sleeping pill usage and increased risk of cancer.

➢ Toxic metals -of course you aren't voluntarily consuming these, but we are all exposed to them at some level. It's been said that cadmium for example causes more cancers than all the other toxic metals combined. An HTMA test or a stool test can give insight into your toxic metal status.

➢ mammograms. For this, I feel a page on its own needs to be devoted to this topic...

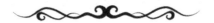

<u>A word on mammograms:</u> Women over 40 are constantly reminded to have mammograms done, for the early prevention of cancer, even if they have no family history of breast cancer. The problem with this is that mammograms are highly ineffective, and lead to astoundingly large numbers of misdiagnosis which not only lead to needless biopsies, but (according to Dr. Samuel Epstein, M.D., Chairman of the Cancer Prevention Coalition and Professor Emeritus of Environmental and Occupational Medicine, University of Illinois School of Public Health, Chicago,) is a prominent cause of breast cancer due to the heavy radiation load delivered each time a woman undergoes screening. He states:

"Mammography is a striking paradigm of the capture of unsuspecting women by run-away powerful technological and global pharmaceutical industries, with the complicity of the cancer establishment, particularly the ACS, and the rollover mainstream media."

He is not alone in his view. This article from the Journal of the Royal Society of Medicine, states:

"There is so much over diagnosis that the best thing a women can do to lower her risk of becoming a breast cancer patient is to avoid going to screening, which will lower her risk by one-third."[1]

If we want to look closer at statistics, *For every breast-cancer death prevented in U.S. women over a 10-year course of annual screening beginning at 50 years of age, 490 to 670 women are likely to have a false positive mammogram with repeat examination; 70 to 100, an unnecessary biopsy; and 3 to 14, an over diagnosed breast cancer that would never have become clinically apparent.[2]*

As Dr. Peter Gotzsche, MD (author of Mammography Screening: Truth, Lies, and Controversy) states: *"Screening saves probably one life for every 2,000 women who go for a mammogram. But it harms 10 others. Cancerous cells that will go away or never progress to disease in the woman's lifetime are excised with surgery."*

Furthermore, a large number of women have the genetic 'oncogene AC' which increases their susceptibility to developing cancer from even short periods of x-ray exposure such as what mammograms give.

Yet, despite the statistics and overwhelming evidence of its inefficacy and dangers, women are still made to believe that mammograms are a necessity. Isn't that a sad reality, especially when safer options (such as thermography) exist but are rarely promoted in most conventional medicine circles.

[1] http://jrs.sagepub.com/content/108/9/341.long
[2] Welch HG, Passow HJ. Quantifying the benefits and harms of screening mammography. JAMA Intern Med 2014;174:448-454

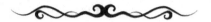

ALTERNATIVE TREATMENTS & PROCESSES

This section will be controversial to some, especially those indoctrinated in conventional medicine who, for reasons of either ignorance, politics or other agendas, refuse to admit the connection between nutrition and cancer, or the lives that alternative cancer treatments have saved. We already know that chemotherapy is harmful, and has a dismal success record. It only makes sense therefore to be open to other treatment methods that have shown effectiveness - for the advancement of medicine, and the saving of lives.

I'll begin this section with a few fitting quotes, followed then by a look at some alternative treatments and processes.

"To the cancer establishment, a cancer patient is a profit center. The actual clinical and scientific evidence does not support the claims of the cancer industry. Conventional cancer treatments are in place as the law of the land because they pay the best, not heal the best. Decades of the politics-of-cancer-as-usual have kept you from knowing this, and will continue to do so unless you wake up to their reality."
- Lee Cowden, MD

"...as a chemist trained to interpret data, it is incomprehensible to me that physicians can ignore the clear evidence that chemotherapy does much, much more harm than good."
- Alan C Nixon, PhD, former president of the American Chemical Society

"The five year cancer survival statistics of the American Cancer Society are very misleading. They now count things that are not cancer, and because we are able to diagnose at an earlier stage of the disease, patients falsely appear to live longer. Our whole cancer research in the past 20 years has been a failure. More people over 30 are dying from cancer than ever before... More women with mild or benign diseases are being included in statistics and reported as being 'cured'. When government officials point to survival figures and say they are winning the war against cancer they are using those survival rates improperly."
~ Dr John Bailer, 20 years on staff of the U.S. National Cancer Institute and editor of its journal, speaking at the Annual Meeting of the American Association for the Advancement of Science in May 1985

322

"But nobody today can say that one does not know what cancer and its prime cause [may] be. On the contrary, there is no disease whose prime cause is better known, so that today ignorance is no longer an excuse that one cannot do more about prevention. That prevention will come no doubt, for man wishes to survive. But how long prevention will be avoided depends on how long the prophets of agnosticism will succeed in inhibiting the application of scientific knowledge in the cancer field.
In the meantime, millions of men must die of cancer unnecessarily."
~Dr. Otto Heinrich Warburg, medical Nobel Prize winner

"I am tired of research groups parading around the few 5 - 9% of the survivors and saying we are doing so well. The survival rates from chemotherapy and radiation are hardly any better than they were when President Nixon waged the war against cancer back in 1972. We need to talk to the other 90% who are not here today. It is becoming evident that the system is very bias. Research money is only going towards a cure that can be controlled and make money. Prevention and alternatives are essentially not funded. If a "cure" was found today, would we send all the cancer researchers home tomorrow? Doctors who really care and practice "Do No Harm" are having their licenses taken away for not practicing conventional medicine, even though most of their patients do not have cancer. This paradox is killing so many people, even the researchers. "
~Samuel S. Epstein, M.D., Chairman of the Cancer Prevention Coalition

✓ Antineoplaston Therapy: (antineoplastons are made up mostly of peptides and amino acids that can turn off the genes that cause cancer. For more information you can look up Dr. Burzynski, or watch his film *"Cancer is Serious Business"* which, as quoted by Tony Robbins **"Anyone who is dealing with cancer and/or the effects of treatment - you owe it to yourself to see this documentary"**. (The documentary film at http://go.thetruthaboutcancer.com/ is also worth watching for anyone struggling with answers to cancer)

Despite the FDA deeming Dr. Burzynski's work illegal for many years, the US government then went on to try to steal his patents. Just one example of its effectiveness is that the treatment is the only cure for brainstem gliomas (which are supposedly 'incurable') - this has been tested in FDA approved trials and cures up to 50% of cases (while conventional treatment cures %0).

- ✓ Anti-angiogenesis treatments: (a growing field of medicine now being widely accepted in the treatment of cancers. By blocking the process called angiogenesis (the growth of blood vessels; and in this context stopping tumors from growing their own blood supply), tumors can be stopped from spreading and growing larger). If you'd like more information on this field and how it can specifically work with certain cancers, visit www.angio.org and www.scienceofcancers.org

- ✓ The Journey Process (as written and taught by Brandon Bays)

- ✓ For breast cancer, the book "Saving Tatas" by Christine Austin is packed with tips and guidance and is highly recommended.

- ✓ Emotional Healing and Clearing Exercises as presented throughout this book

- ✓ The Dalian Method (created by Mada Eliza Dalian)

- ✓ Investigate your mineral and heavy metals status through HTMA testing (www.htmatest.com). Extremely low molybdenum for example can be linked to cancer, as can be levels of toxic metals. Cadmium has one of the highest correlations to cancer of all heavy metals.

- ✓ GAPS Diet Protocol (as defined and written about by Dr. Natasha Campbell-McBride)

- ✓ Hydrogen Peroxide: It's accepted that cancer cells die in an oxygenated environment, and hydrogen peroxide (H_2O_2) helps bring oxygen to the cancer cells, while at the same time the cancer cell is not able to break down the H_2O_2, killing it. The key is getting enough H_2O_2 inside the cancer cell, and for this reason, fasting (both food and water) for a few hours before taking it can help with its absorption. Despite what many critics say, 35% food grade (make sure it's food grade and not the 3% pharmaceutical grade) can kill cancer! Add a few drops to a glass of water each day, or add a cup to a bathtub of warm water and soak in it for up to half an hour (allowing it to be absorbed through your skin).

- ✓ Phage Therapy (effective in protecting cancer patients (who have a weakened immune system) from bacterial infections, even antibiotic-resistant ones, without being harsh on the rest of the body.

- ✓ Gerson Therapy - developed in the 1920s to treat a variety of illnesses including cancer based on its whole body holistic healing approach using natural foods, fresh juices, and improving the body's natural ability to heal itself. As one avenue, Dr. Max Gerson was able to successfully treat many cases of terminal cancer using raw liver juice, a rich source of Vitamin A. Despite numerous success stories and his testimonial

to success in 1946 before a US congressional committee, his achievements were ignored. (The 2006 film Dying to Have Known is worth watching for more information on the effectiveness of this treatment).

✓ pH Therapy and Cesium Chloride. Understanding that cancer is a symptom of acidosis, the key in controlling cancer is creating an oxygenated and alkaline environment in which cancer cannot thrive. The use of cesium chloride (under the strict guidance of an expert trained in its application) helps achieve this environment. Specifically, cesium is able to get inside the cancer cell, making the cancer cell alkaline; starving the cancer cell of food (glucose); neutralizing lactic acid and which in turns limits cancer cell replication.

✓ Laetrile (a.k.a. Amygdalin): (although controversial, the subject of a large-scale cover-up back in the 1970s, and originally written off as a quack, numerous studies have since supported its efficacy in stopping the spread of cancer). Watching the film at www.secondopinionfilm.com will give you great insight into Laetrile.

✓ Hoxsey Treatment (another effective cancer cure that the FDA has tried to suppress and keep hush hush). In addition to a healthy diet and positive energy, the treatment uses an external formula (bloodroot, zinc chloride, antimony sulfide) and an internal tonic (red clover blossom, licorice root, buckthorn bark, burdock root, stillingia root, poke root, barberry root, Oregon grape root, cascara sagrada bark, prickly ash bark, wild indigo root and sea kelp). According to James Duke, Ph.D of the US Department of Agriculture, all of the Hoxsey herbs have known anticancer properties and have long been used by Native American healers to treat cancer. The 1987 film "How Healing Becomes a Crime" explains the treatment and its cover-up in further detail.

✓ Essiac Tea: here again is another 'treatment' that the cancer industry refuses to acknowledge has any merit or scientifically based evidence, and yet has been proven over decades to be effective on numerous cancer patients. The tea is made using the following 4 herbs: burdock root (cut), sheep sorrel herb (powdered), slippery elm bark (powdered), and Turkish Rhubarb root (powdered). The quality of these herbs is paramount to their effectiveness. Boil the herbs hard and uncovered for 10-20 minutes, then cover and steep for about 10 hours. Heat the mixture up again to steaming (not boiling). Drink (up to a couple ounces 3 times per day) and / or refrigerate.

✓ Finally, the Therapies Resource Section at the back of this book lists a number of alternative and natural therapies that can offer varying degrees of effectiveness in the battle against cancer.

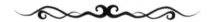

DIABETES

Diabetes results when the body cannot produce or properly use insulin, a hormone needed for glucose metabolism. Since all human tissues need a steady supply of glucose, diabetes can affect every organ, leading to heart disease, kidney failure, even blindness. Type 1 Diabetes, also called juvenile onset diabetes, affects 10% of diabetes cases. In this autoimmune disease the body does not produce enough insulin and so insulin must be taken daily. Despite being labeled as incurable, research into the potential of beta cell regeneration (destroyed or impaired beta cells are the reason insulin is not produced) is showing great promise. A number of natural substances have been shown to help with beta cell regeneration, including: flaxseed, berberine, chard, curcumin, genistein, and nigella sativa.

90% of diabetes patients however are Type II (adult onset diabetes). These people have adequate amounts of insulin but the body cannot use the hormone properly. An appropriate diet can prevent, delay or even reverse the consequences of Type II.

What kind of diet? Going on a low fat diet (ideally plant based) is best. I said low fat NOT 'no fat' as healthy fats are important and necessary for proper functioning in other areas. This low fat diet is key for diabetes - in fact doing so can help you get off medication. I'll explain why.

We have mitochondria in our cells - mitochondria burn fat. When we eat fat, the mitochondria in our cells actually decrease. This makes it even harder to burn fat, and so fat accumulates. As fat accumulates, insulin does not signal properly. Insulin is the natural hormone that allows glucose to enter the cell (think of it as a key that allows glucose into the cell)...and so, glucose cannot enter. Where does it go? It stays in the blood, creating high blood glucose levels...and diabetes. Medication and/or insulin is then given to the patient as treatment. The irony is that insulin is a hormone that actually makes you fat and increases weight even further – leading to more of the very thing that it's trying to prevent. If you want to get off that medication, the answer is simple. Lower the fat in your cells. As you reduce the fat in your cells, the insulin receptors start working again. Now glucose comes out of the blood and into the cell, and as a result, blood glucose levels drop.

The following pages give a basic protocol for effectively treating diabetes.

FOODS TO CONSUME MORE OF

✓ Given the explanation above, focus on low fat, plant based foods. A Paleo diet is ideal for reversing diabetes. In fact, Mark Sisson, author of the bestselling health book 'The Primal Blueprint', states that the low-carb Paleo way of eating "is the BEST way to fix type 2 diabetes."

✓ Additional foods that can help heal include: oats, barley, peas, lentils, low fat dairy, avocado, apples, pears, oranges, garlic, beans, chicken breast, mushrooms, yogurt, blackstrap molasses, apple cider vinegar (daily)

✓ Eat bitter melon (a vegetable-fruit that contains the enzyme AMPK (which helps transport glucose from the blood into the cells) and charantin (gives a blood-glucose lowering effect) and polypeptide-p (an insulin-like compound). Can be eaten raw, cooked, juiced, or as tea.

✓ Eat high fiber

✓ Supplement with chromium, magnesium, zinc, B complex, glucomannan (for hormonal support), cinnamon (its ingredient methylhydroxy chalcone polymer helps improve insulin sensitivity), vanadium, fenugreek, (helps reduce cholesterol and blood sugar levels), huckleberry (helps promote insulin production), spirulina, berberine, purslane, and for mitochondrial support take carnitine, CoQ10, alpha lipoic acid. Natural sea salt and ionic mineral supplements can also help restore necessary mineral balance.

✓ Magnesium (mentioned above) may be especially important. A Harvard study found that diabetics taking 320mg of magnesium for 16 weeks significantly improved their fasting blood sugar levels and their HDL cholesterol.

✓ As diet is the root cause of Diabetes (and specifically microbes and parasites that begin a chain reaction that weakens our immunity and our organs (including the pancreas which produces insulin), we really need to focus on cleaning up our diet, killing off damaging microbes, ad giving our cells and organs a fighting chance. The GAPS diet (www.gapsdiet.com/The_Diet.html) therefore can also be very beneficial in controlling and reversing diabetes.

THINGS TO CONSUME / USE LESS OF

✓ Red meat, butter, saturated fats, processed foods, trans fats

✓ High glycemic foods such as potatoes, soft drinks, white flour, and refined sugars

✓ Keep your carbs low (and the ones you do eat, keep high quality). Constantly consuming carbohydrates over time makes insulin less and less effective, leading to insulin resistance and carbohydrate intolerance, and in turn, diabetes. Lowering your carbs and getting macronutrients from protein sources and healthy fats is important for reversing diabetes.

✓ Protein (keep your protein intake moderate)

✓ The amino acid cysteine (interferes with absorption of insulin)

✓ Limit your alcohol consumption, and avoid tobacco

LIFESTYLE

✓ Regular physical activity is very important

✓ Learn about healthy food choices

✓ Work on reducing stress

✓ Focus on the nutrition guidelines presented above

PART 5:

ARTICLES

DO YOU HAVE THE GUTS TO TRANSFORM YOUR LIFE?

(By Aga Postawska)

The father of Western Medicine, Hippocrates, famously taught that "All disease begins in the gut." And if you don't know who Hippocrates was, well let me tell you, he knew his stuff.

With his famous theory of health, if a person has symptoms of disease or other forms of physical discomfort, the first place to look to identify the source of the problem should be the gut. However, in the modern medical system, there is a tendency to look everywhere but the gut.

Today, many scientists and doctors are returning to the foundation of Western medicine and beginning to examine what Hippocrates was talking about all this time, the gut and its relationship to overall health. They are finding much value in these early teachings and many agree that all disease truly does begin in the gut. Many diverse conditions can be traced back to their origin in an imbalance or disorder of the gut, including:

- Digestive disorders: bloating, constipation, diarrhea, gas, acid reflux, colitis, irritable bowel syndrome (IBS), food sensitives and intolerances

- Brain disorders: chronic headaches, brain fog, depression, bipolar disorder, autism, Parkinson's disease, ADHD

- Skin conditions: acne, psoriasis, eczema, rosacea

- Metabolic conditions: insulin resistance, diabetes, obesity, Hashimoto's, hypothyroid

- Autoimmune disorders: lupus, fibromyalgia, rheumatoid arthritis, chronic fatigue syndrome, allergies

It may seem strange that such a diverse set of symptoms and conditions are related to just one organ in the body. To understand how this can be, we will take a closer look at the gut, its function in the body and how it is crucial to your thriving physical and mental health and well-being.

What Is The Gut?

The "gut" is a common name that refers to the gastrointestinal tract. In a broad sense, this includes the whole pathway that food takes through the human body, from in mouth to out anus. However, for our purposes, we use the "gut" to refer to the lower gastrointestinal tract, which includes your

small and large intestines. These important organs serve two key functions in the body:

> **1.Nutrient absorption:** The intestines are largely responsible for absorbing the products of digestion and delivering these nutrients into the bloodstream where they are distributed throughout the body. The gut essentially feeds your entire body.

> **2.Defense:** The intestinal lining is an important part of the immune system, forming a barrier that prevents harmful microbes, pathogens, allergens, undigested bits of food, and anything else foreign from entering the bloodstream.

Additionally, the beneficial intestinal flora, or "good bacteria" that live in the gastrointestinal tract also play a critical role in digestion and preventing the overgrowth of pathogens or "bad bacteria" in the gut. Anywhere from 70%-80% of your immune system is in your gut!

This intestinal barrier is about 9 meters long (that's 30 feet or the length of a tennis court!). It needs a lot of surface area to bring in all the nutrients necessary to feed and fuel your body. To maximize on space, its surface is covered with villi, little finger-like structures, if you look at your gut lining under a microscope it kind of resembles a shag rug from the 70's.

Your Body Is Your Temple, And Your Gut Is Your Fortress Wall

Many people are familiar with the saying, "Your body is your temple." With that analogy, your gut can be considered the protective fortress wall, protecting your temple from invaders. Your health depends on the integrity of your intestinal lining. Similar to the way in which your skin protects you from the outside world, your intestinal tract is the "skin" that serves as a barrier to protect your internal systems from the outside world. Technically, the inside of your gastrointestinal tract is still the outside of your body.

A Leaky Gut

An easy way to understand your gut lining is to picture it as cheesecloth, with small holes perfectly sized to allow the essential nutrients from food, such as vitamins and minerals, to pass through and into your bloodstream. These little openings are protein structures called junctions, and it is important that they remain strong and the correct size.

Disturbance to the lining can weaken and loosen the junctions and create holes that are too big. This is like stretching your cheesecloth until it looks resembles more a fishnet stocking.

331

With loosened junctions, harmful substances such as toxins, pathogens, allergens and undigested food particles (including poop!) can enter the bloodstream and cause a wide array of health problems. This condition is called intestinal *hyper-permeability*, or in plain English, "leaky gut." A leaky gut allows toxins and other harmful substances to circulate through your bloodstream.

When toxins, allergens, microbes and undigested foods enter your bloodstream they cause inflammation and an immune reaction as your system tries to neutralize them. This leads to popular autoimmune disorders; as foreign proteins pass the intestinal wall undigested, the immune system attacks these proteins, and anything that resembles them, including your own natural proteins (your body), causing the immune system to basically attack *you*, the very thing it is set out to protect in the first place.

Gluten is largely responsible for triggering immune responses in the body. More specifically the gliadin proteins in gluten activate something called zonulin in the body, which regulate intestinal permeability. Now the once tight junctions in your intestines become leaky. Your body, in an attempt to protect you from the gliaden, attack your antibodies. These antibodies can get a bit confused and end up attacking the transglutaminase tissue in the intestinal wall which then adds to more intestinal permeability.

Similar triggers of zonulin are caused by cholera as a result of eating feces in contaminated food or water. But in this case you're causing the same intestinal permeability as cholera but with an innocent looking breakfast bagel.

The immune system can also begin to attack the villi on the lining of the small intestine (remember those shag rug fingers in the intestinal wall that absorb nutrients?). As the villi become blunt they can no longer be as effective in absorbing the essential nutrients you need to thrive. That's why you see malabsorption and nutritional deficiencies in people with leaky gut and celiac disease. Once these villi get worn down, they cannot grow back.

Nutrient deficiencies now begin to occur as these blunted villi (and the leaky gut) aren't as effective at pulling in the nutrients to feed your body. Your organs, muscles, glands and tissues cannot function properly when starved of the nutrients they need. This deficiency along with chronic inflammation begins to wreak havoc on the body, and the perfect environment for chronic dis-ease begins to unfold.

In addition to most autoimmune disorders, leaky gut is also directly linked to common gastrointestinal issues, such as abdominal bloating and cramping, excessive gas, food sensitivities, Crohn's disease, colitis and bowel cancer, and Irritable Bowel Syndrome.

Leaky gut is also at the root of the problem of normal day-to day symptoms of discomfort like joint pain and migraines; it can contribute to adrenal

fatigue and mood disorders including anxiety and depression; skin conditions like eczema, and even seasonal allergies and even more serious health conditions like neurological and nervous system disease including MS, fibromyalgia, autism, depression, and bipolar.

Looks like what Hippocrates said a little over 2000 years ago, "All disease begins in the gut," is beginning to make sense.

Causes Of Leaky Gut

There are many things that contribute to leaky gut syndrome, however the most important factors in our modern world are the following:

1. A SAD Diet (Standard American Diet) consisting of processed foods, refined grains, refined sugars, genetically modified foods, wheat and gluten containing grains, hydrogenated vegetables oils, artificial sweeteners and flavorings, preservatives, and excessive alcohol consumption

2. Gut dysbiosis, which is a deficiency in beneficial flora, the "good bacteria" and an overpopulation of pathogenic flora, the "bad bacteria," including bacteria, parasites, yeast and fungi

3. The overuse of antibiotics, including prescribed medications and antibiotics found in animal products, birth control, as well as overuse of nonsteroidal anti-inflammatory drugs (NSAIDS) such as ibuprofen and other cytotoxic drugs

4. Environmental toxins: chemicals in personal hygiene products and cleaning products, chlorinated water, pesticides and fungicides on the food your eat, air pollution

5. Chronic stress.

At-Home Leaky Gut Test

While this test does not provide a definitive diagnosis, it can help you to assess the health of your gut. Give yourself one point for every symptom you have from the list on the following page. If you have 3 or more points, you have a higher risk of having leaky gut syndrome.

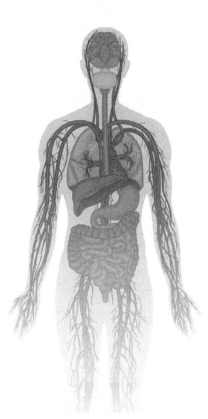

SYMPTOMS IN THE GUT

- ☐ Constipation
- ☐ Diarrhea
- ☐ Excessive gas
- ☐ Abdominal bloating
- ☐ Burping
- ☐ Irritable Bowel Syndrome (IBS)
- ☐ Food intolerances and sensitivities

SYMPTOMS IN THE SKIN

- ☐ Acne
- ☐ Eczema
- ☐ Psoriasis
- ☐ Rashes
- ☐ Itchy skin
- ☐ Hives
- ☐ Rosacea

OTHER ISSUES

- ☐ Joint pain
- ☐ Muscle pain and weakness
- ☐ Seasonal allergies
- ☐ Asthma

SYMPTOMS IN THE BRAIN

- ☐ Brain fog
- ☐ Chronic headaches
- ☐ Migraines
- ☐ Anxiety
- ☐ Depression
- ☐ Bipolar disorder
- ☐ Autism
- ☐ Parkinson's disease
- ☐ Attention Deficient Hyperactivity Disorder (ADHD)

AUTOIMMUNE DISORDERS

- ☐ Celiac disease
- ☐ Rheumatoid arthritis
- ☐ Lupus
- ☐ Type 1 Diabetes
- ☐ Crohn's disease
- ☐ Colitis
- ☐ Hashimoto's disease
- ☐ Chronic fatigue syndrome
- ☐ Fibromyalgia
- ☐ Any other autoimmune disorder

METABOLIC DISORDERS

- ☐ Diabetes
- ☐ Obesity
- ☐ Insulin resistance
- ☐ Difficulty losing or gaining weight

The Gut Flora

The intestinal microbiota, gut flora, or microbiome, is a complex ecosystem of microorganism species that live in your intestinal tract. There are around 100 trillion microorganisms in your intestines – that's more than *ten times* the number of your own human cells! You are outnumbered 10 to 1! And that's a good thing.

The metabolic activities performed by these microorganisms are so important to the body that they are considered as an entire organ on its own. If you added them up altogether they would weight anywhere from 3- 5 pounds.

The microbiome serves as a layer of protection to our gut lining and also provides the intestinal cells with proper fuel, such as butyrate, so that the lining can heal itself and maintain its integrity.

The beneficial bacteria also help us out with thousands of metabolic processes everyday- and still counting! They are involved in at least 20,000 functions in the digestive system alone. Each different strain of bacteria performs its own set of functions that helps us in our day-to-day lives. There's *Lactobacillus acidophilus* that among many things helps us metabolize sugars and breakdown casein and gluten while *Lactobacillus plantarum* reduces inflammation and supports intestinal barrier function.

It's very similar to how we work with dogs in the work force to assist us. These different strains are like the different species of dogs - a Husky is used to pull a sled through snow up North, a German Shepard is the favourite canine for police work. They each have their specific beneficial role that helps make our lives a lot easier.

Scientists are beginning to isolate specific strains of bacteria and their specific roles in our health from pathogenic obesity and diabetes promoting bacteria to helpful bacteria that relieve symptoms of stress, anxiety, depression, and even autism.

Important Functions Of The Gut Flora

The gut flora, or the microbiome, is a critical contributor the human immune system. As mentioned before 70%+ of your immune system lies in your gut. When the friendly bacteria dominate the gut, they also take up the most space, making it nearly impossible for the pathogenic bacteria, viruses, and fungi to take up residence. It's as if all the condos have been sold and they've got to move on over to the next neighbourhood. The beneficial bacteria also train the immune system to distinguish harmful pathogens from beneficial bacteria and stimulate the production of antibodies. To continue the analogy of your body as your temple, the gut lining is your fortress wall, and your gut flora are your army of soldiers defending those walls.

Gut flora also assist in the digestion of foods that your own gut cannot break down, extracting additional nutrients to be used by the body, providing a major source of useful energy. They help the body to absorb essential dietary minerals such as calcium, magnesium and iron and even synthesize some nutrients needed by the body, such as most of the B vitamins and vitamin K. They also provide fuel for the intestinal cells in the form of butyrate, essentially butter fat, which keeps them strong and held together in tight junctions. That's right, your intestines love butter fat!

Gut flora also influence your mood by producing 95% of the serotonin and half of the dopamine in your body. These "feel good" hormones improve your mood, memory, sleep and self-esteem, making it essential in preventing and fighting depression and other emotional disorders.

Gut Dysbiosis

Dysbiosis refers to a microbial imbalance in the body. In your gut, this means that you have too many bad bacteria which have outcompeted your good bacteria. The balance of your internal microbial ecosystem is largely determined by your diet.

An unhealthy diet (including processed foods, sugar, alcohol and refined grains) kills off the good guys and feeds the pathogenic microorganisms, allowing them to dominate the gut. Overuse of antibiotics, birth control, pain killers, and excessive alcohol consumption are also factors in dysbiosis.

When your gut is dominated by the "bad" guys, also nicknamed the *Homer Simpson* bacteria, you are more likely to be lazy, fat, and sick because the pathogenic bacteria create toxins that cause inflammation and weight gain, fog up your mind, make you lethargic, and make you crave sugary junk foods.

When you are in this state of imbalance, you can experience symptoms such as fatigue, headaches, brain fog and digestive issues. The longer the state of imbalance continues, the more severe the symptoms become. Gut dysbiosis has been associated with inflammatory bowel disease, chronic fatigue syndrome, obesity, cancer and colitis.

A study at the University of Kansas looked at people suffering from Irritable Bowel Syndrome - 100% of them were also suffering from gut dysbiosis, and when they were given probiotics, their symptoms improved.

As you may have noticed by now, many of the symptoms of gut dysbiosis are similar to those caused by leaky gut. In fact, these conditions often occur together and contribute to each other.

The Gut Brain Connection

The gut doesn't just absorb food and protect you/ The GI tract also has its own independently working nervous system called the enteric nervous system.

Your gut is directly connected to your brain via the vagus nerve and in your gut there are as many nerve endings as there are in a cat's brain, containing some 100 million neurons, and 500 million nerve cells- that's more than in either the spinal cord or the peripheral nervous system. It's no wonder our gut is nicknamed "The second brain."

Through this connection, the gut flora can directly influence the brain function. We already discussed how good bacteria can produce beneficial hormones such as serotonin; conversely, pathogenic microorganisms in the gut create harmful substances and neurochemicals that alter brain function in a negative way.

This imbalance in your gut microbe is inevitably connected to the brain and can show up as brain fog, behavioural issues, and mood disorders such as depression, anxiety, and even autism.

Recent research has found that behaviour conditions of autism are greatly affected by the gut flora. Children with autism have a less diverse population of probiotics in their gut - they are missing anywhere from 200-400 species. It's now believed that it's actually a *lack* of bacteria that seems to be at the root of these conditions. The more diverse your gut flora, the more healthy you are.

Animal studies reveal that autism-like behaviours can be reversed with the proper beneficial bacteria. In these studies mice with altered gut flora exhibited hallmark diagnostic symptoms of autism such as communication deficits. Once treated with a specific bacteria, *bacteroides fragillis*, the abnormality is corrected.

Healing Your Gut

So as you can see your gut microbiome, digestive health, mental health, and overall health are intimately intertwined. How much are you, *you*, and how much are you your *bacteria*? Interestingly enough, the more in-depth we study the microbiome, the more that boundary between the two blurs.

Not only was Hippocrates onto something when he said *"All disease begins in the gut."* You know what else he said? *"Let they food be thy medicine and they medicine be thy food."*

To start healing the gut, the first place to turn to is the food on your plate. The food you eat not only provides nourishment for your body and building blocks to assist in repairing and damage control but it also feeds the bacteria in your gut thus influencing its diversity and composition. With every bite of food you take, you take a vote for who you want living in your belly, the good guys or the bad.

The easiest and most effective place to start is your diet and incorporating the 4 R Protocol: Remove, Replace, Repair, and Repopulate.

REMOVE
The first step to healing a leaky gut and dysbiosis is to adopt a gut healing diet and remove offending foods and toxins from your diet. This includes:

- wheat and gluten containing foods, dairy, sugar, corn, and soy
- genetically modified foods
- coffee, alcohol, soda's and carbonated drinks
- processed and refined foods
- hidden food sensitivities which act as stressors on your digestive tract

All of these foods irritate the gut in some form and create an inflammatory response which is exactly what you want to be staying away from when on a gut healing protocol.

REPLACE

Now that you've removed the gut offenders from your diet focus on replacing them with nutrient dense, fresh, whole foods such vegetables, greens, fruits, clean organic sources of animal protein, nuts and seeds, and healthy fats such as ghee, coconut oil, olive oil, and bone broth. You want to flood your body with the nutrients it needs to repair and flourish.

Grains and legumes are quite difficult for your body to digest. They contain lectins and phytonutrients which can cause inflammation, prevent nutrient absorption, and further damage the gut. During a gut healing protocol it's a good idea to limit your grain and legume consumption, and completely eliminate gluten containing grains, until your digestive tract is functioning optimally and can actually break these foods down.

REPAIR

There are essential nutrients and supplementing these into your daily regime can help support the rejuvenation of your gut lining and overall gut health. These nutrients include digestive enzymes, l-glutamine, betaine hydrochloride, zinc, vitamin C, magnesium, omega 3 fatty acids, cod liver oil, and quercetin.

REPOPULATE

To rebalance your internal microbial ecosystem you need to eliminate the pathogen residents in your gut - the bad bacteria, parasites, and fungus. A parasite cleanse and candida regime is worth looking into as well as incorporating foods and supplements that help fight these intruders such as garlic, oregano oil, coconut oil, and activated charcoal.

Incorporate plenty of probiotic rich fermented foods into your diet such as sauerkraut, kombucha, kefir, and kimchi. There are dozens of fermented dishes to choose from and all of them you can make at home for pennies. These foods are critical components to a healthy gut as they provide your body with the appropriate diversity of friendly bacteria as well a concentrated dose of nutrients that support the overall healing and detox of your body.

Looking Past What's On Your Plate

Your food is the strongest form of medicine and your lifestyle choices are just as powerful. To truly restore balance to your internal ecosystem and

health, and keep it that way, you will need to look past your plate and at your environment, and behaviour.

Chronic stress plays a huge role in deteriorating your health. Not only does it cause a great deal of a headache, it ignites inflammation throughout your entire system, causes intestinal permeability, suppresses the growth of your heathy bacteria while allowing the pathogenic microbes to thrive and dominate your gut.

Focus on healthy stress management techniques such as meditation, exercise, journaling, gratitude, getting out in nature, connecting with loved ones, and scheduling in regular down time to recharge your batteries.

When you think about toxins and pollution, often we think of the dirty world out 'there'. The car exhausts and city pollution. However, your home can actually be more toxic. Chemicals masquerade themselves in your water supplies, personal hygiene products, cleaning supplies, and even in the air your breath. Most of these chemicals are highly toxic, are known to cause cancer, and also disturb the core of your wellness, your gut.

Ditch the chemicals and go green. Try out 'do it yourself recipes' for soaps, shampoos, cleaning products, perfumes, toothpaste, nearly every chemical laden product you have at home can be swapped out using inexpensive natural products such as baking soda, borax, vinegar, coconut oil, lemons, and essential oils. By doing so, not only are you avoiding unnecessary toxin exposure you are also helping the sustainability of our planet. What's good for Gaia, is inevitably good for you too.

Restoring your gut is not another fad diet, it's a total lifestyle makeover. Stick with these changes and you will create a fertile haven for blossoming health that lasts a lifetime. Now that you know what you need to do, I'll ask you what I ask my clients…

Do you have the guts to transform your life?

H.T.M.A. AND THE IMPORTANCE OF TESTING YOUR MINERAL LEVELS

(by Rick Fischer)

The delicate balance of minerals in our bodies has far reaching effects on health, both physically and mentally. Mineral levels (and ratios between minerals) can effect everything from weight (thyroid activity), energy levels (adrenal activity), digestive problems, personality (reactivity to stress and conditions including schizophrenia, paranoia, anxiety, addictive behaviour and even depression), susceptibility to heart attack, osteoporosis, and inflammation), and a wide range of other symptoms. While blood tests will miss many of the mineral dysregulation markers behind these conditions, H.T.M.A. (Hair Tissue Mineral Analysis) is a screening test that picks up very accurately these stored mineral levels and imbalances.

> *"[HTMA] may be the most important health test that exists... Only when you and your doctor know for sure your mineral status and important ratios can you adapt your diet, minerals and supplements to work toward proper balance."*
> ~Dr. Robert Thompson, MD (author of The Calcium Lie, deemed to be in the top 5 percent of US physicians)

HTMA uses hair (ideally from the scalp) to analyze a variety of minerals and heavy metals stored in the body. Unfortunately, when it comes to testing mineral levels, all too commonly physicians still rely on blood testing – a horrible flawed approach. A diagnosis is then made based on the results of that blood test with neither patient nor practitioner understanding that blood testing does not accurately pick up on stored mineral imbalances. Blood testing will only show high mineral levels immediately after or during acute exposure (and can be useful for hour by hour monitoring), but ignores long term stored and bio-unavailable levels. Blood testing also fails to assess key ratios between minerals which, even more important than any individual mineral level by itself, are the essential indicators that must be examined to properly determine the extent of any mineral deficiency or toxicity problem, and the subsequent supplementation and correction program. Hair Tissue Mineral Analysis not only picks up mineral toxicity levels that the blood doesn't show, it also provides very accurate ratios (discussed further below) from which then, and only then, can proper dietary, supplementation, and corrective advice be given. Without this vital information, any supplementation program is being done blindly.

> The blood is homeostatic, and regulated to stay within a certain range at the expense of tissue levels. It is merely a transport system. Our biochemistry happens at the cellular level, not the blood transport system! This is why medical science misses most deficiencies (ie: potassium, magnesium..) until it's too late. HTMA much more accurately reflects the metabolic process occurring within the cell.

When toxic amounts of a mineral accumulate in the body, they do not stay in the blood. The blood, due to its homeostatic nature, must by necessity

remove excess toxins and minerals quickly. Some of this excess gets excreted in urine (and urine analysis will therefore show what's being excreted). Much of the excess amount however largely gets stored, in a bio-unavailable form that the body can't use, in the cells and tissues. This explains why, all too often, heavy metal and mineral toxicity results based on blood serum testing return levels showing normal, even when toxic amounts are stored in the body's tissues. The doctor says you're fine, despite the possibility of severe dysregulation still occurring in (and affecting) the body (and mind). Misdiagnosis from blood serum tests, as a result, is unfortunately astoundingly common. HTMA on the other hand is able to pick up these stored toxic amounts, giving an accurate indication of the levels of toxicity while offering an evidence based approach to rectifying a number of serious chronic and acute conditions that can result from mineral imbalances.

HTMA is a powerful diagnostic tool that provides telling indicators behind a wide range of conditions, including: fatigue and adrenal problems, thyroid issues and weight gain, blood sugar problems, depression, sudden or severe changes in perception and/or personality, hormonal imbalances, stress, addictions, schizophrenia, osteoporosis, heart attack, hypoglycaemia, liver and kidney problems, PMS, and even skin problems.

Why Hair (H.T.M.A.) Is Superior To Blood For Mineral Testing

Above I mentioned how the blood works quickly to remove excess minerals, and this excess gets stored in tissues. As minerals (and metals) are being mobilized and transported, the hair picks up on these levels and provides a much more accurate reflection of the cellular and tissue levels of mineral and metals.

HTMA offers the following key benefits:

* sampling is simple and non-invasive
* mineral levels are much more accurately detected in hair than in blood
* Blood serum tests are misleading because excess minerals are not stored in the blood, they are stored in tissue!
* Since hair is a non-essential, excretory, storage sitof the body, the body tends to deposit more excess minerals and dangerous metals here than in many other tissue areas of the body.
* hair remains stable for biopsy for months or even years
* it is extremely cost effective, accurate, and reliable

Examples of why HTMA is superior to blood for understanding mineral levels.
Example 1: A blood test can show a perfectly 'healthy' level of copper even in the presence of copper toxicity in the tissues (very common).
Example 2: Forty days after acute lead exposure, lead is undetectable in the blood, though it's still in the body.
Example 3: When blood calcium drops, calcium is removed from bone to replenish the blood - meaning the blood calcium can appear within

normal range even though bones are being demineralized and osteoporosis is developing.

Example 4. An intracellular magnesium loss or potassium loss may be occurring at the cellular level even when the blood shows normal or high.

Example 5: Even the more advanced RBC (red blood cell) test for magnesium lacks logic. Roughly only 1% of the body's magnesium is in the blood - almost all of it is in the mitochondria of the cell - and red blood cells don't have mitochondria! A person can be depleted of magnesium before it shows up in a blood test.

Sample Scenarios That Show How HTMA Can Be A Life Saving Tool

Scenario 1:
A physician recommends to an elderly female to take Calcium supplementation in order to prevent osteoporosis. She has low magnesium levels (as many people do), yet the doctor has not verified this through testing. By increasing her calcium supplementation, this increases the ratio of calcium to magnesium in the body. A high calcium to magnesium ratio results in the calcium not being properly deposited in the bone, and instead it gets stored in cells and tissues, leading to a hardening of the arteries (calcium plaque) - leading to possible stroke or heart attack - and a further weakening of the bone. This vital calcium to magnesium ratio can only be properly determined through an HTMA test, and the magnesium level should first be known before given any calcium supplementation is given.

Scenario 2:
A young, healthy female has a copper IUD inserted. A few months later her adrenals burn out, her personality changes, and she becomes numb to her relationship. Her physician recommends a blood test, which shows elevated copper, and subsequently her IUD is removed. A second blood test later then shows a 'normal' copper level; she is advised she's now fine, and subsequently divorces her husband because she realizes she no longer 'feels anything'. This not uncommon scenario plays out all too often with physicians failing to recognize that excess bio-unavailable copper is stored in tissues (primarily the liver and the brain), and not the blood. After the IUD is removed, blood levels quickly return to normal, and subsequent blood testing completely ignores stored bio-unavailable copper in the tissues which can lead to severe psychological changes. This stored copper increases calcium levels (which leads to a calcium shell effect that numbs feelings leaving a person dead emotionally), lowers magnesium and increases sodium (both of which in turn increases the stress response and negative aspects of ones personality, along with anxiety, anger, and panic), and can lead to wide range of psychological problems. Had an HTMA test been done, the patient would have understood that, contrary to what the blood test showed, her copper levels were still high, and a proper, corrective detox and nutritional balancing protocol could have been advised based on her specific mineral levels as determined by the HTMA.

Scenario 3:
A middle aged male suffers from chronic fatigue. Years of traditional testing and lifestyle / dietary adjustments have been unsuccessful. An HTMA test is then performed, which shows the patient has an extremely low level of magnesium. Such a low level of magnesium puts this patient at very high risk for a sudden fatal heart attack, not to mention increased feelings of stress, anger, and depression. Should this same patient, for any number of reasons, start taking high dose Vitamin D (as is commonly recommended for immune function and overall maintenance of good health), this patient is putting himself at even greater risk for a heart attack as Vitamin D lowers magnesium even further. Thanks to the specific findings of the HTMA, the patient is able to begin a proper magnesium and mineral supplementation program that not only increases his energy, but also lowers his risk of early death.

Why Is HTMA Not More Common?

HTMA is a form of advanced nutrition science that threatens both the politics and finances of the health ("disease") care system. Money is not made by selling 'awareness' or natural healthy foods high in mineral content, but rather in pharmaceutical drugs that can be patented and sold for large profits - many that then cause side effects which then require more pharmaceutical drugs - a system that perpetuates profits at the expense of the public's health. In 1985 and again in 2001, two studies were picked up by the Journal of the American Medical Association that on the surface seemed to dismiss the findings of HTMA. These studies however violated most all acceptable protocol for testing, including ignoring the most basic principles for how to cut the hair itself and even using an illegally operating unlicensed mineral testing laboratory. Nonetheless, those bias studies cast an unnecessary doubt over HTMA among those who simply didn't understand it or take the time to research it further. As a result, those behind the studies have disgracefully impeded the progress of medicine, the health of people, and a greater understanding of natural based healing and testing methods which, contrary to the aforementioned bias studies, has been proven over and over again to be extremely accurate when performed as intended.

A widely watched 'Nightline' expose on hair analysis subsequently tried to dispel the benefits of HTMA by doing their own test. However, instead of using human hair, they submitted DOG hair, without mentioning this to the testing lab. Since the results came back odd compared to what should have been expected (for a human), the show suggested HTMA was a fraud!

Another reason, and perhaps most important, as to the greater lack of acceptance in the medical community of HTMA, is that doctors themselves simply have not received any proper training on assessing HTMA charts. Understanding HTMA charts is not as simple as just looking at a mineral level. An advanced understanding of mineral ratios and their various effects on physical and personality changes is required. However most practitioners do not receive this training. Rather, as has happened often, they will open an account at a testing lab (as any M.D. is easily able to do, run hair tests

on patients, and then prescribe supplements based on simply looking at mineral levels as being high or low. (As an illustration of this, let's assume a patient shows a high Mg level with an extremely low K level. Looking simply at Mg, Mg would therefore not be recommended. However, with a deeper understanding of how to interpret HTMA, the low K represents an increased burn rate of Mg, leading to Mg deficiency, and thus Mg for this patient is required!). In the end, incorrect interpretations of HTMA results has led to poor improvement in patients, and doctors therefore dismiss HTMA as not being an accurate tool. In effect, they have dismissed a very accurate screening tool based on their own lack of understanding how to use it.

As a result of bias and flawed studies and doctors who were not able to help patients through HTMA due to their own lack of understanding how to use it, the toll has been taken, and many in the medical community who have not taken the time to research HTMA further simply shy away from it. There are however thousands of peer-reviewed references that support HTMA, decades of research behind mineral interrelationships and balancing, and those who understand the benefits of HTMA (including various heads of government, world class athletes who have access to the very best medical care, forward thinking doctors and health practitioners, as well as the US Environmental Protection Agency) choose HTMA as the primary method of heavy metal testing and mineral screening.

Not All HTMA Testing Is The Same
Of course, for HTMA testing to be both accurate and affective, not only are specific and standard testing procedures required, but also required is an understanding of what the results mean. Unfortunately, not only do some labs not follow proper procedure (for mineral testing), but also damaging to the reputation of HTMA is the mis-interpretation of results by physicians who are not properly trained in understanding the sometimes very powerful effects (both physical and psychological) of mineral patterns and ratios. Interpreting results involves FAR more than just looking at the individual mineral levels, as will be explained further below.

Trace Elements Inc (TEI) and Analytical Research Labs (ARL) are distinctly different from other medical labs in the way they both test and interpret results, and thus in this author's opinion, are the only two recommended labs for HTMA. Most other medical labs analyze mineral levels in isolation, independent of other mineral levels. Doing so ignores one of the most important benefits of HTMA, that being the specific ratios and patterns between dynamically interconnected minerals that indicate dysregulation and/or health concerns. To illustrate an example of this, consider a chart that shows high Magnesium. Looking at magnesium independently, some labs (and physicians too) will assess this to mean that magnesium levels are adequate and there is no need for supplementation. However, when one looks further and understands the importance of ratios, one may see that there is also a high level of Sodium to Potassium, which in turn can lead to an intracellular loss of Magnesium (into the blood - which then shows as a high Mg level), and is in fact a sign of current or impending magnesium deficiency.

This underscores the importance of physicians being properly trained in understanding the dynamic connection between minerals. It is not as simple as looking at one mineral level alone to determine if one is toxic or deficient, and yet, a surprisingly high number in the medical field are not adequately trained to understand this.

Another reason why patients may receive a misdiagnosis from HTMA is the way the lab itself runs the test. For example, almost all other labs (including one used by a large percentage of physicians and which markets itself as a specialist and pioneer in essential and toxic elemental testing) wash the hair sample beforehand. The problem with such practice is that washing the hair beforehand undermines the validity of both sodium and potassium levels, by depleting each. Many of the key ratios (including the Ca/P, Na/K, Ca/K, Na/Mg) are then thrown off and the results become largely invalid.

If you are considering having HTMA done, ensure that the lab does NOT wash the hair beforehand - TEI and ARL being the only labs that correctly follow this protocol. Incomprehensibly this is common practice in the majority of labs worldwide, and washing the hair can remove 15% or even more of the mineral content (especially potassium and sodium as mentioned). This will significantly throw off key ratios. Equally important, ensure that the person analyzing your results understands the interconnection of minerals and both the physical AND psychological effects common for each of the key mineral ratios and patterns. If the practitioner offering you an HTMA is not able to tell you about the various mineral ratios, patterns, hidden toxicities, and effects both physical and psychological, it would be wise to rethink where you get your test done.

What Are The Key Mineral Ratios?

More important than individual mineral levels are the ratios between certain minerals. Over decades of research and thousands of cases, certain conditions can be clearly determined by the extent of a mineral ratio. Some of the key ratios are mentioned here.

Metabolic Type Ratio (Ca/P)
The ideal Calcium to Phosphorus ratio is 2.6:1. Above 2.6 represents a slow metabolizer experiencing stages of stress burnout and a slowing of the adrenals and thyroid. Below 2.6 represents a fast metabolizer experiencing intense stress and a tendency for magnesium and calcium loss.

Stress Ratio (Na/K)
The ideal Sodium to Potassium ratio is 2.4:1. The higher this number, the more intense the person's stress condition, and with it, a tendency for negative psychological and 'short fuse' reactions, fight or flight, and anger. A high ratio of sodium to potassium is also associated with asthma, allergies, lethargy, kidney and liver problems. The higher the number, the more likely the patient is also losing magnesium. As copper levels rise, this ratio increases. Vitamin D also has a similar effect by lowering the Potassium level, further increasing this ratio (in other words, a person with a high Na/K ratio should NOT be taking Vitamin D!). A low ratio on the other hand can be a reflection of adrenal burnout, and at very low levels can lead to heart

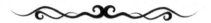

attack and cancer and, like a high ratio, liver / kidney disorders. The balancing of this ratio is essential, especially for anyone dealing with copper toxicity who, at high levels of copper or copper mobilization through detox, is greatly affected by the negative psychological aspects of a high Na/K which create reflex 'short fuse' reactions that bypass higher cortical intellect functions.

Thyroid Ratio (Ca/K)
The ideal Calcium to Potassium ratio is 4.2:1. Both calcium and potassium play an important role in thyroid activity. A high ratio of calcium indicates a slow thyroid (and symptoms such as weight gain, fatigue, cold hands and feet, depression, lack of sweating, and tendency towards constipation...). A low Ca/K ratio indicates a faster thyroid (and symptoms such as excessive sweating, irritability, nervousness, and loose or frequent bowel movements during stress). To help with weight loss, diet and exercise will help, but it will be an uphill battle against a slow thyroid if the Ca/K ratio is not first addressed).

Adrenal Ratio (Na/Mg)
The ideal Sodium to Magnesium ratio is 4:1. Sodium levels are directly associated with adrenal function. A higher ratio represents hyper-adrenal activity (with symptoms including inflammation, aggressiveness, impulsiveness, diabetes, hypertension, Type A personality), while a low ratio represents adrenal insufficiency (leading to fatigue, depression, hypoglycaemia, poor digestion, changes in weight, and allergies).

Hormone & Energy Ratio (Zn/Cu)
The ideal Zinc to Copper ratio is 8:1. A higher level of zinc reflects progesterone dominance and copper deficiency (with symptoms that may include anemia, arthritis, neurological disorders, cardiovascular disorders, amenorrhea, and more). A higher level of copper on the other hand indicates copper toxicity and estrogen dominance with symptoms which may include skin problems (such acne, psoriasis, eczema), emotional instability, "spaciness", detached behaviour, schizophrenia, PMS, reproductive problems, prostatitis, menstrual difficulties including amenorrhea, diminished feelings, depression and fatigue.

Blood Sugar Ratio (Ca/Mg)
The ideal Calcium to Magnesium ratio is 7:1. Hypoglycemia occurs as the ratio moves in either direction away from the ideal and, at both very high and very low calcium levels, mental and emotional disturbances are common. A high ratio of Ca/Mg also leads to increased insulin secretion, increased risk of muscle spasms, increased risk of blood clotting, and heightened anxiety. A very high calcium ratio as can result from copper toxicity can lead to the numbing of feelings and a detachment from reality.

How Are Mineral Levels Inter-Related?
All minerals are either antagonistic or synergistic to certain other minerals. Meaning when one mineral goes up, it may raise or lower other connected minerals. While endless scenarios could be painted with various minerals, here is a one very basic circuit. As copper goes up, calcium increases while zinc and potassium drop. The heightened calcium can end up creating a

"calcium shell" that numbs emotions, while the low potassium will increase both the Ca/K ratio (slowing of the thyroid) and the Na/K ratio. A high Na/K ratio leads to negative aspects of personality including increased anger, anxiety, panic, fears, a shortening of one's fuse, and a decrease in the functioning of the higher cortical mind. Meanwhile, magnesium will also drop as a result. The drop in magnesium increases risk of such things as diabetes, inflammation, and heart attack, while increase panic, denial, and the sense of stress. In turn, the heightened calcium with the lowered magnesium leads to a high Ca/Mg ratio, resulting in an increase in insulin, low blood sugar, and increased risk of muscle spasms and blood clots. Each of these increases stress which in turn further increases the Na/K ratio, increases the copper level, and lowers magnesium, and the cycle continues to spiral.

When correcting any condition through nutrition, or when taking supplements, we must recognize that nutrients do not operate independently from other nutrients. Having a clear picture, as presented through HTMA, is essential prior to supplementation, and makes supplementation and corrective guidance much more practical, meaningful, manageable and safer. Understanding one's mineral levels should be an essential first step to any dietary, weight loss, or health restoration program.

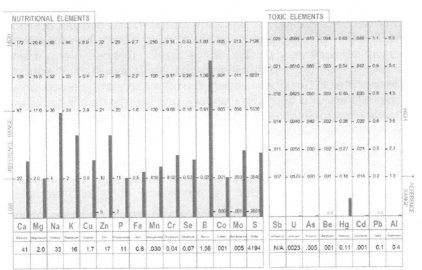

Sample image of a basic HTMA chart

"Any health practice or dogma, by way of rigid restriction or forced application, that takes not into consideration a person's bio-individually unique nutrient or bio-mechanical structural status, risks eventual damage to one's system. Taking into account a person's physiological limitations and their nutritional deficiency and toxicity profile through evidence-based testing is essential for designing intelligent and safe movement and dietary protocols." ~ Rick Fischer

COPPER TOXICITY

(by Rick Fischer)

Copper Toxicity. A silent epidemic that very few have heard of. Most doctors have no understanding of it. Yet it's an epidemic that has shattered the lives of countless women, and relationships. It is time the world wakes up to this condition, because the lives of our young women especially are most at risk. I have made it my personal mission through ongoing research and the creation of www.coppertoxic.com, the Internet's #1 support and education site on the topic, to bring much needed awareness to copper toxicity, to educate medical professionals on the devastating effects that copper dysregulation can cause and how to correctly test and treat it, and to help other women navigate their way through the often very long-term healing process.

What Is Copper Toxicity?

Copper toxicity is a build-up of bio-unavailable copper in the body that gets stored primarily in the liver and then subsequently in the brain and other organs. As copper accumulates it initially gets stored in the liver, causing the most common early symptoms of brain fog and fatigue. At high levels of accumulation however, the mind start racing and the adrenals may 'burn out'. Following adrenal burnout copper levels then spike even further as ceruloplasmin production declines. Copper is now being deposited in the brain and other organs, and this in turn leads to neurotransmitter imbalances causing brain function and perception to become altered, and depression, anxiety, and pseudo-bipolar conditions can result, even schizophrenia, and paranoia. Copper does not act alone however. As minerals are interconnected, the rise in copper lowers zinc and magnesium while raising sodium and calcium. One of the effects of copper toxicity is what's known as a "calcium shell" - a high buildup of bio-unavailable calcium that blocks the person's feelings and deadens emotions, making a person become emotionally numb and detached from reality. Awareness is diminished. Meanwhile zinc also drops as a result of high copper. This drop in zinc weakens the neocortex (the part of the brain which allows humans to reason and express higher conscious feelings such as love, and compassion). At the same time, the sodium to potassium ratio increases as a result of the rise in copper, and this causes negative aspects of personality to come to the surface, as well as past fears, anxiety, the fight or flight response, and a shortening of one's 'fuse'; and the person acts out based on those influences. The psychological connection of copper toxicity is just as important to understand as is the physical. In extreme cases, especially when the sodium to potassium ratio is high, the rebalancing of copper can only be accomplished once an underlying emotional issue is first dealt with, and this can be a catch 22 when the patient is unaware or unwilling to acknowledge this connection.

Ultimately, the body may shut down physically as a result of adrenal burnout, and the patient's mind is left is a state of detached reality based on numbed higher consciousness emotions, stimulated negative emotions, and altered memory and perception. Copper plays a key role in many patients who develop schizophrenia, paranoia, and Alzheimer's.

How Do You Get It?

Why is copper toxicity so prevalent? People can have high copper levels for many reasons, including drinking water from copper pipes, adrenal insufficiency, and occupational exposure. However the incidences of copper toxicity in recent decades is growing rapidly due to 3 main factors: the "birth" of birth control, the vegetarian diet fad, and the in utero passing down of copper from generation to generation. While a copper IUD directly feeds copper into the body, the birth control pill raises estrogen. Estrogen increases copper retention in the body. In both cases the body's copper level increases. This is one of the primary reasons why, in the past 5 decades, we have seen a large spike in the prevalence of high copper individuals. At the same time, the trend towards vegetarian diets also leads to copper excess. Vegetarian diets are high in copper and low in zinc. Zinc (primarily found in meat sources at least terms of highest absorption) is needed to keep the copper level balanced. Without adequate zinc, copper is allowed to spiral out of control. Ironically, those with high levels of copper have a harder time digesting meat protein. Liver and digestive function are affected as bio-unavailable copper increases, leading to declining bile function and subsequent difficulty digestion meat which can then feel unpalatable. This subconsciously leads a lot of people to finding reasons to adopt vegetarian/vegan diets - the very thing that will make their health even worse. Furthermore, copper excess in the mother is passed down in utero to her baby. This new life then starts life with a higher than normal level of copper, and a greater tendency to later in life develop symptoms related to copper excess. This effect compounds with each successive generation, and without addressing this, we are putting the health of our children at risk.

Stress is an additional factor that must be mentioned. As bio-unavailable copper increases it weakens the adrenals which then leads to even more bio-unavailable copper eventually building up. Stress is also one of the biggest contributors to zinc loss. Zinc is needed to keep copper in balance. So not only do the weakening adrenals create a spiraling effect on copper, but so too does the loss of zinc, both of which are caused by stress, both of which further increase stress, and all of which increases copper further.

How Do You Test For It?

"Disruption of the copper-zinc ratio is an overlooked contributor to intractable fatigue that follows excessive reliance on a plant-based diet. The result is toxic accumulation of copper in tissues and critical depletion of zinc through excretion.

This condition usually goes unrecognized because copper levels in the blood can remain normal. Also, most doctors are unprepared to meet with extreme zinc deficiency and its baffling effects on many systems of the body. Hair mineral analysis, competently used, is the tool which can unravel the complexities of this growing problem." ~Laurie Warner, M.A., C.N.C.

One of the things most concerning for me is the complete lack of understanding among most practitioners on how to test for and measure copper toxicity. Most doctors still rely on blood testing, while many patients are led to concern themselves with their blood test results. They have no understanding that bio-unavailable copper accumulates in soft tissue and not the blood, not to mention blood is homeostatic by nature and will always work to remove excess toxins and metals (copper included). As a result many highly copper toxic individuals will be told they are fine based on blood test results showing "normal". My plea to practitioners who want to help copper toxic individuals is to STOP diagnosing based solely on blood testing. The misdiagnoses that result from such a narrow minded view of testing can shift a person's entire life trajectory, and lead to often decades of additional healing work. People's lives are at stake, and we need to step away from outdated medical ideas that misrepresent and adopt more effective and holistic testing (and healing) strategies. H.T.M.A. (Hair Tissue Mineral Analysis) is by far the best way to test for copper toxicity, and yet, because most have not been trained in how to interpret the results of HTMA data, this powerful screening tool is still, by those too ignorant to study it properly, considered pseudo-science and largely dismissed. HTMA interpretation is complex, and extends far beyond just looking at individual mineral levels on a chart. Even the copper level in a copper toxic person may show normal on an initial HTMA test. This is because the toxicity can be hidden, sequestered in the organs until a certain stage of adrenal recovery is achieved at which point the copper then begins being released and shows up later. However, unlike blood testing, HTMA provides key mineral ratios which indirectly can indicate copper toxicity. Even more important than the copper level itself are these various ratios between other minerals, and only by understanding these various other mineral ratios and levels can proper diagnosis, mineral balancing and healing be addressed.

What Can Be Expected During Detox?
People often run into difficulty when they begin to 'detox' the copper, especially because most practitioners out there really have very little understanding of the psychological effects of copper, and the detox process can actually make the person far worse. A detox that focuses simply on supporting the liver (the obvious first place to look at for heavy metals and adrenal fatigue) can make one feel both physically and mentally better while in reality copper is mobilized in the body and further impairs the brain's perception. Added to this, a high increase in zinc (as part

350

of the detox) can significantly increase anxieties. Zinc helps mobilize copper, creating a temporary hypoglycemic state which boosts adrenal secretion and in turn increases anxieties. Panic attacks are also common. How this plays out depends largely on the individual's unique background and level of suppressed and subconscious hurts and fears.

As one eliminates copper through detox (even a proper detox), patients will often experience the effects of copper "dumping". The dumping is simply the elimination of copper. Typical symptoms of a copper dump include severe depression, uncontrollable anger, anxiety, panic attacks, and sleep disturbances, as well as increased headaches, paranoia, increased awareness of fears, decreased libido, fatigue, and digestive problems. Often the symptoms are frightening and very uncomfortable, and if the patient is unaware of what is happening they often stop treatment as it is too unbearable. By understanding that copper dumping and the associated symptoms are part of the detoxification process, patients (and their partners) are better able to endure what they are experiencing. Dumping usually occurs in cycles, and life can feel like quite a roller coaster for some time. Detoxing does not happen quickly, and can usually take 6 months to several years until the health of the mind and body are restored.

It should be noted that aerobic exercise, stimulant drugs, and increases in stress while detoxing can further exacerbate symptoms of copper elimination. These activities increase metabolic rate and cellular energy production which in turn can trigger copper dumps from cellular storage. Detoxing, when not monitored correctly, will mobilize copper from storage sites and increase the negative aspects of personality as well as increase the calcium shell even further. The danger is that the patient feels a return in their energy, and without proper guidance and education behind what may be occurring psychologically, the patient may believe at a certain point they are fine, unaware of what it has done to their perception and mind, or the risks their remaining copper level will pose down the road for their children.

Why Is Copper Sometimes Called The Emotional Mineral?

Copper, at a normal healthy level, helps in the release of endorphins that contribute to love and euphoria. The great misinterpretation of this is that, as copper levels get higher and higher, so too do feelings of love and euphoria. The truth is, copper at high levels creates the exact opposite! Copper in fact enhances all emotional states in humans – and predominantly, the negative ones. Copper stimulates the diencephalon or old brain. Zinc on the other hand is needed for the new brain (cortex) – the brain associated with the "higher emotions" such as reasoning, compassion and love. As zinc drops and copper rises, these higher emotions are weakened and the person tends to revert to using the old brain, also called

the animal/lizard brain or emotional brain – triggering a wide array of negative emotions and behaviors. Copper toxicity causes "excessive emotions of many types such as anger, rage, frustration and others." Copper, at high levels, leads to loss of libido, detachment from loved ones, and diminished feelings of love and compassion – leading time and again to the copper toxic individual losing interest in and feeling the need to end key relationships. Often, the more intense the relationship, the more intense the opposing reaction.

> *"The overall psychological effect of excess copper is a loss of emotional control and awareness accompanied by diminished feelings and numbness.... I would venture to say that divorce courts are loaded with people who's relationships were destroyed by copper toxicity."*
> ~ Dr. Rick Malter, Ph.D.

Copper's Connection With Other Key Minerals And Vitamins
Copper toxic individuals will usually display the following patterns when it comes to their vitamin and minerals levels:

Elevated Calcium: As bio-unavailable copper increases to high levels, a phenomenon known as the "calcium shell" is formed. This high level of bio-unavailable calcium is the body's ultimate defense against the stress caused to it by the copper and other stress inputs, and this leads to the aforementioned numbing and deadening of feelings.

Low Zinc: We've already looked at the important role zinc has in the brain, helping the functioning of the neocortex. Zinc deprivation also destroys the cells in the hippocampus (the part of the brain associated with recording and integrating meaningful memories, experiences, and emotions). *"Any deficiency in mossy fiber cells, or of zinc or histamine in the [hippocampus] cells, might result in schizophrenic behaviour."*[1] As copper increases, zinc decreases. This also leads to increased anxiety, lightheadedness, and detachment. Zinc deficiency is one of the greatest and least known dangers of the vegan diet.

Low Magnesium: Magnesium is the calming mineral, and as copper rises, magnesium decreases, further exacerbating irritability, inability to handle stress, and poor concentration.

Elevated sodium: Sodium is the primary stress, and the higher sodium rises over potassium, the shorter one's fuse becomes, and the fight or flight response is intensified. Later on, sodium will drop as aldosterone declines.

Low Potassium: rising bio-unavailable copper lowers potassium, increasing the aforementioned sodium to potassium ratio.

Low Vitamin B12: While copper may not directly lower B12, B12 deficiency is common is many copper toxic individuals, especially those who are vegetarian / vegan. In fact, B12 deficiency is inevitable for the vegan/vegetarian unless otherwise supplemented. Decades of studies show that B12 deficiency is common in patients with emotional

[1] Pfeiffer Ph.D, MD. Mental and Elemental Nutrients, USA, 1975

disturbances and mental illness. The late Dr. Victor Herbert from Mt. Sinai Hospital blamed B12 deficiency for the hospitalization of many patients in mental institutions.

Low Vitamin C: The adrenal glands require large amounts of Vitamin C, and as copper stresses the adrenals more, the greater the need for Vitamin C in order to help eliminate the excess copper. Stress depletes Vitamin C from the tissues, especially from those of the adrenal cortex. Dr. Carl Pfeiffer, Ph.D., M.D., a pioneer in the field of biological psychiatry, describes in one of the chapters from his groundbreaking and classic book Mental and Elemental Nutrients, the strong connection between excess copper and schizophrenia. In this book he states *"In the schizophrenic extra Vitamin C is needed to get rid of the accumulated copper... Any biological state which elevates the serum copper is likely to increase the need for C. The schizophrenic state, late pregnancy, excessive smoking of tobacco and, particularly, the use of the contraceptive pill produce states of elevated copper.... as all research to date has shown, drugs or situations which cause a rise in serum copper demand extra ascorbic acid."*

If I suspect I may be copper toxic, what should I do about it?

The first step is to properly determine if indeed you have excess copper. HTMA is by far the best way to assess this, as only through HTMA can the various key indicators of copper toxicity be seen. A simple blood test, which most doctors will offer, is NOT the answer as it does not accurately show stored copper levels (bio-unavailable copper is stored in tissues, not blood). Even the copper level on an HTMA can be misleading at first glance (especially because one can be copper toxic (high bio-unavailable copper) despite a low level showing visually, and this is why it is imperative to understand the mineral ratios and patterns that indicate copper toxicity, as easily evidenced on an HTMA chart. A high soft tissue calcium level, a low potassium level and a very high Ca/K ratio are major mineral effects of elevated copper.

Treatment will usually involve gradual supplementation with magnesium, potassium, Vitamin B6, Vitamin B12 (if vegetarian), Vitamin A, whole Vitamin C molecule (NOT synthetic ascorbic acid), light zinc (sometimes), manganese, MSM, chromium, taurine, a return to (at least even a light) meat diet for vegetarians, reducing stress, examining one's programs, fears and past hurts (which copper brings to the surface), and restoring the liver and adrenals with liver and bile and gentle adrenal support, all as part of a full copper detox process. Without adequate adrenal function, ceruloplasmin (Cp) production remains low and Cp is needed to bind to copper to make it bioavailable. Detoxing must be done slowly and monitored, as otherwise the effects of copper dumping can be severe and frightening to the individual or people around them. The detox protocol therefore should only be implemented once a thorough understanding of mineral levels has been performed through HTMA, and ongoing monitoring

of the detox process must be done by someone who understands the various physical and psychological symptoms that can occur during detox.

We truly need a paradigm shift in the way we look at health. We cannot continue to blindly believe that diet and nutrition do not play key roles in our health (minerals after all are the very spark plugs of life) - yet most doctors receive very little training in this area. The field of psychology also needs to catch up and understand that minerals, including copper, play a profound role in determining one's personality, with personality and behaviour changing based on mineral levels. We also cannot continue to pretend that vegan diets and birth control usage do not come without dangerous side effects, when each one directly raises one's level of copper (and it's therefore no surprise that the majority of people who have severe copper toxicity are either vegan and/or using birth control, especially the copper IUD). Women deserve to be fully informed of the dangers of birth control use, and currently almost all OB/GYNs continue to deny any such connection between birth control and symptoms of copper excess exists. Nor can we count on 'doctors' to help this condition when the vast majority of those who pretend they know how to 'fix' it only make matters worse by having no idea how to test for it, nor how to safely treat it. The suffering of people affected and the astounding lack of awareness is only perpetuated as a result.

The graphic on the following page offers a simplified overview of copper toxicity and its many implications, based on the author's more in depth research of copper which is available at www.coppertoxic.com.

354

Physical & Psychological Implications of Copper Toxicity

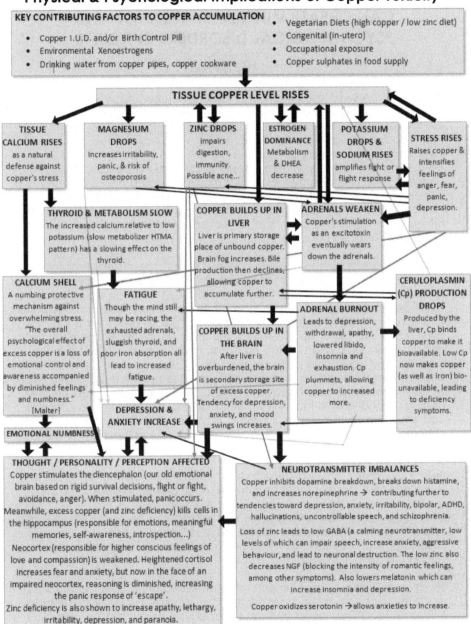

KEY CONTRIBUTING FACTORS TO COPPER ACCUMULATION

- Copper I.U.D. and/or Birth Control Pill
- Environmental Xenoestrogens
- Drinking water from copper pipes, copper cookware
- Vegetarian Diets (high copper / low zinc diet)
- Congenital (in-utero)
- Occupational exposure
- Copper sulphates in food supply

TISSUE COPPER LEVEL RISES

TISSUE CALCIUM RISES as a natural defense against copper's stress

MAGNESIUM DROPS Increases irritability, panic, & risk of osteoporosis

ZINC DROPS impairs digestion, immunity. Possible acne...

ESTROGEN DOMINANCE Metabolism & DHEA decrease

POTASSIUM DROPS & SODIUM RISES amplifies fight or flight response

STRESS RISES Raises copper & intensifies feelings of anger, fear, panic, depression.

THYROID & METABOLISM SLOW The increased calcium relative to low potassium (slow metabolizer HTMA pattern) has a slowing effect on the thyroid.

COPPER BUILDS UP IN LIVER Liver is primary storage place of unbound copper. Brain fog increases. Bile production then declines, allowing copper to accumulate further.

ADRENALS WEAKEN Copper's stimulation as an excitotoxin eventually wears down the adrenals.

CALCIUM SHELL A numbing protective mechanism against overwhelming stress. "The overall psychological effect of excess copper is a loss of emotional control and awareness accompanied by diminished feelings and numbness." [Malter]

FATIGUE Though the mind still may be racing, the exhausted adrenals, sluggish thyroid, and poor iron absorption all lead to increased fatigue.

ADRENAL BURNOUT Leads to depression, withdrawal, apathy, lowered libido, insomnia and exhaustion. Cp plummets, allowing copper to increased more.

CERULOPLASMIN (Cp) PRODUCTION DROPS Produced by the liver, Cp binds copper to make it bioavailable. Low Cp now makes copper (as well as iron) bio-unavailable, leading to deficiency symptoms.

COPPER BUILDS UP IN THE BRAIN After liver is overburdened, the brain is secondary storage site of excess copper. Tendency for depression, anxiety, and mood swings increases.

DEPRESSION & ANXIETY INCREASE

EMOTIONAL NUMBNESS

THOUGHT / PERSONALITY / PERCEPTION AFFECTED Copper stimulates the diencephalon (our old emotional brain based on rigid survival decisions, flight or fight, avoidance, anger). When stimulated, panic occurs. Meanwhile, excess copper (and zinc deficiency) kills cells in the hippocampus (responsible for emotions, meaningful memories, self-awareness, introspection...) Neocortex (responsible for higher conscious feelings of love and compassion) is weakened. Heightened cortisol increases fear and anxiety, but now in the face of an impaired neocortex, reasoning is diminished, increasing the panic response of 'escape'. Zinc deficiency is also shown to increase apathy, lethargy, irritability, depression, and paranoia.

NEUROTRANSMITTER IMBALANCES Copper inhibits dopamine breakdown, breaks down histamine, and increases norepinephrine → contributing further to tendencies toward depression, anxiety, irritability, bipolar, ADHD, hallucinations, uncontrollable speech, and schizophrenia.

Loss of zinc leads to low GABA (a calming neurotransmitter, low levels of which can impair speech, increase anxiety, aggressive behaviour, and lead to neuronal destruction. The low zinc also decreases NGF (blocking the intensity of romantic feelings, among other symptoms). Also lowers melatonin which can increase insomnia and depression.

Copper oxidizes serotonin → allows anxieties to increase.

"Virtually all MDs, including psychiatrists, still have not heard of this health problem. They practice medicine and psychiatry with an incredible lack of awareness that such a serious health problem even exists. They claim to be practicing "evidence based medicine", yet they are practicing without the most basic evidence – real laboratory data showing the presence of excess (toxic) copper that has a profound effect on both the physical and mental health of the vast majority of their patients." ~ Dr. Rick Malter Ph.D

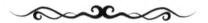

HOW IN-UTERO AND CHILDHOOD ENVIRONMENTS CAN CREATE MINERAL IMBALANCE AND PSYCHOLOGICAL DISORDERS IN ADULTS

(by Rick Fischer)

As parents we want the best for our children - raising them healthy, self-aware, confident, feeling worthy, and raised in an environment that instills every possibility for their own future success. Often this includes not having them repeat the same hard mistakes we as adults have made. Our words, love, encouragement and lessons in life all can help in this endeavor. However, there are at least two deeper undercurrents than run in all of us that can so easily sabotage even the most dedicated efforts of parents. Beliefs, and mineral patterns. That's right, mineral patterns. As we'll examine in this article, beliefs can literally alter mineral levels in the body, while mineral levels can have a profound effect on how one views the world and, consequently, one's beliefs.

What happens between parents in Vegas might stay in Vegas, but what happens in childhood might stay with that child for life. Children are imitators, they often learn by copying what they see others doing around them, especially their parents. In those early formative years, from age 0 to 7, children are like sponges, absorbing things that as adults we might not even realize we say or do. The interaction they see between mommy and daddy, their exploration of the world around them, the messages they receive, and their own interpretation of those messages, create their beliefs. Some are empowering, some are disempowering. Sometimes, when the message is so disempowering (or traumatic), the child creates coping mechanisms to bury the emotional pain. (As we'll get into later, this can show up in the person's mineral pattern). These mechanisms can remain with the person for life, subconsciously keeping the individual from a life more fulfilled.

Before we delve into the all-important mineral connection, let's look at some innocent situations that can create disempowering beliefs in a child.

Situation 1: A child is learning to tie his shoelaces as he and mommy are about to go somewhere. In a rush to leave, mommy innocently says "here I'll do it for you." Through this, the child picks up a belief that he's not good enough to do things himself.

Situation 2: Daddy was never around as the child grew up. As a toddler's world revolves only around herself, the little girl grows up feeling she's not fully lovable (I'm not good enough for daddy to love me, that's why he's never around); or abandoned, or believing that important men will always leave her (as her daddy did). She then grows up with an underlying fear of abandonment, following in her mom's footsteps as a single mom, abandoning anyone who comes too close before they might abandon her.

<u>Situation 3:</u> Every time the child cries or asks a question, the parents shhh the child. The child grows up feeling his or her voice isn't important, and is afraid to ask for what s/he wants.

As parents it's so important to be aware of these potential incidences, and counter any innocent mis-step with immediate positive reinforcement. This positive reinforcement (and challenging any negative beliefs the child may verbalize) is so vital in these early developmental years. Otherwise, the child unconsciously searches for evidence to back up the disempowering belief, and the more evidence it gathers, the more the belief becomes ingrained. (The same of course goes for empowering beliefs). Just as a child will want to do something again for which it's rewarded, the child will seek to avoid any future experiences that will lead to the negative emotional pain it felt during the disempowering moment. It's easier for a child to accept (and adopt) the negative repressive belief than it is to not understand why something happened, and thus the negative belief is so easily adopted.

Now let's fast forward to adulthood. With enough supportive and empowering guidance during childhood, the adult now has the tools to question his or her environment and thoughts. Limiting (or difficult) patterns may begin appearing in life (such as in finances, relationships, health, etc), but with enough awareness, reflection and searching, often the underlying cause of these patterns can be traced back to their origin, worked through, and resolved. But what happens if the awareness isn't there --- or disappears?

The awareness behind certain decisions and actions can become numbed when stress or pain (physical, mental, emotional, or a combination thereof) becomes too much to tolerate. To understand this dynamic, one needs to understand the interrelationship minerals have with each other and the relationship those minerals have with stress. This work and understanding is based on the foundational work and research of Dr. Hans Selye (acknowledged as the 'Father' in the field of stress research); Dr. Carl Pfeiffer, M.D., Ph.D. (physician, biochemist, founder of orthomolecular psychiatry, and who did some of the most important early research in the fields of schizophrenia and trace metals), Dr. Paul Eck and Dr. David Watts who's life works revolved around the establishment and utilization of HTMA to better understand mineral patterns and ratios and their corresponding health effects both physically and psychologically), and Dr. Rick Malter, Ph.D (nutritionist and child psychologist who for over 40 years through the use of HTMA data has further developed the understanding of how copper and other minerals affect one's psychology).

As stress increases, mineral levels within the body are affected. For example, stress will increase sodium, calcium and copper while decreasing magnesium. While physically a high ratio of calcium relative to magnesium can lead to muscle tightness and spasms, unstable blood sugar, and increased risk of heart attack, psychologically this high Ca/Mg ratio increases addictive behavior and cravings, increased risk of alcoholism, and co--dependency in relationships. In fact, a high Ca/Mg ratio,

especially when seen along with a high sodium to potassium ratio (which we'll look at next), is a common pattern seen in addicts and alcoholics as well as in their co--dependent partners who stay with, or return, to their abusive partners.

Sodium is the primary stress mineral, and as stress rises, the ratio of sodium over potassium becomes greater. As this Na/K ratio increases, it not only 'burns' magnesium leading to an even higher Ca/Mg ratio and more of the aforementioned symptoms, it also intensifies anxiety, fear, depression, low self-esteem, entitlement, loss of emotional control, agitation to the slightest irritation, fight or flight, and denial. It also increases the person's "Judge" (inner tyrant) while shrinking the person's "inner child" (true self)[1]. The rise in these negative feelings and loss of emotional control will lead to a need to numb feelings. Sometimes the person will turn to an external method such as alcohol or addiction. Alternatively, the body's own natural defense might kick in naturally and numb the person before they even become aware of what's happened to them. This natural defense is called the 'Calcium Shell'.

The calcium shell is a high level of tissue calcium that accumulates as the body's ultimate defense against stress. This calcium level, along with the aforementioned ratios, can easily be spotted on a Hair Tissue Mineral Analysis test/profile. The calcium shell serves to block feelings, deaden emotions, and diminish awareness so that the person does not have to 'deal' with some underlying pain or stressor that led to the calcium shell formation in the first place.

> *"In alcoholic or other dysfunctional families, there seems to be a strong tendency for a child to develop a calcium "shell" as a natural self-protective mechanism which helps to constantly deaden feelings of vulnerability and anxiety ...By adversely affecting glucose metabolism, the high Ca/Mg ratio also tends to predispose the individual to a higher risk of alcoholism or other addictions. Thus, TMA profiles allow us to observe and explain how psychological stress within a dysfunctional family can affect critical mineral patterns which then increase the person's risk to repeat the addictive and dysfunctional behavior. Over an extended period of time from childhood to adolescence, a high Ca/Mg ratio may become chronic and entrenched. Psychologically, a chronic high Ca/Mg ratio tends to be associated with denial or covering up a problem with which the individual cannot or will not deal."*
> ~ The Journal of Orthomolecular Medicine Volume 9, Number 2, 1994

In the past half century the increasing use of birth control has had a silent yet profound effect on the psychological health of the population. By way of increasing estrogen, copper retention in the female body is increased. Copper, as it rises to bio-unavailable levels, further increases stress, while lowering magnesium and increasing calcium (leading again to a greater tendency toward the high Ca/Mg traits previously mentioned). The use of copper IUDs and vegetarian diets have a similar effect - both directly raising the copper level in the body. When copper in a bio-unavailable form becomes too great in the body, it overloads the liver leading to adrenal fatigue and eventually impacts neurotransmitter balances in the brain, leading to a variety of psychological conditions including depression,

schizophrenia, paranoia, and with the calcium shell, a sense of apathy and detachment. (Perhaps this offers a clue as to why statistical rates of conditions such as depression and ADHD have been rising consistently over the past few decades). What mothers need to be aware of, even if they themselves are not aware of exhibiting obvious symptoms, is that copper gets passed down in-utero via the placenta to their fetus, and their child then begins life with an elevated copper level, and is pre-disposed to an increased risk for mental and physical health concerns as they grow up. In fact, 60 years ago the world's population as a whole had far lower levels of calcium and copper in their bodies than they do today. With each new generation this copper 'toxicity' problem becomes worse and as a result children are becoming more and more predisposed to conditions such as ADHD, depression, anxiety, bi-polar reactions, adrenal disorders (as excess copper weakens the adrenals[2]), liver problems, and other psychological disorders. In fact, high copper levels break down histamine, and this high copper low-histamine trait is found in over half of all schizophrenics. Behavioral symptoms in high-copper histapenia include paranoia and hallucinations in younger patients, but depression may predominate in older patients.[3]

> *"To illustrate one example of how powerfully a simple mineral can both affect as well as treat a person: An 18year old schizophrenic patient had a hair copper level of 41 mg% (normal is 2.5 mg%). She hallucinated and attempted suicide twice while in the Scottsdale Camelback Mental Hospital in Arizona. When her copper was brought back into the normal range with a nutritional balancing program, her symptoms disappeared and she has remained well ever since."*
> ~Dr. Malter, PhD

Another example of how mineral balancing can affect personality is the case of a 9 year old boy exhibiting extreme ADHD symptoms. He was a 'fast oxidizer' with a very low sodium level relative to potassium (a trademark commonly found in ADHD children) along with excessive levels of heavy metals and a high level of latent (hidden) copper. Over a roughly seven month period under the careful monitoring through HTMA and nutritional balancing (by Dr. Rick Malter, Ph.D), his copper dropped to near normal, the heavy metals were eliminated, and his sodium and potassium came back into better balance. The result - the child's behavior improved dramatically, with a substantial decrease in hyperactivity.

These examples show how the simple adjustment of mineral levels can profoundly affect one's personality.

As parents it's so important to understand the effect that copper (and other minerals and metals as well) have on children, detect any imbalances in childhood, and correct such imbalances naturally before the 'medical system' places them on anti-depressants, stimulants, and other dangerous psychotropic drugs. HTMA is the best lab test to detect such imbalances. Correction of imbalances is easier to do in childhood. Left undetected, imbalances can get worse. If you live in a home with copper piping and your child is drinking tap water, this will lead to a further increase of copper. If you have a daughter, as she reaches adolescence and her estrogen rises,

this will further raise her copper levels. Stress that your child experiences in childhood and adolescence will also increase copper. Left undetected, this can manifest years later in any number of conditions including adrenal burnout and / or a calcium shell which, as mentioned, numbs the person and decreases the awareness of what's happened to them.

Another thing that can happen in adulthood is the recurrence of memories associated with minerals patterns that were created earlier in life. Take for example a child with strict parents who were always scolding him, or a young girl in an early relationship with an abusive partner. Both of these situations caused the person tremendous stress, which would have created a particular stress--induced biochemical mineral pattern. Years later, when that same mineral pattern is recreated either through stress, nutritional balancing or some other life event no matter how innocent, those painful past memories and thoughts can be triggered and brought to the surface. This is very similar to how the scent of something like homemade cookies can bring back happy memories of vacations at grandmas, or a song triggers painful memories from a past relationship. A similar thing occurs with mineral patterns, yet this trigger happens in the subconscious and the person is not aware of why they suddenly may feel a certain way.

Beliefs and emotional issues developed in childhood can not only exacerbate the extent of mineral pattern / problem, but can also block the correction the mineral imbalance. A person with a copper toxicity issue (or other extreme mineral or heavy metal imbalance) may be unaware (or unwilling) to look at what happened to them due to their calcium shell, toxic metal levels, as well as their high Na/K ratio which inflates their Judge over their Inner Child. Emotional issues can in effect block the correction of the Na/K, copper level, and other ratios (as well as override the effect of supplementation) as "the issues are imprinted in the brain and nervous system at a sub-cortical cell and tissue level" [Malter]. In other words, mineral patterns (and numbing mechanisms) that developed in childhood from stressful events (or the child's interpretation of events) can create a mineral pattern that then becomes entrenched.

> *"As an adult, if we find ourselves overreacting to stressors in our life with a heightened stress response – an argument with our spouse, a bill we weren't expecting, a car that swerves in front of us on the highway – our inflammatory response stays on high, and this leads to physical disease and neuroinflammation, and mental health disorders. Mental and physical health disorders are a result of both the toxic stress response that developed in childhood, intertwined with our behavior - how we react to the adversity around us now - and together this becomes embedded deep into our biology. "*
> ~Donna Jackson Nakazawa

Inevitably as adults we create not what it is we say we want, but rather what we subconsciously believe we deserve. Let's say a woman finds the love of her life - something she's always consciously wanted. Or as another example, she wins the lottery. However, entrenched in her subconscious is the belief that she isn't worthy of such love, that she'll be abandoned, that

360

she doesn't deserve to be rich, whatever the subconscious belief may be. Of course no one would consciously ever try to ruin such a relationship, or lose the lottery winnings. But the conscious doesn't run the show, the subconscious does. If the loyal & loving man of her dreams shows up yet she subconsciously believes 'men' will leave, or hurt her, because that's what her father did, she'll subconsciously create a story (or condition) to inevitably lose him. She'll eventually look for, or somehow create, evidence that supports her subconscious programming that 'it's too good to be true'. Somehow, unless brought into awareness, addressed, and healed, she will subconsciously take actions that will sabotage the relationship, or the money, or whatever the case may be. Something even as simple and good-intentioned as adopting a healthy vegetarian diet could be a subconscious way of hurting oneself by starving oneself nutritionally, building up that copper, and eventually leading to the formation of a calcium shell that, beyond the person's awareness, sabotages that person's life in some way yet aligns with some unconscious belief that was manifested in childhood.

It's my hope that all parents explore this topic further for the love and well-being of their children. We cannot control how a child interprets events (even identical twins with the same DNA can interpret the exact same event in different ways, leading to completely different outcomes in their lives). However, we can control consistently giving empowering messages to our children, we can control setting good examples for them that they will want to follow, we can control the water they drink from and the balanced diet they eat growing up, we can choose to proactively investigate their mineral levels through HTMA when they are young and adjust through diet and nutritional balancing to give them the greatest chances for optimum mental and physical health as they mature; and we can choose as adults to incorporate relaxation techniques and lessen the stress in our own lives, to investigate our own mineral levels and ratios to better understand how they may be affecting our own thoughts and actions, and to do all we can to shrink our 'Judge' (through balancing Mg, Na, Cu, K, and Ca especially) and rediscover our own Inner child - our true self.

---

1 The concept of the Judge is taken from the work of Dr. Rick Malter Ph.D. and his book Shrinking the Judge: Freeing the Inner Child. The Judge is the negative voice, the ego not willing to reason, the 'inner tyrant' that disempowers and criticizes. The Inner Child is the part of our consciousness that is playful, innocent, open, uncomplicated, and connected to our higher self, truth.

2 As adrenals weaken due to rising copper and stress, ceruloplasmin (Cp) production declines. Cp is a carrier protein that binds to copper to make it bioavailable. The weaker the adrenals, the less Cp is produced, and the more copper becomes bio---unavailable, raising the level of stress on the body, and exacerbating a vicious cycle.

3 http://www.orthomolecular.org/library/jom/1999/articles/1999---v14n01---p028.shtml

ADRENAL FATIGUE

(by Rick Fischer)

Adrenal conditions are largely ignored in Western medicine, despite a tremendous number of health problems stemming from adrenal insufficiency and burnout. Stress is very often at the root of such disorders. This article looks at how the 3 stages of stress (developed by Nobel prize nominee Dr. Hans Selye, the "father of stress research" and who coined the term 'stress') lead to increasing stages of adrenal insufficiency. Further we look at some of the most common health symptoms (physical and psychological) that can result during each stage.

The adrenal glands consist of two parts, the medulla and the cortex. When a threat or stressor occurs, the medulla sets off the flight or fight response along with increasing the body's blood sugar, blood flow to muscles and the brain and lungs, increasing the rate of breathing, and pouring out adrenaline. The cortex produces cortisol (an anti-inflammatory hormone) and regulates immune, metabolic, and mineral balancing functions.

Stressors come in all shapes and sizes, and can include any of the following: direct physical threat, physical trauma, emotional trauma, toxic and heavy metal toxicity, lack of sleep, anxiety, poor diet (including over-consumption of sugars and refined carbs and/or deficiencies in Vitamins B and C), coffee, alcohol, infections and illness, prescriptions drugs, pregnancy, and excessive exercise. It's important to note that, when it comes to emotional stressors, the body reacts the same whether the threat is real or just imagined. Worry about some future event that may never even happen, for example, can create stress and over-tax the adrenals.

Let's return for a moment to the work of Dr. Hans Selye, who's widely accepted model of General Adaptation Syndrome explains the 3 stages of stress - alarm, resistance, and exhaustion. These 3 stages further align with his work around maladaptive stress syndrome (MSS). Just as with stress, MSS has 3 stages as well - alarm, suppression, exhaustion - yet these stages deal specifically with adrenal function. Let's take a look at what happens in each of these stages.

The first stage of stress is the alarm stage. This is known as the fight or flight reaction, and a burst of adrenaline and cortisol is released. Strength and energy increases in order to deal with the event at hand. This corresponds with the first stage of MSS, known as MSS1. When the stress is dealt with quickly, the body is able to return to normal rather quickly in a healthy manner (usually within a few hours). With today's fast-paced hectic lifestyles, most people find themselves in a fairly constant MSS1 state.

If the stress is not properly dealt with however, then stress turns into the resistance stage. The unresolved stressor/threat keeps the body continually

'on-guard' in a state of emergency and eventually reduces the body's ability to effectively defend itself. Adrenaline release subsides, but cortisol continues to be released in high amounts, along with neurotransmitters epinephrine and norepinephrine. When this ongoing defense attempt continues, disease sets in, and the sufferer becomes prone to symptoms such as fatigue, concentration lapses, and irritability. In terms of the adrenals, this is the suppression stage of MSS2. The adrenals are getting worn out and additional common symptoms include depression, anxiety, lack of appetite, and even possibly diabetes (due to insulin resistance). Progesterone decreases, while androgen production increases, leading to an increase in estrogen and testosterone.

The third stage of stress is the exhaustion stage (corresponding with the exhaustion stage of MSS3). The body has run out of resources to maintain it's energy, and the body 'crashes'. This is experienced as adrenal exhaustion or "adrenal burnout". Mentally, physically, and emotionally, the person has nothing left. Blood sugar levels decrease, cortisol production drops, stress tolerance drops, illness sets in, and the body collapses. The immune system is suppressed, feelings of depression increase (as serotonin activity has been compromised), and fatigue is apparent. Individuals at the burnout stage exhibit serotonin depletion (affecting reduced appetite, reduced sexual urges, poor sleep, and reduced memory) and/or dopamine (reward driven part of the brain) depletion. Other common conditions that occur with MSS3 include chronic fatigue, fibromyalgia, atypical depression, apathy, hypoglycaemia, light-headedness, lack of focus, and irritability. The immune deficiency caused by severe stress (such as the death of a spouse) can result in cancer or other fatal diseases (underscoring the importance of recognizing the cause of one's stress and moving toward releasing it). At this stage, after adrenal exhaustion, the hippocampus part of the brain becomes very vulnerable, and both thinking and memory are likely to become impaired - further increasing anxiety and depression. It's common for individuals suffering from low adrenal function to withdraw from certain areas of life. Another thing that occurs with many adrenal burnout patients is that prolactin levels drops, and with this drop are corresponding low serotonin and oxytocin levels. All these factors can really play havoc on close relationships as the patient begins functioning in a depressed state of apathy and dis-attachment.

According to the book 'The Everything Guide to Adrenal Fatigue' by Dr. Maggie Luther, the following are the common and true symptoms of adrenal gland dysfunction:

> difficulty getting up in the morning
> strong salt cravings or strong sugar cravings (usually one or the other, not both)
> daytime fatigue that is not relieved by any amount of sleep
> lowered or no libido
> difficulty handling stress, decreased productivity

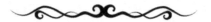

- ➤ increased emotional symptoms including anxiety, irritability, depression
- ➤ trouble recovering from illnesses, chronic infections
- ➤ lightheadness when standing quickly, ongoing ringing in the ears
- ➤ worsening of symptoms if meals are skipped
- ➤ lack of focus, "brain fog", memory loss
- ➤ exhaustion in the morning, crashes in the early afternoon, energy bursts after dinner at night

(Other common symptoms may include headache, nausea, vomiting, dehydration, confusion, frustration, insomnia, joint pain, weight loss (after burnout), and decreased appetite.)

What is interesting is how the list above resembles the symptoms of copper toxicity. Copper toxicity, while certainly not the only cause of adrenal burnout, is nonetheless a primary contributor. Copper toxicity is a buildup of high amounts of bio-unavailable copper in the body, a silent epidemic affecting millions and, most predominantly, women. Copper piping, birth control usage, vegetarian diets, and estrogen all contribute to rising levels of copper in the body. A high level of bio-unavailable copper is a stressor on the body, and directly affects (weakens) the adrenals. What are the primary symptoms of copper toxicity? Not surprisingly, they are almost identical to those of adrenal burnout! The primary symptoms of late stage copper toxicity include:

- ➤ fatigue and exhaustion
- ➤ mood swings
- ➤ depression, PPD, irritability and anxiety
- ➤ brain fog and spaciness
- ➤ concentration and memory problems
- ➤ withdrawal and decreased libido
- ➤ lowered immunity
- ➤ hormonal fluctuations and estrogen dominance
- ➤ bi-polar, paranoia and schizophrenia
- ➤ insomnia

Copper toxicity and adrenal burnout go hand in hand, each contributing to the other, and each exhibiting very similar symptoms, physically and psychologically.

Before beginning the discussion on ways to improve the adrenals, the following salient points written by Dr. Maggie Luther in her book 'The Everything Guide to Adrenal Fatigue' very effectively describe a few of the key issues regarding adrenal burnout symptoms. The following excerpts are from her book, which, for anyone dealing with adrenal fatigue or burnout or wanting to understand this condition better, is a highly recommended and comprehensive book on the topic.

Regarding insomnia:
"One main contributor to poor sleep quality is the health of your adrenal glands. When you push yourself during the daytime, eventually you burn out your adrenals, which can cause a disturbance to the natural rhythm of the sleep-wake cycle. Eventually cortisol spikes are seen prior to bed, around 10P.M., or in the middle of the night between 1-3A.M., causing insomnia."

Regarding irritability:
"Irritability is a feeling that often stems form not being able to do something. This state of feeling commonly comes from unaccomplished goals, inability to finish a task to completion prior a deadline, or having unrealistic deadlines. Some individuals also experience simultaneous challenges with emotional expression, often stemming from childhood. This can also contribute to feelings of irritability. When your adrenal system is fatigues, you revert to more immature states."

Regarding brain fog:
"Brain fog, mental fatigue, and inability to focus are common symptoms of an undernourished cellular and mitochondrial system, weakened nervous system, and heightened stress response. Over time, the acute effects of cortisol, which includes improving your ability to focus and helping with retention of short-term memory, flatlines and your brain becomes overwhelmed with the amount of cortisol and neurotransmitters bombarding it, day in and day out."

So, what's the answer to healing the adrenals? Well, it really depends on what stage of MSS you're at. A person with exhausted adrenals will naturally want to find ways to boost their energy, through stimulants such as coffee, or ginseng. However, this is can be counterproductive as it is akin to taking a whip to an exhausted horse - you'll make the horse move a bit, but eventually the horse will just collapse. Instead, the adrenals need to rest, long enough to rejuvenate. Generally, regardless of stage, and in addition to resting, steps that will support the adrenals include:

✓ identifying and removing/rectifying any factors such as heavy metal toxicity, food sensitivities, parasites…and of course stress
✓ restoring and repairing healthy gut function
✓ improving liver function

Let's take a closer look at each stage in turn.

In MSS1, you can still get away with stimulating the adrenals, in healthy ways, though of course it is always best to let the adrenals rest. At this stage however, you could get away with using stimulating herbs such Asian Ginseng (energizing, boosts vitality in the aged), American Ginseng (slightly less stimulating and can help balance the adrenals), Eleuthero (energizing, boost mental clarity, supports immune function and emotional resilience during stress), spices, and even limited caffeine when necessary (though never fully advisable). The aforementioned being said, it's important to

remember that the more the adrenals are stimulated without enough recovery time, the more likely you are to progress into MSS2.

During MS2, you would certainly want to avoid stimulating herbs. Therapy needs to center around calming down the adrenals. Asian ginseng is not advisable as it is too stimulating. American ginseng is a slightly better alternative as it is not as stimulating, though it too at this stage is best avoided. Holy basil (promotes a more balanced stress response and keeps adrenals from overreacting), schisandra (supports immune system while calming the heart and spirit), Ashwaganda (an adaptogen that can be both stimulating and relaxing), licorice (great to use when cortisol production is high, though it should be avoided in people with high blood pressure), rhodiola, wild yam and milk thistle can all be be beneficial at this stage. Just as with MSS3, relaxing therapies, stress management techniques and lifestyle management for better balance need to be adopted.

At MSS3, the key is to let the adrenals fully rest. They need to be 'put to bed' so to speak. Stimulating supplements, hard exercise, and stress will all exacerbate the condition and will not allow your adrenals the recovery that they need. Focus on scaling back your activities, getting at least 8 hours (or more) sleep per night, emphasizing stress reduction activities such as massage, light yoga, deep breathing, taking time to smell the flowers... and understand that this stage of adrenal exhaustion will take a longer term committed effort in order to heal. This is the time to simplify your life as much as possible. Eat plenty of fresh, whole foods, with extra emphasis on magnesium (calming) and potassium, while avoiding sodium (the primary stress mineral). More complete dietary guidelines are available on page 91.

In closing, a cautionary note on using adrenal formulas when copper toxicity is the cause of the adrenal exhaustion. Adrenal formulas can certainly assist the adrenals and can sometimes offer a fairly quick return to energy. However, the adrenal boost can mobilize copper that has been stored in the liver and/or brain, and this mobilization can lead to an increase in negative detox symptoms, both physical and psychological. For this reason the person's minerals levels should be monitored through HTMA during the process of copper elimination and adrenal restoration. HTMA also provides a powerful indicator of adrenal strength through the sodium to magnesium ratio. Balancing this ratio can also help in the improvement of adrenal issues.

Adrenal burnout is the culmination of long-term chronic stress. Correcting this condition takes time (figure anywhere from 2 – 6 months while following a full restorative program), so please be patient (and kind to yourself) with your progress.

The Darker Side of Vitamin D

(By Rick Fischer)

I used to be a big believer in the benefits of supplementing Vitamin D until I learned how dangerous it really can be. We're sadly all conditioned to believe, through what our doctors, nutritionists, and the media tell us, that Vitamin D is healthy, especially as it's the "sun vitamin", and it's hyped in health and medical articles as being a cure for almost everything under the sun. Indeed Vitamin D certainly has health benefits, and there is no shortage of information out there that supports that view. However, there is also a dark side to Vitamin D that very few talk about or understand, and it needs to be brought to light. It's not talked about because very few individuals (doctors included) understand the interrelationship between minerals (and vitamins). It's almost all but completely ignored in medical school, yet this mineral interrelationship is at the very foundation of our health. When one comes to understand the effect that excess Vitamin D has on other minerals (as this article explains), we then begin to see its more dangerous side. The truth is, the recent herd mentality fad of blindly supplementing Vitamin D pills is putting millions of people (in fact, the vast majority of the population) at high risk for everything from weight gain and heart attack to decreased energy and even depression. Chances are, if you're popping vitamin D pills, you're putting your health at risk.

"Healthy people have been popping these pills, but they should not continue taking vitamin D supplements unchecked. At a certain point, more vitamin D no longer confers any survival benefit, so taking these expensive supplements is at best a waste of money."
~Muhammad Amer, M.D., M.H.S (lead researcher at John Hopkins)

First it's important to understand that the Vitamin D we get from the sun (which is in a sulfate form) affects the body differently from isolated synthetic oral Vitamin D supplementation. What I'll be referring to in this article is oral Vitamin D supplementation...which really, isn't even a vitamin, but an immunosuppressive steroid[1]! When we're exposed to the sun (UVB), the skin synthesizes Vitamin D sulfate. This sulfate form is water soluble, is able to travel freely in the blood stream, strengthens the immune system, protects against cardiovascular disease, helps against depression, assists with detoxification, and nourishes the brain. Sunshine Vitamin D therefore really is healthy for us, as long as we maintain intelligent exposure. The supplement form of Vitamin D3 however is un-sulfated, not water soluble, and requires LDL ('bad cholesterol') to be transported. The un-sulfated supplement form does not offer the same benefits as the sulfate form, although the supplement form is great at transporting calcium through the body which the sunshine form doesn't do - at least, not initially. The sulfated form, after offering it's other benefits in the body, 'drops' the sulfate and then, in its newly un-sulfated form, is able to assist with calcium and bone health. So basically the sunshine version offers the best of both worlds, whereas the supplement version misses out on a lot of the benefits...and...as you'll learn in this article, comes with dangerous

consequences. Specifically, Vitamin D directly lowers Potassium and Vitamin A levels and raises Calcium levels. Let's look at the implications of this.

The balance between Calcium and Potassium affects thyroid performance. The higher this ratio, the slower the thyroid. As calcium rises and potassium drops, the Ca/K ratio increases, leading to a slowing of the thyroid, and potentially, weight gain! Another consequence of low Potassium as a result of Vitamin D supplementation is a higher Sodium to Potassium ratio. As the Na/K ratio increases, inflammation and the stress response increase. As one's stress increases, Magnesium, drops. In other words, taking excess Vitamin D leads to magnesium depletion. Magnesium deficiency in turn leads to increased risk for heart attack, especially in the face of high stress and a high Calcium level (which Vitamin D also contributes to). The lowered Magnesium also contributes to diabetes (as Magnesium helps regulate insulin). The consequences of high calcium relative to low magnesium also lead not only to psychological concerns and heightened anxiety, but also unstable blood sugar levels and craving of all kinds (including various addictions). The irony is magnesium is needed to raise Vitamin D levels - yet by taking all this vitamin D that we're being told to take we're only lowering magnesium further and actually impairing the goal of raising Vitamin D! If you really want to raise your body's natural vitamin D level, work on boosting your magnesium - it's a key cofactor required to bind Vitamin D to its transport protein.

Vitamin A is necessary to decrease inflammation. However Vitamin D lowers Vitamin A (both in the liver and in the blood). Vitamin A deficiency in turn impairs iron utilization and transport, and it's well known that Vitamin A deficiency is a cause of iron anemia[3]. Taking synthetic Vitamin D, which lowers Vitamin A, therefore contributes to this anemia. Even more dangerously, both Magnesium and Potassium are necessary for the body's anti-inflammatory response, and yet, as we've already looked at, Vitamin D lowers both these essential minerals. Without the necessary anti-inflammatory response, a host of disease processes arise, and arteries also become damaged. Calcium and cholesterol then get drawn to these sites of arterial damage and plaque builds up, leading to atherosclerosis (hardening of the arteries). Furthermore, Vitamin A is necessary for the production of ceruloplasmin, a protein that binds to Copper to make it bioavailable. Unfortunately, Vitamin D lowers Vitamin A which lowers ceruloplasmin which makes copper bio-UNavailable. This in turn leads to many of the negative side effects associated with copper toxicity, while also raising bio-unavailable calcium - weakening the bone matrix and contributing to a higher risk of osteoporosis. Yes, contrary to the lies we're told by Vitamin D proponents, too much Vitamin D at best has a negligible effect on bone density or, as has also been shown, may actually increase the risk of bone loss and osteoporosis, not to mention increase the risk of kidney stones[1]!

"Until now we haven't worried about giving people extra vitamin D because we thought "it might help anyway and of course (as it's a vitamin) doesn't do you any harm". With our increasing knowledge, we

368

should now know better....One 2015 randomized study of 409 elderly people in Finland suggested that vitamin D failed to offer any benefits compared to placebo or exercise - and that fracture rates were, in fact, slightly higher......One study involving over 2,000 elderly Australians, which was largely ignored at the time, and the one just published found that patients given high doses of vitamin D or those on lower doses that increased vitamin D blood levels within the optimal range (as defined by bone specialists) had a 20-30% increased rate of fractures and falls compared to those on low doses or who failed to reach "optimal blood levels". " ~ Tim Spector, Prof of Genetic Epidemiology [2]

Returning to the issue of soft tissue calcification, the Merck Veterinary Manual says the following about Cholecalciferol (which is essentially Vitamin D, used as a rat poison)... *"Cholecalciferol produces hypercalcemia, which results in systemic calcification of soft tissue, leading to renal failure, cardiac abnormalities, hypertension, CNS depression, and GI upset."* Sure, this is relating to effects in rodents, but it still conveys nonetheless how too much vitamin D leads to calcification, and the dangers therein.

Why then do some people feel good when taking Vitamin D pills? For one thing, the effect is usually a short term benefit at the expense of detrimental effects longer term. For some people, taking Vitamin D supplementation is beneficial - typically the fast metabolizer with high potassium. This however can only be determined by first understanding your unique mineral levels as shown through a Hair Tissue Mineral Analysis (HTMA). Blood testing for this purpose is highly inadequate as blood serum levels can fluctuate day to day and do not accurately represent stored tissue mineral levels. Through HTMA testing we can see if a person is a fast metabolizer (as defined when the Calcium to Phosphorus ratio is below 2.6 and with lower calcium relative to sodium and potassium) or a slow metabolizer (when the Ca/P ratio is above 2.6 and with higher calcium relative to lower sodium and potassium). Over 80% of the population are slow metabolizers, and for these people, who generally already have higher levels of calcium and lower levels of potassium, Vitamin D supplementation can have very adverse effects. Fast metabolizes can benefit from Vitamin D supplementation as it can help bring better balance to their mineral pattern.

What about those serum tests that show almost everyone being deficient in Vitamin D (chances are quite good that your doctor has told you that you are low in Vitamin D)? One problem is that typical testing (along with many studies for that matter) most often tests Vitamin D in the form of 25(OH)D (the storage form of D) and this usually tests low. However there is also the active (calcitriol) form (1,25(OH)2 D3) - very few doctors ever test for this. If doctors test both forms as opposed to just one they would see that Vitamin D deficiency may be less extreme than what it appears to be. If your doctor is telling you that you're low in Vitamin D, demand that s/he first test BOTH the storage and active forms to give you a truer picture. Added to this, most people will still be deemed Vitamin D insufficient when their results come back between 21-29 ng/mL even though those levels have

traditionally been a normal and healthy level. Indeed, too much Vitamin D is just as dangerous as too little, and as this article explains, **"adequate vitamin D prevents heart disease, but too much vitamin D promotes heart disease. The available evidence suggests that the lowest risk of heart disease occurs when vitamin D status is between 20 and 40 ng/mL."**[4] It's only due to what could be considered misinterpretation of a few studies in the early 2000s that then led the public and medical community alike to believe we are all suddenly now insufficient at those levels. Popping back extra D without further inquiry, rather than fixing a supposed condition of insufficiency, is instead today opening the door to a much wider range of health conditions!

"The definition of Vitamin D deficiency needs re-evaluation in view of the fact that low 25(OH)D is found in both healthy and sick individuals... It is reasoned that if low 25(OH)D indicates a current or potential disease state, then increasing 25(OH)D by supplementing with vitamin D should provide some symptom relief and/or protection. So far, there is scant evidence for this hypothesis... Despite the recent increase in vitamin D supplementation, chronic diseases have increased & are expected to continue increasing." [5]

"Taking extra calcium and/or vitamin D without an understanding of how they are interrelated with other vital nutrient minerals can start a cascade of adverse changes in the nutrient mineral system. Unfortunately, for countless numbers of people, their medical doctors lack this essential information and understanding of dynamic scientific nutrition."
~Dr. Rick Malter, Ph.D.

It is shocking the number of physicians that are telling their patients to boost their Vitamin D levels based on (a) not testing both active and storage forms, (b) telling patients they are insufficient when indeed they may not be, (c) not assessing the other cofactors (such as magnesium) necessary to maintain an adequate D level, and (d) suggesting dosages ranging from 5000iu to 50,000iu!!!! In most instances when a client comes to me showing rock bottom potassium in their HTMA, sure enough they have been supplementing with high dose Vitamin D. Please, before you waste money on synthetic Vitamin D (or any other vitamin or mineral supplement for that matter), it's so important that you first understand the risks of Vitamin D (and other nutrients) in terms of how they affect your mineral ratios and the health of your body. As we've seen, even something as "popular" as a Vitamin D pill can have very serious consequences on health. Unfortunately, until HTMA is more widely adopted by mainstream health, these effects will largely go hidden and doctors and nutritionists alike will continue to go on touting Vitamin D supplementation as a cure-all for everything.

"Studies which incorrectly interpret the reason for low vitamin D in patients with chronic disease have been seized upon by the media, and form the basis of massive advertising campaigns – which, along with ill-informed

recommendations by doctors and researchers, have created a perfect storm of misunderstanding and bad advice."
~Amy Proal, Ph.D.

The benefits of taking vitamin D are usually short term, and most studies only track this short-term period. This is why many 'experts' continue to promote the benefits of taking more vitamin D, not connecting the dots to the negative longer term biochemical effects.

"One of the abiding weaknesses of studies on the effects of vitamin D on health is that researchers simply do not follow subjects consuming the secosteroid for a sufficient period of time. Instead, they tend to track subjects over the course of weeks, months, or one or two years, during the period of time when study participants are usually feeling the palliative effects of the steroid. This practice is a mistake as it does not account for the long-term immunosuppressive effects."[6]

If you're concerned about your Vitamin D levels and want to raise it in a safe way, there are natural ways to do this which are far safer than taking synthetic supplementation. First and foremost, check your magnesium level!! You can pop all the Vitamin D in the world, but without adequate magnesium you will still have trouble raising your D levels. This is even more true when we consider that most of the Western world is over-calcified, and as a natural feedback loop the body attempts to lower Vitamin D as a result (to prevent calcium from going higher). Taking isolated Vitamin D pills therefore is not the answer, as it only compounds the calcification issue, which then further depletes magnesium, and in turn promotes the body's need to suppress Vitamin D. In other words, if you truly are Vitamin D deficient, chances are fairly good that it's because you are deficient in magnesium and/or over-calcified! Due to our over-calcified 'epidemic' on the other hand, Vitamin K2 is very supportive not only in assisting proper calcium absorption, but also in the proper utilization of Vitamin D while also protecting against toxicity. Safe sun exposure is an excellent way to naturally raise D, though we should also include a dietary focus, still being cautious though of the lowering effect too much 'vitamin' D will have on potassium and other nutrients. That said, some of the best dietary sources of Vitamin D include:

- ✓ cod liver oil
- ✓ fish - specifically salmon, sardines, herring, mackerel
- ✓ eggs - 1 egg contains roughly 10% DV
- ✓ shiitake and button mushrooms - though a poorer source and ONLY if they have been grown in sunlight
- ✓ other sources include grass-fed butterfat and organ meats, cheese, and bone broth

Still scratching your head that the answer to raising your Vitamin D level could lay with magnesium. Consider the following:

"Hypomagnesemia impairs secretion of PTH and renders target organs refractory to PTH. Reduced secretion of PTH or impaired peripheral response to the hormone leads to low serum concentrations of 25(OH)D3. In addition, the hydroxylase enzyme 25-hydroxycholecalciferol-1-hydroxylase, which is responsible for production of the most active, hormonal form of vitamin D, calcitriol, requires magnesium as its cofactor. Consequently magnesium deficiency impairs calcitriol production." [7]

Or, from this study [8]:

"Intake of magnesium significantly interacted with intake of vitamin D in relation to risk of both vitamin D deficiency and insufficiency... findings indicate it is possible that magnesium intake alone or its interaction with vitamin D intake may contribute to vitamin D status."

Every day, the public gets more and more misled by media and articles written by people who have little understanding of the molecular effect of Vitamin D and it's cascade of effects on a person's mineral profile; or by bias studies or (surely well-meaning) doctors who simply just don't know any different. We really have to start asking if any of those who scream about the epidemic of Vitamin D deficiency have ever bothered to look at a person's magnesium level first? Have they considered that low 'Vitamin' D may actually be an effect of illness or imbalance rather than a cause, and that additional supplementation may moreso 'cause' than 'cure'. Very few people are standing up to write about this side of the story, and it is time that more people come to understand (and take interest in) the effects of that which they put into their bodies, sold to them as 'healthy', but which may potentially be doing more harm than good.

"Vitamin D is far more often a cause, and not a cure for disease. And that discrepancy makes a world of difference. It is the difference between advising the public to supplement with vitamin D and telling people to avoid supplementation at all costs. It is the difference between preventing a disease and speeding its progression, the difference between fighting an epidemic of chronic disease, and watching more and more people fall ill every day. And it's a change that needs to happen right now."
~Amy Proal, Ph.D.

[1] http://www.medicinabiomolecular.com.br/biblioteca/pdfs/Biomolecular/mb-0439.pdf
[2] https://www.sciencealert.com/vitamin-d-tablets-may-be-worse-for-you-then-nothing-at-all
[3] http://pdf.usaid.gov/pdf_docs/Pnacr902.pdf
[4] https://www.westonaprice.org/health-topics/beyond-cholesterol/
[5] https://www.ncbi.nlm.nih.gov/pmc/articles/PMC4160567/
[6] https://mpkb.org/home/pathogenesis/vitamind#fn__2
[7] https://www.ncbi.nlm.nih.gov/pmc/articles/PMC4712861/
[8] https://www.ncbi.nlm.nih.gov/pmc/articles/PMC3765911/
http://nutritionalbalancing.org/center/htma/science/articles/vitamin-d.php
http://bacteriality.com/2009/08/iom/
http://www.traceelements.com/Docs/News%20Jan-April%202008.pdf
http://naturopathconnect.com/articles/magnesium-calcium-potassium-vitamin-d-kerri-knox/
http://www.precisionnutrition.com/stop-vitamin-d
http://www.reuters.com/article/us-health-vitamind-supplements-idUSKBN19B2F0
http://theconversation.com/the-sun-goes-down-on-vitamin-d-why-i-changed-my-mind-about-this-celebrated-supplement-52725

PART 6:

THERAPY

RESOURCE

GUIDE

The following pages present an overview of a vast number of natural treatments and therapies of the Western world (including many also from the East). Some are mainstream while others are less known and more alternative. Some hold vast scientific evidence, while others hold less. However, just as energy meridians and homeopathy are not fully embraced by western medicine, the fact they work is almost indisputable. Even for those therapies where research may be lacking, enough people have benefitted from the therapies included herein that they value mention, as you deserve to at least be aware of the options available to you. These therapies all hold great benefit to healing a variety of conditions. This list, although very comprehensive, cannot and does not cover every single possible treatment and condition. It should however provide a multitude of options for the typical patient seeking a new form of treatment.

Depending on your condition, some of these therapies will work as a stand-alone treatment, while others can work very well as complimentary treatments to your existing care. As these are all natural therapies, there is very little harm in combining multiple treatments together as part of a complete healing regimen, although it is highly advised you always check with your primary care practitioner first before starting or stopping any treatment.

To be clear, there is no promise that the therapies listed here can outright 'cure' all the said conditions; rather, the therapies have shown to be beneficial to varying degrees for the listed conditions. Each patient responds differently and each practitioner treats differently. The purpose in presenting this list is to offer you, the reader, as much opportunity as possible to discover new and effective treatments that may help with your specific condition. This is in no way meant to diagnose or be all-inclusive, rather it is a starting point from which to open new doors to potential healing solutions along your journey. While not all treatments may work for you, you now have at your fingertips a world of new treatment options; and a very easy reference from which to choose therapies that have shown to be helpful. (The index at the back of this book may help make you search easier if you are searching by 'condition').

At the end of this list of therapies you will find a separate Herbs and Supplements Guide to use as a further tool.

Warning: The information given below, as in the rest of this book, should not be considered as medical advice. Rather, it is simply to inform the reader of treatment options available. Always consult a trained physician or therapist before beginning any new treatment.

Treatment:	**ACUPRESSURE**
Description:	Uses physical pressure by hand, elbow, or various devices, applied to trigger points on the body in order to clear blockages along energy meridians.
Can Treat or Help With:	Allergies, Arthritis, Asthma, Bronchitis, Bursitis, Cancer, Chronic Fatigue, Colds, Cerebral Palsy, Circulation, Constipation, Chest Pain, Cramps, Depression, Diarrhea, Deafness, Dizziness, Drug And Alcohol Addiction, Fibromyalgia, Flu, Gout, Headaches, Hypertension, Immunity, Insomnia, Muscle Tension, Mumps, Nausea, Neuralgia, Numbness, Pain, Paralysis, Pneumonia, Relaxation, Rhinitis, Scoliosis, Sinusitis, Stress, Stroke, Trauma, Ulcers, Vertigo...

Treatment:	**ACUPUNCTURE**
Description:	As with acupressure, points along energy meridians in the body are stimulated with the use of fine needles to correct imbalances in the flow of 'qi' (energy).
Can Treat or Help With:	Allergic Rhinitis (Including Hay Fever), Arthritis, Biliary Colic, Depression, Dysentery, Dysmenorrhea, Circulation, Craniomandibular Disorders, Functionality Of Various Areas In The Body, Headache, Hypertension, Induction Of Labour, Knee Pain, Leukopenia, Low Back Pain, Malposition Of Fetus, Improving Mood, Morning Sickness, Muscle Tension, Nausea, Neck Pain, Oral And Facial Pain, Postoperative Pain, Renal Colic, Rheumatoid Arthritis, Sciatica, Sprain, Stress, Stroke, Tennis Elbow, Ulcers...

Treatment:	**AROMATHERAPY**
Description:	Uses the physiological and psychological aromatic benefits of herb and plant essences (oils) to promote healing and wellness through the sense of smell.
Can Treat or Help With:	Anxiety, Arthritis, Cancer, Dementia, Immune and Respiratory Systems, Obesity, Pain Reduction, Tissue and DNA Repair, Stress ...

Treatment:	**AURICULOTHERAPY**
Description:	Based on the premise that the ear reflects a microcosm of the entire brain and thus body. By stimulating the corresponding spot on the correct spot on the ear, conditions affecting the physical, mental or emotional health of the body can be treated.
Can Treat or Help With:	Addiction, Chronic Pain, Detoxing, Nausea, Hypertension, as well as a variety of other ailments

Treatment:	**AYURVEDA**
Description:	In Ayurveda, one of the oldest forms of healthcare in the world, specific nutritional and lifestyle guidelines are suggested in order to balance the energies within our bodies. There are 3 energies ('doshas') referred to in Ayurveda, and each individual has their own ideal balance. Natural health is achieved when our doshas are properly balanced, and this is achieved through practices including diet, exercise, meditation and massage.
Can Treat or Help With:	Allergies, Arteriosclerosis / Atherosclerosis, Celiac Disease, Depression, Epilepsy, Fibromyalgia, Gallstones, Headaches, Hypertension, Irritable Bowel Syndrome, Multiple Sclerosis, Ulcers...

Treatment:	**BACH FLOWER REMEDY**
Description:	These liquid-based remedies contain minute dosages of flower material mixed in a 50:50 brandy and water mixture. As the flower essences contain unique vibrational or 'energetic' properties, various flower essences can be safely used by everyone to promote wellness.
Can Treat or Help With:	Remedies Focus Primarily On Balancing Body And Mind Through Improving Emotional And Mental States Such As Stress, Anxiety, Depression, Anger, Fear, Guilt, Worry, And Many Other Disturbing Feelings...

Treatment:	**BIOFEEDBACK**
Description:	Precise instruments are used to electronically measure physiological activity such as brainwaves, heart function, breathing, muscle activity, and skin temperature. The feedback helps pinpoint sources of blockages and pain, and allows for the desired physiological changes to occur.
Can Treat or Help With:	Anxiety, Cardiac Arrhythmias, Cerebral Palsy, Chronic Pain, Digestive Disorders, Edema, Epilepsy, Headaches, High Blood Pressure, Hypertension, Low Back Pain, Low Blood Pressure, Migraines, Pelvic Pain, Paralysis, Raynaud's Disease, Stress, Stroke, TMD, Torticollis...

Treatment:	**BOWEN TECHNIQUE**
Description:	A system of gentle movements performed by a therapist on the superficial and deep fascia – the largest and richest sensory organ in the body. Using very gentle non-manipulative movements, blockages are released and energy flow is stimulated. Rather than focusing on treating a specific condition, it stimulates the body's own healing resources to achieve healing through balance and harmony.
Can Treat or Help With:	ADD, Arthritis, Carpal Tunnel, Chronic Pain, Digestive Problems, Drug Detox, Fibromyalgia, Headaches, Herniated Disc, Infertility, Menstrual Pain, Migraines, Musculo-Skeletal Conditions Of The Spine And Limbs Including Acute, Chronic, And Post Trauma/Surgery, Neurological Conditions Such As Cerebral Palsy, Stroke, Muscular Dystrophy, Multiple Sclerosis, Parkinson's, Pain And Inflammation, Pelvic Imbalances, Repetitive Stress Injury, Respiratory Conditions, Rotator Cuff Injury, Sacroiliac Pain, Sciatica, Scoliosis, Sprains, Strains, Tennis Elbow, TMJ, Whiplash...
Treatment:	**CHAKRA BALANCING**
Description:	Chakras are the energy vortexes through which energy flows, and they are

	responsible for our physical, mental, and spiritual well-being. We each have 7 main chakras located along the central line of our body from the base of the spine to the top of our head. When a chakra is blocked, it can negatively impact our physical and emotional health. Balanced chakras lead to feelings of calm, peace, and positive energy. As each chakra works with corresponding organs, it is easy for the chakra practitioner to tell which chakra(s) are blocked based on where the illness shows in the body.
Can Treat or Help With:	(1st chakra): lower back pain, diarrhea, knee pain, gout, anger, fear, spinal cord dysfunction, lethargy, scoliosis, rectal cancer, fibromyalgia, arthritis... (2nd chakra): infertility, kidney stones, urinary tract infections, sexual addiction, impotency, appendicitis... (3rd chakra): nightmares, aggression, ulcers, feelings of victimization, bulimia, obesity, anorexia, indigestion, irritable bowel syndrome, heartburn, hepatitis... (4th chakra): heart attack, poor circulation, angina, high blood pressure, asthma, weak immune system, hypertension, cancer (lung & breast), pneumonia, upper back problems... (5th chakra): laryngitis, thyroid disease, anxiety, hyperactivity, bronchitis, hoarseness, mouth ulcers, chronic neck pain, TMJ... (6th chakra): spaciness, migraines, forgetfulness, inability to meditate or visualize, poor eyesight, tension, brain tumors, stroke, tinnitus, Parkinson's disease, seizures... (7th chakra): confusion, headaches, MS, hallucinations, mental illness, cerebral palsy...

Treatment:	**CHELATION THERAPY**
Description:	This detoxification therapy involves an intravenous drip being administered which uses chelating agents to remove harmful toxins and heavy metals. Alternatively, oral administration is also done. (Many serious health conditions can be caused by high metal levels in the body, and while the problem is quite common, it very often goes properly undiagnosed).
Can Treat or Help With:	Symptoms Of Heavy Metal Poisoning Including: Anxiety, Brain Fog, Depression, Emotional Highs And Lows, Forgetfulness, Headaches, Mental Racing, Mood Swings, Muscle And Joint Pain, Physical Fatigue, Reproductive Problems, Skin Problems, Unsteady Gait...

Treatment:	**CHIROPRACTIC**
Description:	Joint adjustment and manipulation using predominantly manual therapy to resolve joint dysfunctions / subluxations. Most often, emphasis is on the spinal column which, when brought back into correct healthy alignment, allows the body to heal itself while reducing pain.
Can Treat or Help With:	Arthritis, Back Pain, Bursitis, Carpal Tunnel Syndrome, Disc Conditions, Fibromyalgia, General Joint Pain, Headache, High Blood Pressure, Migraine, Neck Pain, Repetitive Stress Injuries, Sciatica, Sleep Disorders..

Treatment:	**COGNITIVE BEHAVIORAL THERAPY (CBT)**
Description:	Through working with a psychotherapist or other mental health counselor, unhelpful thoughts and behaviors can be identified and changed, allowing the patient to respond more effectively to challenging situations and releasing thoughts that may be hindering good health.

Can Treat or Help With:	Anxiety, Eating Disorders, Personality Disorders, Substance Abuse, Psychotic Disorders...

Treatment:	**COLON HYDROTHERAPY**
Description:	Uses enemas to eliminate waste and toxins from the colon, cleansing the walls of the large intestine and inducing therapeutic healing.
Can Treat or Help With:	Allergies, Arthritis, Asthma, Bloating, Candida, Colitis, Constipation, Diarrhea, Fatigue, Flatulence, Mental Fogginess, Headaches, Hemorrhoids, Leaky Gut, Low Energy, Weight Problems, And Various Circulatory, Immune, And Inflammatory Conditions...

Treatment:	**COLOR THERAPY (aka CHROMOTHERAPY)**
Description:	Uses color (in the form of light, visualization, verbal suggestions, or other tools) to balance the body's energy on physical, emotional, spiritual, and mental realms.
Can Treat or Help With:	Addictions, Aggressive Behaviour And Violence, Burns, Cancer, Bulimia Nervosa, Depression, Eating Disorders, Insomnia, Lung Conditions, Neonatal Jaundice, Rheumatoid Arthritis, SAD (Seasonal Affective Disorder), Scar Tissue...

Treatment:	**COUNSELING / PSYCHOTHERAPY**
Description:	Interactive processes with a mental health professional (psychiatrist, psychologist, clinical social worker, licensed counselor, or other trained practitioner) that explore thoughts, feelings and behaviours to improve the individual's functioning and well-being.
Can Treat or Help With:	Addiction, Alcoholism, Anxiety, Behavioural Problems, Bipolar Disorder, Child Abuse

	Issues, Depression, Emotional Issues, Low Self-Esteem, OCD, Personality Disorders, Phobias, Post-Traumatic Stress Disorder, Schizophrenia...

Treatment:	**CRANIOSACRAL THERAPY**
Description:	This gentle, hands-on bodywork releases restrictions in the soft tissues surrounding the central nervous system, regulating the flow of cerebrospinal fluid and aiming to restore whole body health.
Can Treat or Help With:	ADD/ADHD, Autism, Brain And Spinal Cord Injuries, Central Nervous System Disorders, Chronic Fatigue, Chronic Neck And Back Pain, Fibromyalgia, Migraines And Headaches, Motor-Coordination Impairments, Orthopedic Problems, Post-Traumatic Stress Disorder, Scoliosis, Stress And Tension-Related Disorders, TMJ Syndrome

Treatment:	**CRYOTHERAPY**
Description:	Uses either low freezing temperatures (either locally or generally) to achieve medical therapy. With localized cryotherapy, freezing temperatures are used to deaden an irritated nerve. Whole body treatment on the other hand is systemic, activating biochemical, hormonal, and immune processes and giving the nervous and circulatory systems a boost.
Can Treat or Help With:	Cancer (Especially Prostate, Liver And Cervical) And Tumors In Other Areas Including The Kidneys, Spine, Lungs, And Breasts, Pre-Cancerous Skin Moles And Skin Tumors, Fibromyalgia, Improving Joint And Muscle Function, Multiple Sclerosis, Rheumatoid Arthritis, Skin Conditions Like Psoriasis And Dermatitis, Sports Injuries.

Treatment:	**CRYSTAL HEALING**

Description:	The unique internal structure of each crystal variety resonates at a certain frequency, the resonance of which when applied properly can help to balance the body's energy systems and stimulate healing.
Can Treat or Help With:	Depression, Headaches, Imbalanced Chakras, Insomnia, Low Energy, Low Libido, Negativity, Poor Concentration...

Treatment:	**CUPPING**
Description:	In this ancient form of Chinese alternative medicine, local suction is applied to the skin in order to mobilize blood and energy flow , draw out pathogenic factors, and promote healing.
Can Treat or Help With:	Anxiety, Back Pain, Cellulite, Fatigue, Migraines, Muscle Pain (Especially In The Back And Shoulders), Neck Pain, Respiratory Conditions, Rheumatism, Stiff Muscles...

Treatment:	**CURANDEROS AND PLANT HEALING**
Description:	Although not yet understood or accepted by mainstream modern medicine, the medicine men (shaman or curandero) of ancient cultures have relied for thousands of years on native plants, many of them entheogenic (bringing out the divine within us) for a wide range of healing. Given thousands of years of success, it would be wrong to not include here and educate the reader on potential benefits that may be found by pursuing this avenue. With over 40,000 species of plants, the Amazon rainforest is home to nature's largest pharmacy. The curandero of the Amazon view a person's health based on the combined condition of the physical, spiritual, and psychological state, and all 3 areas must be addressed for proper healing. When removing a person from the diversions of modern society (technology, social connection, material possessions, etc) and creating an environment free of conflict or

	interruption, the patient is able to find a clearer path to health and spiritual well-being. This is combined with a specific healing diet and administering a number of delicately prepared and specially selected native herbs and plants that show astonishing healing benefits. I list just a few of these below, with the caveat that many of these are highly dangerous if not taken under the direct and expert care of an experienced healer. Always consult with an experienced curandero or herbologist before beginning any of these treatments.
Can Treat or Help With:	Coca: altitude sickness, asthma, broken bones (pain killer), fatigue, headaches, internal bleeding (slows down), malaria, rheumatism, ulcers Tahuari: antibacterial, antifungal, antiparasitic, diabetes, immune booster, respiratory problems, rheumatism, ulcers, urinary tract infections Ajo Sacha: arthritis, bacterial infections, flu, inflammation, pneumonia Chuchuhuasi: arthritis, back pain, menstrual pain, muscle soreness, rheumatism, skin cancer Abuta: digestive problems, diuretic, internal bleeding, menstrual cramps Aloe Vera: one of the world's most widely accepted herbal remedies, it works great for healing burns, wounds, & rashes. Sangre de Grado: used widely across South America for skin injuries (cuts, rashes, bites, scrapes). Also used as a remedy for cancer, diarrhea, digestive problems from cholera and AIDS, eczema, hemorrhoids, internal inflammation, irritable bowel syndrome, ulcers, and vaginal infections Clavo Huasca: arthritis, digestive problems, fever, muscle aches, rheumatism, toothaches Graviola: cancer, intestinal parasites Chanca Piedra: dysentery, hepatitis, jaundice, liver cancer, prostatitis, urinary tract infections Pampo Oregano: depression, dizziness,

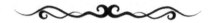

epilepsy, heart palpitations, hysteria
Ayahuasca: this highly alkaline plant is
considered the cornerstone of many
Amazon healing methods. The properly
prepared brew is consumed as part of a
sacred ceremony. It strongly purges the
body of toxins while inducing a lucid dream-
like state allowing the skilled curandero to
reach & interact on a spiritual level with the
patient.
San Pedro: this cactus has been used for
thousands of years in spiritual ceremonies,
generating a vivid and illuminated state of
altered consciousness and deepening the
effects of other medicinal plants. The high
alkaloid properties of San Pedro also help
fight off cancer and other chronic illnesses.
Toé: although potentially deadly if not
administered properly, the healing benefits
can help control Parkinson's Disease and
treat asthma, bronchitis, wounds, burns, and
rashes. Toé also has the highest levels of
alkaloids of any in the plant world.
The site 'thesacredscience.com' offers
great information for those interested in
learning more.

Treatment:	**DALIAN METHOD**
Description:	This ground breaking healing system uses the wisdom of the body, the chakra system, and the light of one's own consciousness to identify and permanently remove causes of energy blockages (from fears, emotions, and subconscious belief patterns held in our cells) that in turn can heal pain and disease.
Can Treat or Help With:	Addictions, Anxiety, Asthma, Cancer, Cystitis, Chronic Pain, Crohn's Disease, Depression, Emotional Healing (forgiveness, self-love...) Fear, Fibromyalgia, High blood Pressure, Past Traumas, Post Surgery Recovery, Relationship Issues, Repressed Thought Patterns, Thyroid Conditions, Ulcers, Weight challenges

Treatment:	**DETOXIFICATION**
Description:	Also known as 'detox', it is the ridding in our bodies of all harmful toxins, resulting in a healthier body and sense of well-being. (Detoxification can include such therapies as colonics, chelation, fasting, infrared saunas and diet).
Can Treat or Help With:	Cancer, Cardiovascular Disease, Degenerative Diseases, Heavy Metal Toxicity, Immune Function, And A Host Of Other Innumerable Symptoms That Could Be Caused By Toxins Built Up In Our Bodies.

Treatment:	**EARTHING (aka Grounding)**
Description:	The simple act of walking barefoot or placing your bare feet on the earth. The Earth is energized with free flowing negative electrons that, when we absorb them, balance out our positively charged bodies. It is a powerful non-dietary way of increasing antioxidants in our bodies. The best places for earthing / grounding are bare soil, grass (especially moist), sand (beach), and even concrete or brick (as long as it's not painted). 'Earthing sheets' can also be purchased which offer similar benefits.
Can Treat or Help With:	Adrenals, Blood Pressure, Circulation (thins blood), Chronic Pain, Energy, Headaches, Inflammation, Injury (speeds healing), Muscle Tension, Pain management, Psoriasis, Sleep (improved), Snoring, Stress, Tendonitis, Well-being (feeling)...

Treatment:	**EMOTIONAL FREEDOM TECHNIQUE**
Description:	EFT (Emotional Freedom Technique), also referred to as acu-tapping, is method of releasing dysfunctional beliefs. EFT is a meridian based energy healing system working on the premise that "the cause of all negative emotions and beliefs is a

	disturbance in our body's energy system." Negative emotions cause disruptions in our flow of energy along these meridians, leading to the development of pain or disease. By tapping on specific areas along the meridian channels while making a specific statement, negative memories, emotions, and beliefs which block the natural flow of energy can be released.
Can Treat or Help With:	Addiction, Anxiety, Depression, Disease (of any kind) caused by negative emotions, Emotional Issues, Insomnia, Pain, Phobias, Stress, Trauma...

Treatment:	**FAR INFRARED SAUNA**
Description:	Unlike conventional saunas which heat the air, far infrared saunas use an energy that heats the body directly, without heating the surrounding air. Not only is this more comfortable for some people, but the infrared rays are able to penetrate several inches into the body's tissues, stimulating healing. It's also estimated that sweat from an infrared sauna contains 17% toxins (as compared to just 3% from regular sweating).
Can Treat or Help With:	Arthritis, Asthma, Autism, Chronic Fatigue Syndrome, Chronic Pain Conditions, Fibromyalgia, Heart Disease, Lowering Blood Pressure, Muscle & Joint Pain, Jaundice, Psoriasis, Relaxation, Sports Injuries, Stress, Toxin Build-Up (Helps With Detoxification), Weight Loss...

Treatment:	**FASTING**
Description:	The intermittent or long-term abstinence from food and/or water. (Please note that, as with most of the treatments mentioned here, fasting should only be done under proper supervision. Fasting, although it may sound simple, can be dangerous if overdone).

Can Treat or Help With:	Addictions, Allergies, Arthritis, Atherosclerosis, Detoxification, Digestion, Reducing Blood Sugar And Blood Pressure, Immunity, Inflammatory Bowel Diseases, Psoriasis, Rheumatoid Arthritis, Weight Loss...

Treatment:	**FELDENKRAIS METHOD**
Description:	Rather than treating specific injuries, illnesses, or attempting to alter the body's structure, the Feldenkrais method uses the awareness of touch and movement patterns of the body to restore our natural abilities to move easily and with minimal effort. Mindfulness in our movements leads to improved posture, balance, co-ordination and well-being.
Can Treat or Help With:	Cerebral Palsy, Chronic, Recurring, Or Acute Pain Of The Back, Neck, Shoulders, Hands, Hip, Leg, Or Knees, Multiple Sclerosis, Stroke, Performance Enhancement In Athletes, Ease Of Movement In The Elderly, Relaxation, Vitality...

Treatment:	**FLOATING**
Description:	Lying down in a sensory deprivation tank of Epson-salt-dense water. Due to the extremely high amount of salt, the body floats effortlessly on the surface, while all forces of gravity on the musculoskeletal system and nervous system are eliminated and all senses receive minimal input. Complete body relaxation is achieved.
Can Treat or Help With:	Adrenal Fatigue, Anxiety, Arthritis, Bursitis, Back Pain, Blood Pressure (helps decrease), Circulation, Immune function, Inflammation, Insomnia, Magnesium absorption, Muscle Tension, Neck Pain, Osteoporosis, Relaxation, Stress...

Treatment:	**FREQUENCY SPECIFIC MICROCURRENT (FSM)**
Description:	Uses specific electrical frequencies that

	support tissue healing, increasing the capability of cellular tissue repair while reducing systemic inflammation and pain.
Can Treat or Help With:	Disc And Facet Injuries , Herpes, Inflammation, Muscle Pain, Myofascial Pain, Nerve Pain, Scar Tissue, Shingles, Tendon And Ligament Repair, Various Diseases...

Treatment:	**GERSON THERAPY**
Description:	A natural treatment that boosts your body's own immune system to heal various degenerative diseases. An abundance of nutrients from thirteen fresh, organic juices are consumed every day, providing your body with a super-dose of enzymes, minerals and nutrients. These substances then break down diseased tissue in the body, while enemas aid in eliminating the lifelong buildup of toxins from the liver.
Can Treat or Help With:	Allergies, Arthritis, Cancer (Including Melanoma, Lymphoma, Breast, Ovarian, And Duke's C Colorectal), Diabetes, Heart Disease, Migraines, Systemic Lupus Erythematosus, Various Degenerative Diseases...

Treatment:	**GUIDED IMAGERY**
Description:	A process of directing thoughts, via verbal, mental, or virtual suggestion, to a more positive, healthy, relaxed state. When you use creative imagination to visualize certain healing scenarios, your body tends to respond as though what you are imagining is real.
Can Treat or Help With:	Anxiety, Cancer, Headaches, Immunity, Lowering Blood Pressure And Cholesterol, Pain Management, Post-Operative Healing, Quitting Smoking, Side-Effects Of Chemotherapy (Such As Nausea, Depression, And Fatigue), Stress, Weight Loss...

Treatment:	**HAIR TISSUE MINERAL ANALYSIS**
Description:	A sophisticated laboratory screening test which measures the mineral and toxic heavy metal content of human hair, reflecting imbalances and toxicities within the body. While blood testing only shows the fluctuating levels of circulating minerals, HTMA offers a much more accurate reading of stored tissue levels. These stored levels are very often behind a number of often undiagnosed serious physical health and mental conditions.
Can Treat or Help With:	While the hair mineral analysis alone doesn't treat any conditions, deficient or toxic heavy metal levels can commonly lead to the following conditions: Acne, Allergies, Adrenal Fatigue, Anemia, Anxiety, Arthritis, Brain Fog, Cancer, Chronic Fatigue Syndrome, Depression, Diabetes, Fears (Increase In), Headache, Heart Attacks, Irritability, Kidney Disorders, Libido (Decreased), Lowered Immunity, Mood Swings, Multiple Sclerosis, Nervousness, Osteoporosis, Panic Attacks, Phobias, Psychosis, Schizophrenia, Urinary Tract Infection...

Treatment:	**HERBALISM / HERBOLOGY**
Description:	Uses plants and plant extracts to stimulate and restore the body's natural healing ability.
Can Treat or Help With:	Allergies, Angina, Anxiety, Arthritis, Asthma, Chronic Fatigue, Depression, Fibromyalgia, Headaches, High Blood Pressure, Immune Deficiency, Indigestion And Other Bowel Conditions, Infections, Insomnia, Migraines, Prostate Enlargement, Reproductive Problems, Stress... (see also: Curanderos & Plant Healing, as well as Herb & Supplement Guide at end of this chapter)

Treatment:	**HOMEOPATHY**
Description:	A system of medicine that uses highly diluted substances, usually in tablet form, in order to trigger the body's natural healing response. It uses the principle of 'like cures like'. In other words, a substance that ails you in high dose can be used to treat symptoms when taken in a very small dosage. It can be used to help treat almost any condition for which you would normally see a GP.
Can Treat or Help With:	Amenorrhea, Anxiety, Arthritis, Back Pain, Bell's Palsy, Bronchitis, Circulatory Disorders, Cold Sores, Crohn's Disease, Cystitis, Depression, Eating Disorders, Fears, Fibroids, Hay Fever, Gout, Herpes, High Blood Pressure, Infertility, Irritable Bowel Syndrome, Kidney / Liver Dysfunction, Laryngitis, Low Sperm Count, Migraines, Multiple Sclerosis, Neuralgia, Palpitations, Pelvic Inflammatory Disorders, Psoriasis, Sciatica, Sinusitis, Sprains And Sports Injuries, Thyroid Disorders, Tinnitus, Vertigo, Viral Illnesses, Vitiligo...

Treatment:	**HORMONE REPLACEMENT AND/OR SUPPLEMENTATION**
Description:	Hormone replacement therapy ('H.T.') is traditionally thought of in the realm of treating the symptoms of menopause. In this case the hormones being supplemented are commonly estrogen, progestin, and sometime testosterone. However, hormone supplementation can also be a very powerful treatment for adrenal fatigue – a fairly common but lesser understood cause of many negative symptoms. For adrenal fatigue, a saliva hormone test is administered and supplementation often includes hormones such as DHEA, cortisol, progesterone, testosterone, and pregnenolone. In both cases, hormones are administered under guidance in order to raise the certain hormone levels which are lacking.

Can Treat or Help With:	Menopause Symptoms: Hot Flashes, Vaginal Dryness, Mood Swings, Sleep Disorders, And Decreased Sexual Desire... Adrenal Fatigue Symptoms: Chronic Stress, Morning And Mid-Afternoon Sluggishness, Anxiety, Chronic Fatigue, Obesity, Diabetes, Depression, Insomnia, Lack Of Energy, Muscular Weakness, Inability To Handle Stress, Frequent Sighing, Decreased Sex Drive...

Treatment:	**HYPERBARIC OXYGEN THERAPY**
Description:	Involves breathing pure oxygen in a pressurized room where the air pressure is up to 3 times that of normal air pressure. As a result, your lungs can take in more oxygen than otherwise would be possible when breathing pure oxygen at normal air pressure.
Can Treat or Help With:	Anemia (Severe), Back Pain, Bubbles Of Air In Blood Vessels, Burns, Carbon Monoxide Poisoning, Decompression Sickness, Gangrene, Recovery from Stroke, Surgical Recovery, Trauma, Wounds That Won't Heal As A Result Of Diabetes Or Radiation Injury...

Treatment:	**HYPERTHERMIA TREATMENT**
Description:	The use of high heat (either full body or localized) up to 104F. This high heat benefits a number of conditions, increases the body's immune lymph cells and macrophages, and also creates an environment hostile to cancer cells.
Can Treat or Help With:	Autoimmune disease, Cancer, Osteoarthritis

Treatment:	**HYPNOSIS**
Description:	Cooperative interaction between patient and hypnotist whereby the patient responds to the suggestions of the hypnotist in order

	to change thinking patterns and physical conditions of the body.
Can Treat or Help With:	ADHD, Anxiety, Certain Psychological Problems, Chronic Pain, Dementia, Depression, Habit Disorders, Irritable Bowel Syndrome, Nausea And Vomiting In Cancer Patients undergoing Chemotherapy, Psoriasis And Other Skin Conditions, Rheumatoid Arthritis, Stress...

Treatment:	**INDIAN HEAD MASSAGE (CHAMPISSAGE)**
Description:	A flowing sequence of rhythmic massage movements focusing primarily on the top half of the body from upper back to scalp in order to relieve stress and tension in body & mind.
Can Treat or Help With:	Anxiety, Clenched Jaw, Eyestrain, Headache, Insomnia, Migraine, Stiff Neck, Stress, Tense Shoulders, Tiredness...

Treatment:	**KATI VASTI**
Description:	Involves keeping a warm, thick medicated Ayurvedic oil on the lower back or other parts of the spine for 30 to 40 minutes. This is usually followed by a massage and steam and performed for 5 to 7 days as prescribed by the Ayurvedic practitioner.
Can Treat or Help With:	Back Pain, Intervertebral Disc Prolapses, Lumbago, Lumbar Spondylosis, Sciatica, Spinal Curvature, Spinal Tuberculosis, Various Other Conditions Of The Back Affecting The Spine, Vertebrae, Muscles And Nerves...

Treatment:	**LIGHT THERAPY**
Description:	Involves sitting or working next to a bright light device called a light therapy box which mimics natural outdoor light. Your eyes should be open but not staring directly at the light.

Can Treat or Help With:	Depression, SAD (Seasonal Affective Disorder), Sleep Disorders...

Treatment:	**LYMPH DRAINAGE THERAPY**
Description:	The practitioner, working with flat hands, works through the patient's lymphatic system using all the fingers to simulate gentle wave-like movements. This activates body fluid circulation and stimulates the immune and parasympathetic nervous systems.
Can Treat or Help With:	Adhesive Capsulitis (frozen shoulder), Arthritis, Bronchitis, Burns, Chronic Fatigue Syndrome, Chronic Pain, Edemas (Swelling), Detoxification, Fibromyalgia, Insomnia, Lymphedema, Menieres Syndrome, Migraines, Muscle Hypertonus, Otitis, Regeneration Of Tissue, Sinusitis, Sports Injuries, Stress, Venous Stasis Ulceration, Whiplash...

Treatment:	**MAGNETIC HEALING**
Description:	Placing magnets of various sizes and strengths on the body to help relieve pain or treat disease. It is thought that magnetic fields can increase blood flow, alter nerve impulses, increase the flow of oxygen to cells, and realign thought patterns to improve emotional well-being.
Can Treat or Help With:	Arthritis Pain, Cancer, Circulation, Degenerative Diseases, Headaches, Migraines, Stress...

Treatment:	**MASSAGE THERAPY**
Description:	This term encompasses a vast array of various massage techniques far beyond the scope of this book. Each country and culture seems to have its own unique massage technique. There is also massage for relaxation, and massage for clinical purposes. Here we are discussing purely clinical massage. In this context, we can

	define massage therapy as the manual manipulation of muscles, tendons and ligaments in order to enhance health, function, and the healing process.
Can Treat or Help With:	Anxiety, Back Pain, Cancer, Carpal Tunnel Syndrome, Chronic Fatigue Syndrome, Depression, Dislocations, Emphysema, Fibromyalgia, Fractures, Headaches, Inflammatory Conditions, Kyphosis, Leg Pain, Multiple Sclerosis, Neck Pain, Parkinson's Disease, Post-Surgical Rehabilitation, Scoliosis, Sports Injuries, Sprains And Strains, Stroke, Tendonitis, Whiplash...

Treatment:	**MEDITATION**
Description:	While techniques may vary, the underlying principle is that of quiet thought and clearing the mind in order to create a state of rumination. Meditation allows for connection with our inner source of energy and knowledge. The benefits are numerous, and it is an approach that can be used by anyone.
Can Treat or Help With:	ADD/ADHD, Addiction, Aging, Anxiety, Arthritis, Asthma, Bipolar Disorder, Cancer, Chronic Pain, Circulation, Coronary Artery Disease (Atherosclerosis), Communication, Concentration, Decrease Blood Pressure, Depression, Digestion, Discovery Of Skills And Talents, Fibromyalgia, Grief (Dealing With), Headaches, HIV/AIDS, Hormones (Helps Boost Levels Of Beneficial Hormones), Hypertension, Immunity, Inner Strength, Irritable Bowel Syndrome, Memory (Improves Focus And Slows Aging Of The Mind), Muscle Tension, Organ Transplantation, Panic Attacks, Phobias (Overcoming), Psoriasis, Psychotherapy, Relaxation, Smoking (Quitting), Stress, Sweating, Weight Loss...

Treatment:	**MEGAVITAMIN THERAPY**
Description:	Using vitamins in large amounts (greater than the recommended daily allowance) to help cure or prevent mental or physical disorders.
Can Treat or Help With:	ADHD, Autism, Cancer, Common Cold, Heart Disease, Psychotic Behavior, Schizophrenia, Various Other Symptoms Resulting From Vitamin Or Mineral Deficiencies

Treatment:	**MOXIBUSTION**
Description:	A traditional Chinese medicine technique that involves the burning of in most instances mugwort (a small, spongy herb) on or very near the surface of the skin to stimulate the flow of Qi in the body and promote healing.
Can Treat or Help With:	Allergies, Anemia, Arthritis, Asthma, Back Pain, Cancer, Chronic Fatigue, Cold And Flu, Digestive Problems, Infertility, Irregular Elimination, Headaches, Immunity, Migraines, Nausea, Shock, Ulcers...

Treatment:	**MYOTHERAPY**
Description:	A multi-faceted and effective approach to the treatment and rehabilitation of musculoskeletal pain and associated conditions. Myotherapy includes a thorough assessment followed by various treatment modalities including trigger point therapy, soft tissue massage, manipulation, dry needling, joint mobilization, stretching, nutritional advice, and exercise guidance.
Can Treat or Help With:	Ankle Sprains, Arthritis, Back Pain, Biomechanics (Improvement Of), Carpal Tunnel Syndrome, Chronic Fatigue Syndrome, Fibromyalgia, Headaches, Joint Pain, Kyphosis, Migraines, Multiple Sclerosis, Neck (Chronic And Acute Stiffness Or Pain), Neuro-musculoskeletal Conditions, Patella Tracking Dysfunction, Posture, Sciatica,

	Scoliosis, Shin Splints, Shoulder Pain and/or Impingement, Sports Injuries, Stiffness, Stress, Tendonitis, Thoracic Outlet Syndrome, Vertebral Dysfunction...

Treatment:	**NATUROPATHY**
Description:	A science based practice that promotes wellness by first looking at the unique qualities of each patient and the underlying cause of the disease or dysfunction, and then utilizing natural, non-toxic therapies to restore physiological, psychological, and structural balance. Naturopaths are trained not only in standard medical curriculum, but are also experienced in the sciences of clinical nutrition, botanical medicines, homeopathy, physical medicine, and exercise therapy, among other disciplines.
Can Treat or Help With:	ADHD, Alzheimer's, Anxiety, Arteriosclerosis, Arthritis, Autism, Back Pain, Basal Cell Carcinoma, Carpal Tunnel Syndrome, Celiac Disease, Crohn's Disease, Depression, Digestive Disorders, Fatigue, Fractures, Gout, Irregular Heartbeat, Hemorrhoids, Irritable Bowel Syndrome, Lupus, Menopausal Concerns, OCD, Osteoarthritis, Osteoporosis, Pain, Parkinson's Disease, Pneumonia, Post Herpetic Neuralgia, Psoriasis, Respiratory Tract Infections, Rheumatoid Arthritis, Sciatica, Scleroderma, Sleep Disturbances, Sports Injuries, Sprains And Strains, Ulcerous Colitis, Urinary Tract Infections...

Treatment:	**NUTRITION THERAPY**
Description:	Uses a specially designed diet, devised and monitored by a certified clinical nutritionist, registered dietician or functional doctor, to reduce the risk of developing complications or to help alleviate pre-existing conditions.
Can Treat or Help With:	AIDS, Cancer, Diabetes, Down Syndrome, Heart Disease, High Cholesterol, Kidney Disease, Various Other Symptoms Resulting

	From Intolerances Or Vitamin/Mineral Toxicities Or Deficiencies...

Treatment:	**OZONE THERAPY**
Description:	Ozone (oxygen with a third molecule added) is an antibacterial and antifungal agent and has been used successfully throughout Europe for a number of years in the treatment as well as prevention of a variety of health conditions and diseases. As oxygen levels in our blood decrease with age, chemical reactions necessary for cellular health becomes impaired. Healthy blood ozone levels help protect against viruses, inactivate bacteria, inhibit tumor metabolism, and enhance circulation. Although ozone can be applied topically, it is more often (and effectively) applied systemically via rectal insufflation (introducing oxygen into the body through the rectum) or via autohemotherapy (the withdrawal and reinjection of blood).
Can Treat or Help With:	Acne, AIDS, Arrhythmia, Arthritis, Asthma, Cancer, Cirrhosis of the liver, Constipation, Crohn's Disease, Diarrhea, Emphysema, Fibromyalgia, Fungal Infections, Gastro-intestinal disorders, Glaucoma, Hepatitis, Herpes, Multiple Sclerosis, Parkinson's Disease, Raynaud's disease, Sinusitis, Stroke, Virus Infections, Wound Healing (acceleration of)...

Treatment:	**OSTEOPATHY**
Description:	A health care system that focuses on the whole body and preventative care. The underlying philosophy is that any anatomical abnormality is a sign that disease is present, and when that abnormality is corrected, the symptoms will improve. Although the manual techniques used are quite varied, they center around the free flow and actions of nerves, arteries, veins, lymphatics, and cerebrospinal fluids.

Can Treat or Help With:	Arthritis, Asthma, Autism, Bell's Palsy, Degenerative Disc And Joint Disease, Epilepsy, Fibromyalgia, Headaches, Irritable Bowel Syndrome, Migraines, Musculoskeletal Problems, Sprains And Strains, Tendonitis, TMJ...

Treatment:	**PHYSIOTHERAPY**
Description:	A healthcare profession helping with the remediation of impairments, bodily weaknesses and disabilities through a variety of techniques including massage, ultrasound, and administering special exercises. The goal is to promote mobility, functional ability, reduction of pain, and an improved quality of life. Physiotherapists combine orthopedic, pediatric, and neurophysiotherapy training to address a number of health and injury concerns.
Can Treat or Help With:	Asthma, Arthritis, Back Pain, Brain Injuries, Core Strengthening, Emphysema, Hand Injury, Joint Injuries, Ligament Tears, Muscular Dystrophy, Neck Pain, Pelvic Pain And Incontinence, Parkinson's, Post Heart Attack Recovery, Post-Surgical Rehabilitation, Spina Bifida, Spinal Cord Injuries, Sports Injuries, Sprains And Strains, Tendonitis, Vertigo...

Treatment:	**PILATES**
Description:	A form of exercise that emphasizes core strengthening, flexibility, and awareness to support efficient body movement. It also promotes muscle strengthening, endurance, as well as proper body alignment and posture, coordination, and breathing.
Can Treat or Help With:	Back Pain, Balance Issues, Cancer, Chronic Fatigue Syndrome, Fibromyalgia, Lower Back Pain, Lumbar Stabilization, Pelvic Floor Dysfunction, Postural Alignment, Spinal Problems, Sciatica, Whiplash...

Treatment:	**PLATELET RICH PLASMA THERAPY (PRP)**
Description:	A prolotherapy-related injection therapy whereby a small amount of blood is drawn, and then using a special device, the red blood cells and plasma are separated and the blood platelets concentrated. Platelets are critical to the healing process, containing a number of important growth factors. When they are re-injected at the location of injury, stem cell production is increased and drawn to the area to regenerate damaged ligaments or tendons, initiate the repair or regeneration of bone, and speed the wound healing process. PRP is an effective tissue growth accelerator that is recommended for more serious and chronic conditions when the results from standard prolotherapy aren't optimal.
Can Treat or Help With:	Back Pain, Bone Regeneration, Chronic Joint Pain In Almost All Areas, Neck Pain, Plantar Fasciitis, Osteoarthritis, Rotator Cuff Tears, Tendonitis/Tendonosis, Tennis Elbow...

Treatment:	**PRAYER**
Description:	Believing that there is a greater power than oneself, prayer is the asking or begging for a specific or non-specific outcome through spoken or silent words, or through the mind or heart
Can Treat or Help With:	Various – Non Specific

Treatment:	**PRANIC HEALING**
Description:	Prana is a similar concept to that of chi, which means life energy. In this highly evolved system of energy medicine, prana is used to balance, harmonize and transform the body's energy processes. The pranic practitioner works on the bioplasmic energy body, and therefore physical contact is not required. Energy is transferred from person to another.

Can Treat or Help With:	Colds, Coughs, Fever, Gas Pain, Headaches, Loose Bowel Movements, Muscle Pain, And Various Major Illnesses Of The Eye, Liver, Kidney, And Heart...

Treatment:	**PROLOTHERAPY**
Description:	An injection therapy very effective for chronic musculoskeletal pain. In many cases of chronic pain, the body has become 'accustomed' to the injury and is no longer trying to heal it. For these cases, a dextrose-based prolotherapy solution is injected into the area of injury in order to create a controlled inflammation, the purpose of which is to reawaken the body's natural healing response. Prolotherapy has an 85% success rate for most types of musculoskeletal pain.
Can Treat or Help With:	Arthritis, Back Pain, Carpal Tunnel Syndrome, Degenerated Or Herniated Discs, Dislocations, Fibromyalgia, Ligament Damage, Neck Pain, Overstretching Injuries, Sciatica, Sports Injuries, Tendonitis, TMJ, Whiplash (Chronic)...

Treatment:	**QIGONG**
Description:	Widely understood in China but with limited knowledge in the West, it is the ability to manipulate Qi (vital life force energy) to promote self-healing, prevent disease, and increase longevity. Qigong largely relies on breathing techniques and postures, as well as meditations and guided imagery. Qigong can, through first correcting imbalances that have built up over a lifetime, help correct a number of symptomatic health concerns.
Can Treat or Help With:	Anxiety, Asthma, Arthritis, Back Pain, Cancer, Cardiovascular Disease, Chronic Circulation, Diabetes Type II, Fatigue, Depression, Fibromyalgia, Flexibility, Headaches, Improving Blood Flow And

	Lowering Blood Pressure, Pain, Posture, Respiration, Stamina, Stress...

Treatment:	**RADIONICS**
Description:	A method of healing that uses the sending of energy in order to detect and correct energy imbalances within the patient. A radionics practitioner does not treat any specific condition, but rather focuses on restoring balance which thereby in turn then restores whole body wellness.
Can Treat or Help With:	Correcting Energy Imbalance

Treatment:	**RAPID EYE TECHNOLOGY (R.E.T.)**
Description:	Rapid Eye Technology (R.E.T.) helps replicate REM sleep (in which memories are reactivated, integrated, and can be released) while in an awake state. Although in an awake state, the trauma is not relived - the patient is in full control. A wand or other eye-directing device is used to help rapidly move the patient's eyes in a series of directions while blinking. An RET technician also uses rapid spoken verbal communication to help release core issues - emotions, pictures, and memories.
Can Treat or Help With:	Addiction, Anger, Childhood Issues, Depression, Grief, Healing Family and Relationship Patterns, Releasing Negative beliefs and Emotions, Stress, Trauma...

Treatment:	**REBIRTHING**
Description:	A breath-work therapy that allows patients to re-experience suppressed memories and feelings from the past (no matter how long ago) in order to release them. Breaths are performed in a gentle relaxed rhythm allowing a connection to the divine self. When negative memories and feelings are released, healing can take place.

Can Treat or Help With:	ADD, Addiction, Attempted Suicide, Cancer, Child Abuse, Depression, Eating Disorders, Fibromyalgia, Insomnia, Low Self Esteem, Loneliness, Marital Violence, Multiple Sclerosis, Nervous Disorders, Obesity, Panic Attacks, Rape, Relationship Breakdowns, Sexual Abuse, Various Birth Traumas, Violent Behaviour, Stress...

Treatment:	**REFLEXOLOGY**
Description:	Applying pressure to specific reflex points on the feet, hands and ears (which each correspond to specific organs and systems) in order to affect healing and promote general health.
Can Treat or Help With:	Anxiety, Asthma, Cancer, Cardiovascular Issues, Diabetes, Fatigue, Headaches, Insomnia, Kidney Function, PMS, Sinusitis...

Treatment:	**REGULATED THERMOGRAPHY**
Description:	A painless and non-invasive medical exam that measures body heat at specific points on the body (which in turn are associated with specific organs) both at normal body temperature and then after a cooling phase. A normal body response after cooling would show heating in the neck and head and cooling in the extremities. When the body does not complete this process properly, underlying problems can be detected long before any symptoms appear. It is an invaluable tool for not only the detection of breast and prostate cancer, but also for the evaluation of all organ systems.
Can Treat or Help With:	Detection of: Cancer (especially breast and prostate), Food Sensitivities, Inflammation (causes), and other issues associated with the organs.

Treatment:	**REIKI / ENERGY HEALING**
Description:	A form of spiritual healing whereby the practitioner channels 'universal life energy' to the relaxed patient in order to harmonize body, mind, and spirit and balance chakras. While usually no touch or pressure on the body is involved, sometimes a very light touch may be used.
Can Treat or Help With:	Anxiety, Asthma, Back Problems, Clearing Toxins, Headaches, Strengthens Immune System, Pain, PMT, Stomach Upsets, Stress...

Treatment:	**REGENOKINE (a.k.a. ORTHOKINE)**
Description:	An injection treatment similar to PRP Therapy but with a few differences. A small amount of blood is extracted, incubated at a raised temperature (to increase the anti-inflammatory proteins), then separated into layers in a centrifuge. One of the resulting layers is rich in agents that are believed to protect against arthritis and the degeneration of joints and the breakdown of cartilage. This serum is then injected into the affected area of injury. This treatment was first approved for widespread use in Germany in 2003 and offers an effective treatment option for knee and other joint problems that is less invasive than other forms of surgery.
Can Treat or Help With:	Osteoarthritis, Knee Injuries, Lower Back Pain, Mechanical Problems In Various Joints...

Treatment:	**ROLFING**
Description:	Helps to balance the fascia which surrounds all muscle tissue as well as bone, nerve, organ, ligament, joints and vessels. Over time, due to injury, emotional states, or poor posture, misalignment occurs and the surrounding fascia thickens. With pressure applied in a special sequence and performed over a series of usually 10

	sessions, the fascia is manipulated and proper alignment of the body can be corrected.
Can Treat or Help With:	Arthritis, Asthma, Carpal Tunnel Syndrome, Headaches, Heart Disease, Intestinal Upsets, Lordosis, Low Back Pain, Migraines, Musculoskeletal Pain, Piriformis Syndrome And Pronator Syndrome, TMJD...

Treatment:	**SALT THERAPY (a.k.a. HALOTHERAPY or SPELEOTHERAPY)**
Description:	A therapy used in Eastern Europe for thousands of years for respiratory ailments, it involves inhaling microscopic, negatively ionized salt particles in a temperature and humidity controlled microclimate, often in a salt mine or 'salt cave' environment. The ionized particles are able to penetrate deep into the lung tissues, stimulating allergens, which are then expelled through phlegm or mucus.
Can Treat or Help With:	Allergies, Asthma, Bronchitis, Croup, Emphysema, Lung Disease, Respiratory Infections, Rhinitis, Sinusitis, Sports Performance, Vocal polyps...

Treatment:	**SHIATSU**
Description:	A finger and palm pressure massage that helps restore natural energy flow through the body.
Can Treat or Help With:	Anxiety, Arthritis Pain, Back Pain, Constipation, Depression, Digestion, Headache, Insomnia, Injury Rehabilitation, Neck And Shoulder Pain, Relaxation, Stress...

Treatment:	**SHOCK WAVE THERAPY**
Description:	Shockwave Therapy uses a high intensity sound wave to non-invasively treat a number of musculoskeletal conditions. The

	machine used produces energy pulses that literally break the sound barrier, creating controlled and precise shockwaves that target the area of injury. The therapy is especially effective for re-stimulating the healing process in chronic conditions, or for breaking calcification deposits.
Can Treat or Help With:	Achilles Tendon Pain, Calcium Deposits, Heel Spurs, Low Back Pain, Morton's Neuromas, Muscle and Joint Pain and Injuries, Patellar Tendonitis, Rotator Cuff Disorders, Shoulder Pain, Stress Fractures, Tennis Elbow...

Treatment:	**TAI CHI**
Description:	Combines movements derived from both martial arts, as well as the natural movements of animals and birds, with meditative exercise. It consists of a number of sequential movements that are performed slowly, softly, and gracefully in order to foster the qi (chi, or vital life energy) within the body. When combined with standard treatment, tai chi appears to be helpful for several medical conditions.
Can Treat or Help With:	Ankylosing Spondylitis, Arthritis, Breast Cancer, Fibromyalgia, Flexibility, Heart Disease, Hypertension, Low Bone Density, Parkinson's, Sleep Quality, Stroke...

Treatment:	**THERMOGRAPHY**
Description:	Thermal imaging produces an image (called a thermogram) of infrared radiation within the body. As the radiation a body emits increases with temperature, thermography can easily detect variations in body temperature. Areas of coolness or heat shown on the thermogram represent locations of imbalance or inflammation in the body. With breast thermography, for example, the chemical and blood vessel activity in pre-cancerous tissue leads to an increase in regional surface temperature,

	and this is detectable through thermography.
Can Treat or Help With:	Detection of: Breast Cancer, Carotid Occlusal Disease, Carpal Tunnel, Lung Problems, Muscular Irritation, Sinus Infections, TMJ Issues, Trigger Points...

Treatment:	**TRADITIONAL CHINESE MEDICINE (TCM)**
Description:	TCM is based on the Chinese concepts of 'chi' (life-force energy) and yin-yang (the relation and harmony between all opposites). When energy flows freely through our body, and harmony in our lives and body is restored, so too will wellness. TCM is not a specific treatment per se, but rather encompasses numerous therapies including acupuncture, qigong, moxibustion, massage, herbal medicine, etc.
Can Treat or Help With:	Addictions, Allergies, Amenorrhea, Anxiety, Arthritis, Asthma, Bronchitis, Chronic Fatigue, Colitis, Concentration, Conjunctivitis, Constipation, Depression, Diabetes, Diarrhea, Digestive Conditions, Fatigue, Flu, Headaches, Herniated Disc, Herpes, Immune System (And Related Diseases), Indigestion, Infertility, Insomnia, Irritability, Libido, Low Back Pain, Memory Loss, Menieres Disease, Migraines, OCD, Osteoarthritis, Plantar Fasciitis, PMS, Prostatitis, Psoriasis, Repetitive Stress Injuries, Sciatica, Sinusitis, Stress, Tennis Elbow, UTI, Various Other Neurological And Musculoskeletal Disorders...

Treatment:	**TRIGGER POINT THERAPY**
Description:	A trigger point is a tight area or "knot" in the muscle or fascia that results in referred pain and dysfunction usually somewhere else in the body. For example, on old ankle injury not properly corrected could cause shoulder problems later on. Everything is

	connected to everything else within the body. The treatment involves either pressing, rubbing, or stimulating the trigger point areas for at least 10-15 seconds, usually with the hand, although sometimes other devices may be used, including injections (TPI). Through trigger point therapy, constricted areas in the muscle are released, alleviating pain, correcting neurological muscle imbalances, and restoring function.
Can Treat or Help With:	Chronic and/or referred muscle pain, Fibromyalgia (although TPI not recommended), Myofascial Pain Syndrome, Neurological Muscle Imbalances, Tension Headaches...

Treatment:	**TUI NA**
Description:	A Traditional Chinese Medicine body work treatment used to harmonize yin and yang in the body by manipulating Qi in the energy channels through a "pinch and pull" technique.
Can Treat or Help With:	Emotional Problems, Headaches, IBS, Immobility, Musculoskeletal Problems Such As Neck, Shoulder, And Back Pain, Sciatica, Tennis Elbow, And Superficial Injuries And Trauma...

Treatment:	**WATSU**
Description:	A therapy, performed in warm water, that combines elements of massage, joint mobilization, muscle stretching, and dance in a wide repertoire of basic movements and positions. The patient is held afloat, supported, cradled, and/or stretched throughout the treatment. In the warm water with ears below the surface, the mind turns inward and the spine loosens, allowing the patient to 'let go' and therapy to take place.

Can Treat or Help With:	Anxiety, Arthritis, Cerebral Palsy, Chronic Pain, Fatigue, Fibromyalgia, Headaches, Low Back Pain, Joint Pain, Neurological Conditions, Parkinson's Disease, Post Injury Or Surgery Recovery, Pregnancy Relief, Relaxation, Sleep Problems, Soft Tissue Damage, Stress, Stroke...

Treatment:	**YOGA**
Description:	A form of relaxed concentration that includes (but is not limited to) performing a variety of postures ('asana') that promote inner peace, heightened creativity, stress reduction and the self-awareness of our essential nature.
Can Treat or Help With:	Asthma, Arthritis, Back Pain, Balance And Coordination (Improving), Cardiovascular System, Carpal Tunnel, Concentration, Depression, Diabetes, Flexibility (Increasing), Heart Disease, Hypertension, Insomnia, Irritable Bowel Syndrome, Mood, Multiple Sclerosis, Scoliosis, Relaxation, Strength (Increasing), Stress, Weight Loss...

HERBS, SPICES & SUPPLEMENTS GUIDE

While it would be far beyond the scope of this book to go into a detailed listing of all possible herbs, vitamins, minerals, foods, and supplements for all conditions, I do want to offer you a brief look at some of the areas in which natural supplementation can help with certain injuries and illnesses.   While the list of herbs to treat any number of conditions is very extensive, only a few commonly used herbs are mentioned here for each condition. The intention here is not to give an all-inclusive review of herbal remedies (as that could fill an entirely separate book), but rather that you use this section as a jumping off point to do further research into the world of herbal and nutritional medicine if this is an area that appeals to you. That said, my hope is that this section can offer you some additional answers.

Important: Treating oneself with herbs should only be done under the strict guidance of a licensed medical professional. Before taking any of the supplements mentioned herein, talk first with a qualified medical professional who understands your specific medical condition and background.   Toxic dosing and possible drug interaction are possible if not taken properly, and certain herbs should not be taken if pregnant, the patient has high blood pressure, etc. **This information is intended only as a general reference for further exploration, and is not a replacement for professional health advice.**

CONDITION	COMMONLY USED HERBS/ SUPPLEMENTS
ALCOHOLISM	Goldenseal, Kudzu, Glutathione, Vitamin B5
ALLERGIES	Butterbur, Quercitin, Stinging Nettle
ALZHEIMER'S DISEASE	Ginkgo Biloba, N-Acetyl L-Carnitine, Curcumin, Lemon Balm, Resveratrol, Qian Ceng Ta (Huperzia)
AMENORRHEA	False Unicorn, Pennyroyal
ANEMIA	Bilberry, Dandelion, Yellow Dock, Dong Quai, Nettle, Manganese, Potassium, Pau d'arco
ANGINA	Garlic, Ginkgo Biloba, Arjuna, Hawthorne, Turmeric
ANXIETY	Black Cohash, Lavender, St. John's Wort, Evening Primrose, Lemon Balm, Wood Betony, Passion Flower, Peppermint, Skullcap, Valerian, Kava kava, Linden flower, Fennel
ARTERIOSCLEROSIS	Onion, Hawthorne, Garlic, Carrot (Juice), Cayenne, Chickweed
ARTHRITIS	Alfalfa, Boswellia, Curcumin, Feverfew, Cat's Claw, Ashwaganda, Cramp Bark, Devil's Claw, White Willow, Evening Primrose, Pau D'arco, Cloves, Yucca, Apple Cider Vinegar, Red Clover, Garlic, Cayenne, Du Huo Jisheng Wan,
ASTHMA	Chamomile, Wild Cherry Bark, Nettles, Mullein, Licorice Root, Horehound, Thyme, Cayenne
ATHEROSCLEROSIS	Ginkgo Biloba, Psyllium, Bilberry, Fenugreek, Garlic, Green tea, Citrin
BACK PAIN	St. John's Wort, White Willow, Cramp Bark, Devil's Claw, Boswellin, Curcumin, Horsetail, Maritime Pine Bark, Alfalfa, Burdock, Slippery Elm
BEE STING	Comfrey (poultice), slippery elm (poultice), juniper berry (poultice), yellow dock (tea), Lavender oil, Ledum palustre (homeopathy)

BRONCHITIS	Angelica, Lavender, Cloves, Garlic, Echinacea, Thyme, Marjoram, Barberry, Mullein, Myrrh, Yerba Santa, Comfrey, Colloidal silver, Olive oil extract, Pau d'arco, Black radish, Elderberry, Goldenseal, Cayenne, Horsetail, Lomatium
BURNS	Plantain, Comfrey, Aloe Vera, Lavender, Witch Hazel, Horsetail, Slippery elm, Bayberry, Blackberry leaves, Potassium, Vitamin B complex, Vitamin C, Zinc
BURSITIS	Boswellia, Turmeric, White Willow Bark, Arnica, Bromelain, Horsetail
CANCER	Broccoli, Astragalus, Cardamom, Pau D'arco, Cat's Claw, Burdock Root, Dandelion, Curcumin, Garlic, Beetroot, Maitake, Rosemary, Lei Gong Teng, Graviola, Caraway, Cumin, Resveratrol, Sage, Thyme, Folic Acid, Coenzyme Q10, Germanium, Selenium, Shark cartilage, Green tea, Vitamin C, Inositol hexaphosphate, MSM, Essiac tea, modified citrus pectin, Noni, Olive leaf extract
CANDIDIASIS	Acidophilus, Caprylic acid, Pau D'arco, Copper, Black current seed oil, Flaxseed oil, Garlic, Vitamin B complex, Aloe vera juice, Wild Oregano oil, Maitake tea
CARDIOVASCULAR DISEASE	Garlic, Green Tea, Hawthorne, Ginkgo Biloba, CoQ10, Omega-3, Pomegranate juice, Citrin, Grapefruit pectin, Cordyceps. Cayenne, Resveratrol, Promise oil, Glucomannan, Vitamins E, C, and B5 [Do NOT take ephedra or licorice],
CARPAL TUNNEL SYNDROME	Bromelain, Arnica, St John's Wort, White Willow Bark, Turmeric, CoQ10, Bromelain, Ginkgo Biloba, Rhus toxicodendum (homeopathy), Zhen Gu Shi
CHRONIC FATIGUE SYNDROME	Acidophilus, Ginseng, L-Carnitine, Licorice, Astragalus, Garlic, Echinacea, Goldenseal, Ginkgo biloba, Milk Thistle, Malic acid, Magnesium, Vitamin C,
COLDS	Barberry, Bee Propolis, Ginger, Cinnamon, Elderberry Extract, Astragalus, Garlic, Wild pansy, Goldenseal, Mullein, Catnip, Echinacea, Cat's Claw, Andrographis, Oregano Oil, Thyme, Pau d'arco, Slippery elm, Yarrow, Basil, Apple Cider Vinegar, Eucalyptus oil, Vitamin C, Vitamin A, Zinc, L-lysine

COLIC	Catnip, Fennel, Chamomile
CROHN'S DISEASE	Aloe Vera, Slippery Elm, Ginger, Psyllium, Burdock Root, Fenugreek, Rose hips, Echinacea, L-Glutamine, Vitamin K, Garlic, Evening Primrose
DEPRESSION	Oats, St John's Wort, Lemon Balm, Rhodiola Rosea, Skullcap, Kava kava, L-tyrosine, Vitamin B complex, Zinc
DIABETES	Pau D'arco, Fenugreek, Alpha Lipoic Acid, Bitter melon, Huckleberry, Magnesium, Chromium Picolinate, Garlic, Apple Cider Vinegar, Resveratrol, Dandelion, Goldenseal, Uva Ursi
DIGESTIVE DISORDERS	Fennel, Fenugreek, Ginger, Chamomile, Cinnamon, Catnip, Slippery Elm, Yarrow, Garlic Turmeric, Peppermint, Nutmeg, Coriander, Acidophilus, Aloe vera, Anise seeds,
DYSENTERY	Wild Cherry Bark, Impatiens, Hawthorn Berries, Rhubarb Root
DYSMENORRHEA	White Peony, Turmeric, Passion Flower
ECZEMA	Chamomile, Nettles, Dandelion root, Burdock Root, Neem, Evening Primrose,
EDEMA	Bilberry, Dandelion root, Grape seed Extract, Hawthorn berries, Horsetail, Rose hips
FEVER	Catnip tea, Elderberry tea, Hyssop, Licorice root, Yarrow, Feverfew, Ginger, Vitamin A, Garlic
FIBROMYALGIA	Astragalus, Boswellia, Cayenne, Cat's Claw, Ginger Root, White Willow Bark, Capsaicin, Acidophilus, CoQ10, Vitamin A, Vitamin C
FLU	Catnip, Echinacea, Elderberry, Garlic, Ginger, Yarrow, Barberry, Boneset, Goldenseal, Peppermint, Apple Cider Vinegar, Pau D'arco
FRACTURES	Boswellia, Comfrey, Chlorella Growth Factor, Horsetail, Arnica, Yarrow, Kelp, Boron, MSM, Calcium, Magnesium,

GLAUCOMA	Bilberry, Chickweed, Eyebright, Ginkgo Biloba, Green Tea, Jaborandi, Glutathione, Rutin, Vitamin A, Vitamin B, Vitamin C
GOUT	Alfalfa, Boswellia, Nettles, Devil's Claw, Kelp, Yucca, Bromelain, Turmeric, Vitamin B complex
HEADACHES	Ginger, Quaking Aspen, Cayenne, Rosemary, Eucalyptus, Lavender, Willow, Feverfew, Valerian, Peppermint Oil, Guarana, Kava kava, Primrose oil, Bromelain, Magnesium, 5-HTP
HEART DISEASE	Curcumin, Flax, Garlic, Hawthorne, Cayenne, Gingko Biloba, Ginseng, Green Tea, Omega 3, Resveratrol, American Ginseng, Grapefruit Pectin, Evening Primrose, L-Taurine
HEMORRHOIDS	Aloe vera, Bayberry, Myrrh, White Oak Bark, Butcher's Broom, Catnip, Nettles, Yarrow, Mullein, Goldenrod, Burdock, Witch hazel
HEPATITIS	Artichoke, Shiitake, Reishi Mushroom, Milk Thistle, Licorice, Phyllanthus, Fumitory, Alpha lipoic acid, Glutathione, Dandelion, Goldenseal
HERPES	Coconut, Monolaurin, Lemon Balm, Aloe, Peppermint, Cat's claw, Licorice root, Olive leaf extract, red marine algae, St. John's wort, Garlic, L-lysine, Camu Camu, Vitamin A, Vitamin B complex, Vitamin E, Zinc
HIGH BLOOD PRESSURE	Dandelion, Garlic, Ginger, Reishi Mushroom, Olives, Astragalus, Valerian, Evening Primrose Oil, Rosemary, Mistletoe, Suma, Ylang Ylang, Bilberry, Chives, Omega-3, CoQ10, L-Arginine, Potassium and Magnesium (in order to be in better balance with sodium). [Do NOT take Licorice].
HIGH CHOLESTEROL	Artichoke, Goji Berries, Garlic, Ginger, Apple pectin, Cayenne, Hawthorn berries, Chromium picolinate, Vitamin B complex, Vitamin C, Kelp
HIV / AIDS	Licorice Root, Cat's Claw, Astragalus, Curcumin, Zinc, Selenium, St John's Wort, Green Tea, Aloe Vera, Golden Seal. [Do NOT take Echinacea]
HYPOTHYROIDISM	Kelp, L-Tyrosine, Bayberry, Black cohosh, Calcarea carbonica (homeopathy), Mugwort

INFLAMMATION	Turmeric, Cat's Claw, Pau D'arco, Witch Hazel, Arnica, Aloe vera juice, Bilberry, Boswellia,
INSOMNIA	Chamomile, Passion Flower, Skullcap, Hops, Lavender, Valerian, Kava Kava, St. John's Wort
IRRITABLE BOWEL SYNDROME	Flaxseed oil, Primrose oil, Peppermint, Psyllium, Artichoke, Fenugreek, Hops, Milk thistle, Alfalfa, Aloe vera, Skullcap, Ginger, L-Glutamine, Vitamin B complex
JOINT PAIN	St John's Wort, White Willow, Dandelion, Cinnamon, Burdock, Turmeric
KIDNEY STONE	Wild Carrot, Horsetail, Cornsilk, Dandelion, Aloe vera, Wild yam tincture, Marshmallow root, Cranberry, Uva Ursi, Nettle, L-Methionine, Zinc
LIVER DAMAGE	Beet Root, Milk Thistle, Dandelion, Burdock Root, Turmeric, St. John's Wort, Silica, Yellow Dock
LYME DISEASE	Bromelain, Primrose oil, Garlic, Dandelion root, Ginseng, Echinacea, Horsetail, Red clover
MACULAR DEGENERATION	Bilberry, Zeaxanthin, Astaxanthan, Lutein, Ginkgo Biloba, CoQ10, Shark cartilage, Vitamin A,
MERCURY TOXICITY	Alfalfa, Apple pectin, Garlic, Kelp, Vitamin C, Glutathione, Selenium, Vitamin E, Vitamin B12,
MIGRAINE	Lavender, Skullcap, Feverfew, Rosemary, Magnesium, Ginkgo biloba, Cayenne, Fumitory, Peppermint, Butterbur, Ginger, CoQ10, Calcium Magnesium, TMG, White Willow
MONONUCLEOSIS	Maitake, Astragalus, Cat's Claw, Golden Seal, Olive leaf extract, Acidophilus, Vitamin A, Vitamin C
MOTION SICKNESS / NAUSEA	Ginger, Peppermint tea, Black horehound, Lemon balm, Cinnamon, Clove, Charcoal, Magnesium, Vitamin B6
MULTIPLE SCLEROSIS	Ginkgo Biloba, Rhodiola, Bromelain, Cordyceps, CoQ10, MSM, Vitamin B complex
MUSCLE PAIN	Arnica, Rosemary, St John's Wort, Cinnamon, Lavender, , Black Cohash, Cayenne Pepper

MUSCLE SPRAINS & STRAINS	Bromelain, Curcumin, St John's Wort, Boswellia, Witch Hazel, Chamomile, Chlorella Growth Factor , Comfrey, Chondroitin sulfate, Glucosamine sulfate, MSM, Arnica Montana
NEURALGIA	Devil's Claw, Wood Betony, St John's Wort, Passion Flower
OBESITY	St John's Wort, Hoodia, Psyllium, Green Tea, Aloe vera juice, Amla, Cardamom, Cayenne, Ginger, Cinnamon, Chickweed, Coconut Oil, Fennel, Fenugreek, Guarana, Kelp, Lecithin, Carnitine
OSTEOPOROSIS	Alfalfa, Licorice, Ginseng, Flaxseed, Red Clover, Horsetail, Black Cohosh, Silica, Boron, Kelp
PARKINSON'S DISEASE	Ginkgo Biloba, Turmeric, Cowhage, Brahmi, Dandelion root, Cinnamon, CoQ10, Glutathione, Vitamin B complex
PHLEGM / MUCUS	Fenugreek, Goldenseal, Gumplant, Horsetail, Iceland moss, Andrographis, Lomatium, Eucalyptus oil, Vitamin A
PINK EYE	Eyebright, Chamomile, Fennel Seed, Honey, Calendula, Goldenseal, Vitamin A, Vitamin C, Colloidal silver
PMS	Angelica root, Kava kava, Black cohosh, Dong Quai, Fennel seed, Pau d'arco, Valerian root, Wild yam extract, Acidophilus, Calcium, Kelp, Magnesium, Melatonin, Vitamin B complex, Vitamin E, Raspberry, Pennyroyal
PNEUMONIA	Astragalus, Echinacea, Ginger, Garlic, Barberry, Garlic, Goldenseal, Pleurisy Root, Colloidal silver, Vitamin C, Vitamin A, L-Carnitine
PSORIASIS	Yellow Dock, Oregano Oil, Burdock Root, Oregon Grape, Flaxseed oil, Shark cartilage, Dandelion (poultice), Wild pansy, Primrose Oil
RHEUMATOID ARTHRITIS	Devil's Claw, Collagen, Curcumin, Boswellia, Ginger, Green Tea, Turmeric

SCHIZOPHRENIA	Flaxseed oil, GABA, Garlic, L-Glutamic acid, L-Methionine, Grape seed extract, Zinc, Ginkgo Biloba
SCIATICA	Jamaican Dogwood, St. John's Wort, Turmeric, Arnica, Skullcap, Rue
SINUSITIS	Eucalyptus, Goldenseal, Horehound, Mullein, Turmeric, Ginger, Cayenne, Garlic, Bee Pollen
STRESS	Valerian Root, Eleuthero, Ashwagandha, Holy basil, Ginseng, Licorice, Passion Flower, Lavender, GABA, Vitamin B5, Vitamin C, Magnesium, Chamomile, Catnip
STROKE	Carrots, Bilberry, Garlic, Ginkgo Biloba, Ginseng, Turmeric
SURGERY (POST)	Alfalfa, Echinacea, Goldenseal, Green tea, Rose hips, Zinc, Bromelain, Gotu Kola, Chlorella, MSM Growth Factor, Coq10, Arnica, Acidophilus, Salmon oil, L-cystine, L-Glutamine, Vitamin C
TENDONITIS	Bromelain, Turmeric, Willow Bark, Licorice, Devil's Claw, Arnica
TMJ	Chamomile, Kava kava, St. John's wort, Skullcap, Thyme, Passionflower, Feverfew, Calcium, Magnesium, MSM,
TUBERCULOSIS	Echinacea, Pau d'arco, Fenugreek, Astragalus, Garlic, Ginseng, Barberry, Goji Berry, CoQ10, Colloidal silver, Garlic, Vitamin D3
URINARY TRACT INFECTION	Garlic, Saw Palmetto, Cranberry, Horsetail, Uva Ursi, Parsley, St. John's Wort,
VIRAL INFECTIONS	Echinacea, Olive Leaf Extract, Oregano Oil, Garlic, Elderberry, Astragalus, Licorice
YEAST INFECTION	Grapefruit Seed Extract, Acidophilus, Barberry, Black Walnut, Chamomile, Garlic, Myrrh

PART 7:

CONCLUSION

AFTERWORD

Congratulations! You have completed a remarkable journey over these past 12 weeks, creating more health, wellness, peace, clarity, and direction in your life. If you've followed the information and have taken the daily action steps, you should now be feeling a noticeable improvement in your health, energy, and overall wellness.

The process of creating health is an ongoing lifelong journey and does not end here. You now have the tools and knowledge to bring forward into your future what you've learned. You are free to repeat this 12 week 'program' as often as you wish, in fact I recommend it at least once a year as so much of the information you've learned will soon be forgotten. The more you do it, the more these basic principles of healthy living and positive focus will become a habit in your life.

You deserve to have everything you could dream of wanting in life, and that includes good health. The old saying goes 'I'll believe it when I see it'. Your power lies in turning that around to 'I'll see it when I believe it'. When you believe you can have good health, and take the persistent actions necessary to achieve it, you create an unstoppable force in the universe to manifest it.

Set your intention.

Remain persistent in action.

Remain curious in knowledge.

Trust in the universe.

Breathe.

Wishing you a life of abundance and good health!

I would love to hear from you. Please take a moment to let me know how this Workbook has helped you.

You can send your stories to info@thehealingworkbook.com.

(You can also use the form below, scan, and email it in).

MY STORY OF HEALING

Name: _____ Email: _____ Country: _____

_____

_____

_____

_____

_____

If you would like to offer praise for this book I'd love that too... perhaps your words will inspire someone else out there to pick this book up and start their own healing journey.

_____

_____

_____

_____

(Please indicate below if you give me permission to use your praise in future editions of the book or website).

I _____ give permission to publish my story as written above.

_____
(Signature)

CONTEST

I review and appreciate all stories. Every 3 months my team & I will choose the best story and award a special gift to that person.

INDEX

Hypertension   161, 346, 369, 375-378, 394, 405, 408
Hypnosis   14, 391
Hypoglycemia   341, 346, 351, 363
Imago Therapy   223
Immune System   12, 13, 15, 17, 27, 32, 33, 35, 37, 45, 46, 48, 57, 67, 75, 89, 91, 93, 103, 114, 120, 121, 126, 135, 149, 160, 161, 167, 170, 172, 183, 186, 288, 316, 324, 326, 327, 331, 332, 335, 343, 363, 365-367, 369, 371, 375, 378, 381, 383, 385, 387-389, 391, 393-395, 403, 406
Indian Head Massage   392
Insomnia   44, 66, 87, 91, 120, 137, 156, 161, 364, 365, 375, 380, 382, 386, 387, 389, 391-393, 402, 404, 406, 414
Internal Bleeding   104, 383
Iodine   62, 150, 319
Irritable Bowel Syndrome   80, 120, 214, 330, 333, 337, 376, 378, 383, 390, 392, 394, 396, 398, 407, 408, 414
Jaundice   380, 383, 386
Juicing   134, 135
Kale   6, 28, 68, 77, 78, 91, 203, 276, 291, 294, 298, 299, 303, 308
Kati Vasti   392
Kelp   59, 122, 325, 412-415
Kidney Problems   27, 30, 35, 37, 67, 79, 91, 143, 155, 161, 169, 326, 342, 347, 378, 381, 389-391, 396, 400, 402, 414
Kyphosis   394, 395
Laryngitis   214, 378, 390
Leaky Gut   34, 48, 75, 100, 169, 332-334, 337, 338, 380
Leukemia   58, 143, 375
Leukopenia   375
Light Therapy   392
Liver   6, 12, 27, 28, 35, 48, 49, 65-69, 75, 89, 91, 127, 137, 145, 153, 155, 168, 181, 185, 188, 214, 276, 277, 321, 324, 331, 338, 341, 342, 345, 346, 348-350, 353, 355, 358, 359, 365, 366, 368, 381, 383, 388, 390, 397,

Lordosis   108, 404
Lumbago   392
Lung Problems   37, 214, 224, 317, 318, 378, 380, 381, 391, 404, 406
Lupus   48, 149, 330, 388, 396
Lymph Drainage Therapy   393
Macular Degeneration   414
Magnesium   6, 27, 35, 50, 51, 68, 78, 79, 91, 92, 105, 122, 155-158, 168, 179, 180, 292, 319, 327, 335, 338, 340, 342-348, 352, 353, 355, 357, 358, 366, 368, 370-372, 387, 411-416
Magnetic Healing   393
Mammography   122, 320, **321**
Marine Phytoplankton   126
Massage Therapy   159, 256, 392-394, 404
Meat   33, 49, 58, 60, 61, 76, 91, 92, 102, 103, 121, 145, 150, 181, 276, 287, 297, 300, 303, 313, 320, 328, 349, 353, 371
Meditation   **80**, 83, 90, 220, 235, 241, 243, 244, 339, 376, 394, 400
MegaVitamin Therapy   394
Memory/Memories   48, 79, 81, 82, 99, 101, 156, 242, 259, 262, 335, 349, 352, 360, 363-365, 386, 394, 401, 402, 406
Menieres Syndrome   393, 406
Menopause   390, 391
Menstrual   66, 156, 179, 346, 377, 383
Mental Illness   88, 353, 355, 378
Mercury   66, 75, 87, 100, 146, 172, 173, 186, 414
Migraine   124, 156, **158, 159**, 214, 333, 377-379, 381, 382, 388, 389, 390, 392, 393, 395, 398, 404, 406, 414
Moodiness   28, 48, 65, 87, 89, 126, 288, 333, 335, 337, 355, 364, 375, 379, 389, 391, 408
Morning Sickness   375
Moxibustion   395, 406
MSG   132, 133
Multiple Sclerosis   32, 149, 376, 377, 381 387, 389, 390, 394, 395, 397, 402, 408

SPECIAL GIFT

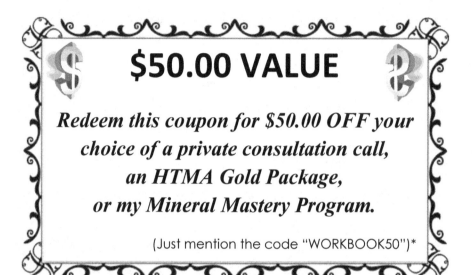

$50.00 VALUE

Redeem this coupon for $50.00 OFF your choice of a private consultation call, an HTMA Gold Package, or my Mineral Mastery Program.

(Just mention the code "WORKBOOK50")*

<u>DETAILS:</u>
The above coupon is my gift to you, a way of saying thank you for purchasing this book and investing in your health.

You can book a private consultation call through my health coaching site www.IntegrativeHealthCoaching.ca

You can learn much more about HTMA and place HTMA orders at www.HTMAtest.com

I also offer an advanced course in mineral-based nutrition at www.MineralMastery.com

*You must have purchased this book and have it with you at the time of redemption to receive this special discount.

ABOUT THE AUTHORS

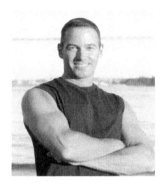

Rick Fischer is a Certified Holistic Health Coach with a background in nutrition, specialization in mineral balancing and Hair Tissue Mineral Analysis, as well as personal training and accountability coaching. He is passionate about helping people discover greater energy, healing, and enjoyment in life through healthy choices – nutritionally, physically, emotionally, therapeutically, and through self-awareness. He learned from an early age the powerful role that mindset plays in healing, using it to heal beyond expectations of doctors after several potentially life-altering serious injuries. Having witnessed the loss of family members and loved ones to negligence within the conventional medical system, conditions that could have instead been cured or ameliorated using safe, holistic approaches, he made a promise to serve others through education and increasing the tide of awareness surrounding holistic wellness. His hope is that, through this work, others can be more empowered and educated in their own healing journeys. His path has led him not only into the world of personal development but also into contact with some of today's most brilliant medical minds. Drawn to the world of holistic healing, he is acutely aware of the answers it holds, and the answers each of us hold within ourselves, to heal.

In addition to his health coaching practice (www.IntegrativeHealthCoaching.ca) Rick is also the creator of the world's number one support site for copper toxicity education and awareness (www.coppertoxic.com). He lives on the beautiful (and healthy) west coast of British Columbia.

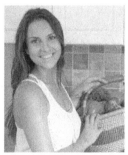

Aga Postawska is a Holistic Health Coach, Reiki practitioner, and Yin Yoga instructor. She has a unique background and skillset developed by her lifelong passion for personal growth, science, holistic health, spiritual development, and experience working in Peru at a shamanic healing centre. She was trained as a Health Coach through the Institute For Integrative Nutrition®.

After transforming her own life and health, she now works with clients to do the same. Aga developed Gut Rehab to empower people to reclaim their health by healing one of the most important organs in the body - the gastrointestinal tract - along with the microbiome. She is also the in-house health coach for Candida Cleanser (candidacleanser.com).

Aga is passionate about awakening the body-mind connection and self-awareness and encourages her clients to look past the food on their plate and explore other realms that impact health such as the energetics of emotion, thought, and spirit. Most importantly she believes the journey to better health needs to be a fun-loving one that nurtures the process of creating an abundance of health and happiness.

Get to know Aga and her work at www.thesomaheart.com.

Made in the USA
Columbia, SC
19 February 2018